MRI

GISTS

EDITION

EDITOR

R)(MR)

Valley, California

McGraw-Hill
MEDICAL PUBLISHING DIVISION

New York   San Francisco   Washington, D.C.   Auckland   Bogotá   Caracas   Lisbon   London   Madrid
Mexico City   Milan   ...   Singapore   Sydney   Tokyo   Toronto

D0322548

MRI for Technologists, Second Edition

Copyright © 2001 by The McGraw-Hill Companies, Inc. All rights reserved. Printed in the United States of America. Except as permitted under the United States Copyright Act of 1976, no part of this publication may be reproduced or distributed in any form or by any means, or stored in a data base or retrieval system, without the prior written permission of the publisher.

Previous edition ©1995 by McGraw-Hill

1 2 3 4 5 6 7 8 9 0   KGP/KGP   0 9 8 7 6 5 4 3 2 1 0

ISBN 0-07-135318-6

This book was set in Galliard by Keyword Publishing Services Ltd.
The editor was Sally J. Barhydt.
The production supervisor was Rohnda Barnes.
The designer was Robert Freese.
Project management was performed by Keyword Publishing Services Ltd.
Quebecor Printing was the printer and binder.
This book is printed on acid-free paper.

Library of Congress Cataloging-in-Publication Data

MRI for technologists/editor, Peggy Woodward – 2nd ed.
  p.; cm.
  Includes bibliographical references and index.
  ISBN 0-07-135318-6
  1. Magnetic resonance imaging.   2. Radiologic technologists.   I. Woodward, Peggy.
  [DNLM: 1. Magnetic Resonance Imaging.   2. Technology, Radiologic. WN 185 M9385 2000]
  RC78.7.N83 M9385 2000
  616.07'548 – dc21   00-032110

Contents

Contributors

Edie E. Cox, R.T.
Odessa, Florida

Luann J. Culbreth, M.Ed.
Manager, MRI Department
Baylor University Medical Center
Dallas, Texas

William Faulkner, Jr., B.S.,
R.T.(R)(MR)(CT)
William Faulkner & Associates
Chattanooga, Tennessee

Roger D. Freimark, R.T.(R)(MR)
Director
Northwest Imaging Forums
Eugene, Oregon

Joseph V. Fritz, Ph.D.
Senior Manager, Clinical Development
Toshiba America Medical Systems, Inc.
Tustin, California

Eric Hohenschuh, B.S.
Director, Licensing
Protarga, Inc.
Conshohocken, Pennsylvania

Yanmin Huang, Ph.D.
Engineering Scientist
Foster City, California

David M. Kramer, Ph.D.
Development Scientist
Toshiba Radiologic Imaging Laboratory
South San Francisco, California

Ralph E. Lee, M.A., R.T.(R)(MR)
Clinical Applications Specialist
Toshiba America Medical Systems, Inc.
Carlton, Texas

Bartram J. Pierce, B.S., R.T.(R)(MR)
MRI Supervisor
Corvallis, Oregon

Rodney Roemer, R.T., H.P.
River Grove, Illinois

Gary M. Schwartz, M.S.
London, England

Michael C. Sweitzer
Product Manager, Delivery Systems
Varian Medical Systems
Palo Alto, California

Alan D. Watson, Ph.D., M.B.A.
Senior Vice President,
Corporate Development
Cubist Pharmaceuticals, Inc.
Cambridge, Massachusetts

Gregory L. Wheeler, B.S., R.T.(R)(MR)
GPW Medical Imaging Consultants
Oakland, California

Preface

Since the publication of the first edition of *MRI for Technologists* in 1995, magnetic resonance imaging has enjoyed great advances in its science. Although the physics of MRI has not changed, our understanding of it has, and that insight is reflected in technological gains that are examined in both old and new chapters of the second edition.

Chapter 5, Imaging Coil Technology, has been updated to incorporate new advancements in the field. Technological progress that has been made in magnetic resonance angiography (MRA) and breast imaging is elucidated in Chapter 9, MR Angiographic Imaging, and Chapter 11, MR Imaging of the Breast. There has been a significant amount of research and subsequent development of MR contrast media since the early 1990s, and this crucial information is covered in Chapter 10, a heavily revised and comprehensive chapter. Safety issues, discussed in Chapter 16, reflect both the comfort level of the industry and the introduction of lower field strength MRI systems. Chapter 18, Evaluation of Magnetic Resonance Imaging Equipment, now includes open MR technology, which enjoys a significant portion of today's market share.

Two new chapters have been added. Chapter 8, Advanced MR Pulse Sequences, describes technologies used in today's MR field. Chapter 19, Perspectives on Future MRI Technology and Applications, gives a panoramic view of what is in store for MRI as seen by investigators and clinicians.

MRI will continue to progress at impressive speeds that will require the continued vigilance of the academics, technologists, radiologists, and clinicians involved in its growth. It is the intent of *MRI for Technologists* to provide an ongoing didactic basis from which all those associated with this field can benefit. For those who are new to MRI, the second edition will prepare you for the use of this exciting technology. For those who are seasoned advocates of MRI, the second edition will give you new perspectives. In either case, without you, this second edition would not have been conceived.

ACKNOWLEDGMENTS

Without past contributors as well as new contributors to *MRI for Technologists*, the second edition would not have been realized. Thus I would like to thank Rodney Roemer, Gary Schwartz, Edie Cox, and Jean Boyle for their contributions to the first edition. Their hard work and talent expressed in that book is gratefully acknowledged.

With appreciation for the important role of their editorial review, hearty "thanks" go to Yanmin Huang, Ph.D., and Joseph V. Fritz, Ph.D., who both contributed to the technical quality of the second edition.

And last but not least, thanks go to my husband, David Stumbos. Without his patient endurance in the scanner, many images used in this edition would not have been obtained. Thanks, David!

Peggy Woodward

CHAPTER 1

Historical Perspective on Nuclear Magnetic Resonance

Rodney Roemer

People have pondered and speculated over the basic structure of matter since the dawn of time. It was Democritus, a Greek philosopher, who in 400 B.C. was first to theorize that all matter consists of both invisible and indivisible particles, which he named atoms from the Greek root word atomos – meaning "uncut."

It was also the early Greeks who first became mystified how certain objects would be attracted or repelled by invisible forces that we now know as static electricity. They first noted and observed that a piece of amber, when rubbed by fur, would attract specific particles or objects. The word "amber" is translated as electron.

Concurrently, in the city of Magnesia in Asia Minor (Turkey), the mysteries of mass further perplexed humans when they observed that when certain rock formations were spun on their axes, they always and immediately returned to their original orientation. These magnetized structures, which are called lodestones, were used for navigational, religious, and magical purposes.

The city of Magnesia is the origin of the term magnetism.

The heart of MRI mathematics that we now use to translate raw MR signals into spatial location first emerged when the brilliant Jean-Baptiste-Joseph Fourier first introduced this very complex mathematical process over 200 years ago while serving Emperor Napoleon of France [Figure 1-1].

Our early ancestors (B.C.) were the first to theorize that there was a relationship between electricity (electron flow) and magnetism (properties of the lodestone). However, its relationship remained unsolved until approximately 2000 years later. In 1819 Hans Christian Oersted accidently discovered that electricity produces magnetism when he noted that a compass needle would deflect in the presence of an electric charge.

Twelve years later, Michael Faraday [Figure 1-2] stated and successfully proved that since electricity can produce magnetism, why not

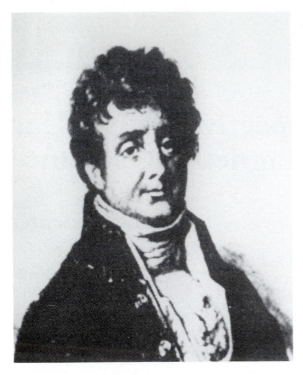

Figure 1-1. Jean-Baptiste-Joseph Fourier, born in Auxerre, France, led a very active mathematical life, which opened the doors to politics. Twice he narrowly escaped the guillotine while serving Napoleon Bonaparte during the French revolution. Among Fourier's most significant contributions to mathematics, science, and engineering are works on series, integrals, applied harmonics, sinusoidal waves, and transformation of energy. Two hundred years later we process MR images using transforms based on his original algorithm, Fourier transforms. (Courtesy of Gauthier-Villars, Dunod Editeur, Paris, France.)

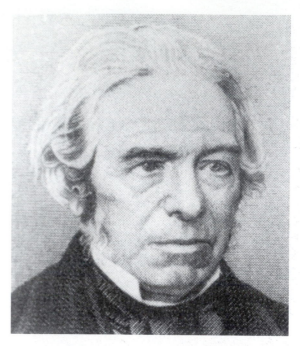

Figure 1-2. Michael Faraday, English physicist, often referred to as the Father of Electricity, postulated that if electricity produces magnetism, maybe magnetism produces electricity. He developed this idea into Faraday's Laws of Induction, one of his many contributions to physics. (Courtesy of Chicago Historical Society.)

the reciprocal? Why can't magnetism produce electricity? This revelation gave rise to Faraday's law of magnetic induction, which is not only the basis of MR signal detection but also is the precursor to modern-day electromechanics. Faraday discovered that magnetic fields traversed through an electrical coil at a 90-degree angle would induce a voltage/current in that coil. He further noted that in order for magnetic induction to be sustained, the magnetic field (or current) had to be interrupted or pulsed. For this contribution, and many others, Michael Faraday is regarded by many as the father of Electricity.

Around the 1860s, Sir James Clerk Maxwell of Scotland discovered that magnetic lines of force could be mathematically expressed. Some of Maxwell's equations also proved that electrical and magnetic fields coexist at 90 degrees to each other. Also, it was noted that an induced magnetic field will spiral perpendicular to and in the opposite direction of the electron flow which produced it, and at the velocity of light – 3.0×10^6 m/s (meters per second) in a vacuum.

It was also Maxwell who calculated the velocity and propagation of electromagnetic

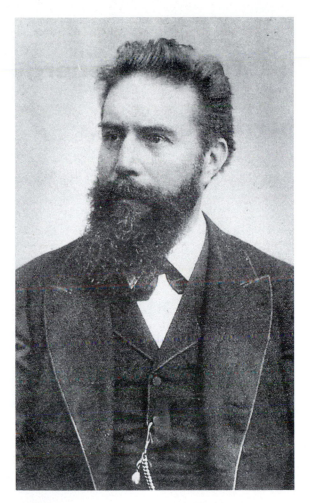

Figure 1-3. In November 1895 Wilhelm Roentgen, a physics professor in Würzburg, discovered mysterious penetrating rays. He called them X, after the mathematical unknown, and the name X-rays is still in use today.

of wave energies corresponding to their properties, began to take form.

The scene was set for Wilhelm Konrad Roentgen to discover high frequency electromagnetic X-rays in 1895 [Figure 1-3] and Frédéric Joliot and Marie Curie the gamma rays (waves) in 1896. Their discoveries soon demonstrated that high frequency wave energies were identifiable, detectable, measurable, and often biologically damaging.

The opening of the twentieth century soon became synonymous with the atomic era. There are many physicists/scientists who collectively set the stage for NMR/MRI, the most significant are the following.

1905 **Albert Einstein:** Conservation law of energy ($E = mc^2$) indicates that mass and energy are one and the same.

1911 **Ernest Rutherford:** Recognized the nucleus.

1911 **J.J. Thompson:** Objective proof of electron's existence.

1913 **Niels Bohr:** Defined the electron geometric patterns and properties; opened door to quantum physics. Related the similarities of our solar system to that of the atom [Figure 1-4].

Otto Stern: Established method to measure a magnetic dipole moment.

Wolfgang Pauli: Coined the phrase nuclear magnetic resonance.

Isidor Isaac Rabi: Devised and performed the first nuclear magnetic resonance experiment.

WORLD WAR II

German/American Albert Einstein [Figure 1-5], then a relatively unknown physicist, proposed and subsequently proved that matter and energy are actually different manifestations yet are one and the same. His famous theory of relativity postulates the equivalence of mass and energy. Einstein's theory of relativity lay dormant for

waves and predicted the existence of other waves in addition to the ultraviolet and infrared regions known to his contemporaries. Eight years later, Heinrich Hertz of Germany discovered that invisible electromagnetic waves do exist and that all electromagnetic waves are identifiable by their characteristic wave frequency values. The electromagnetic spectrum, the categorical arrangement

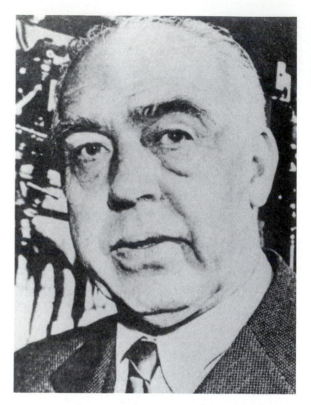

Figure 1-4.   Niels Bohr, Danish physicist, significantly contributed to the field of quantum physics. He received the Nobel Prize in 1922 for pioneering work in atomic physics. (Courtesy the United States Energy Research and Development Administration Technical Information Center, Oak Ridge, Tennessee, no longer in existence.)

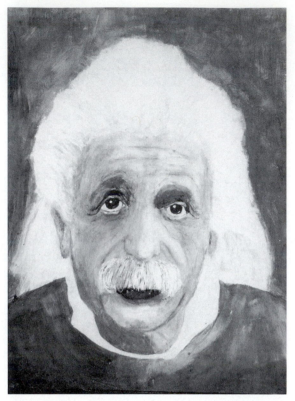

Figure 1-5.   Portrait of Albert Einstein by Tom Olson. (Courtesy the artist.)

years, for there was insufficient sophistication of equipment and/or theoretical vision or knowledge to prove or disprove its authenticity. A spin-off from the conservation of energy formula, $E = mc^2$, the era of atomic energy took on an ominous dimension when Einstein wrote President Roosevelt a letter in 1939 and informed him of the awesome power of the atom. Roosevelt became a believer that a sample of uranium the size of a golf ball had an energy equivalence of several million pounds of coal, and established the Manhattan Project Committee to pursue the development of what would later be called the atomic bomb. As a result, the atomic bomb was developed and five years later it was dropped on Hiroshima, Japan, on August 6, 1945.

POST WORLD WAR II

Some of the technological advances associated with World War II laid the groundwork for utilizing sonography (submarine detection) and nuclear medicine (atomic energy) for human imaging. In 1946 two American theoretical physicists, Felix Bloch [Figure 1-6] and Edward Purcell [Figure 1-7] continued to explore the mystery of the atom. While working independently, they noted that when a test-tube

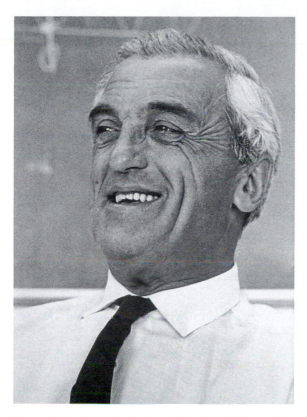

Figure 1-6. Felix Bloch shared the Nobel Prize with Edward Purcell for developing nuclear magnetic resonance (NMR) to measure the magnetic field of atomic nuclei. (Courtesy Stanford University News Service.)

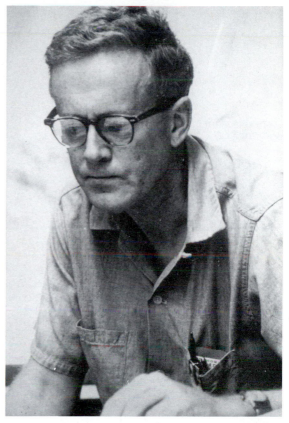

Figure 1-7. Edward Purcell shared the 1952 Nobel Prize for Physics with Felix Bloch. Purcell's NMR detection method was extremely accurate and a major improvement over the atomic beam method originally devised by Isidor I. Rabi.

sample of a pure substance was magnetically energized and RF bombarded the excited atoms themselves would respond by singing their own atomic "tune." These tune signals were detected and recorded into spectroscopic images [Figure 1-8] corresponding to their frequency values. Virtually overnight nuclear magnetic resonance (NMR), the prelude to MRI, was about to be born.

Industry initially benefited from this analytical discovery, as now for the very first time, a pure substance could be analyzed into its frequency components solely from a molecular perspective. Both Bloch and Purcell were the recipients of the Nobel Prize in 1952 for their major contribution in uniquely discovering and implementing the use of atomic energy for analytical purposes.

During the next quarter of a century spectroscopy flourished; more than 1000 NMR units were manufactured and thousands of spectroscopists emerged on an international level. Researchers performed varied and sundry types of in vitro NMR analyses and experiments, but their application for human imaging was viewed as not

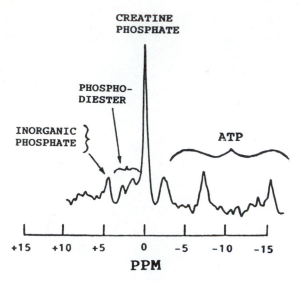

Figure 1-8. Current spectroscopic images recorded as true signals by the nuclear magnetic resonance (NMR) method discovered independently by Bloch and Purcell.

only impossible, but lunatic. This was like comparing a minnow to Moby Dick.

RAYMOND DAMADIAN, M.D.

The world of medical imaging was irrevocably altered when in 1970 a visionary American physician/physicist, Dr. Raymond Damadian, exclaimed to some of his close coworkers that he was going to build a scanner for whole body human imaging. Dr. Damadian suddenly was struck with the idea while performing NMR experiments on rats that he had surgically implanted with malignant cells. He readily observed that the rat tumor tissues would respond to magnetic excitation and, when bombarded by a resonant pulse, would emit two different types of signals as the torqued magnetic dipole moments relaxed to equilibrium. These signals would vary in their image contrast characteristics corresponding to whether the tissue was healthy or diseased [Figure 1-9]. It

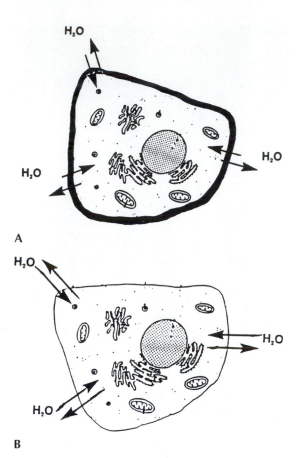

Figure 1-9. The structure of intracellular H_2O in **A** a healthy cell and **B** an unhealthy cell. The healthy cell is smaller and less pervious to the in/out flow of H_2O due to its thicker, relatively impervious membrane. The water movement is more abrupt so the relaxation rates are shorter. The resulting MR signals produce a brighter image. The unhealthy cell is larger and has a thinner membrane more pervious to H_2O. In/out H_2O flow is generally uninhibited and sluggish so the relaxation rates are longer. The resulting MR signals produce a grayer image. Although not widely accepted, the "structural" water theory continues to generate rousting conversations.

was Felix Bloch who named these two relaxation rates T1 and T2 [Figure 1-10], many years prior to Damadian's discovery.

Dr. Damadian also discovered in the early 1970s that the structure of water is the very

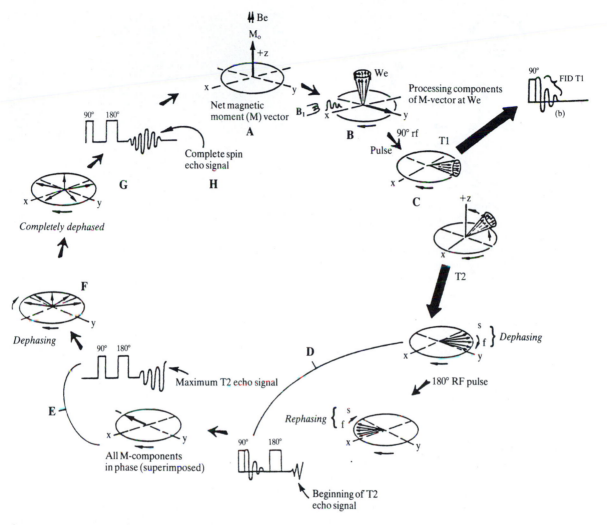

Figure 1-10. An introduction to T1 and T2 relaxation. Free induction decay (FID) is a kind of T1 decay in which the signals are produced without B_1 influence (free) and induces an MR signal in the receiver coil (induction) as a result of its characteristic relaxation decay process (decay).

essence of MRI imaging. He theorized that each water molecule contains a very intense magnetic (north/south) dipole because its hydrogens' orbiting/spinning electrons spend more time orbiting around the bonded oxygen than they spend orbiting the hydrogens [Figure 1-11]. This condition creates an intense regional source of MR signals which Damadian subsequently

proved to be detectable and recordable as a characteristic image.

Damadian, like Roentgen 100 years before him, envisioned the diagnostic value of these new magnetically induced rays. He and his team spent the next seven years designing and building the very first MRI whole body scanner for whole body human imaging [Figure 1-12]. They endured

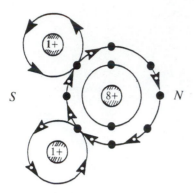

Figure 1-11. A molecule of water consists of two hydrogen atoms and one oxygen atom. Each hydrogen atom is an electron (filled circle) orbiting a proton (1+). Each oxygen atom has six valence electrons (filled circles) orbiting a nucleus of eight protons (8+) and eight neutrons (8n). When two hydrogens and an oxygen are covalently bonded to form a water molecule, not only does each hydrogen electron orbit its own single-proton hydrogen nucleus, it also orbits the larger oxygen nucleus. As the two orbiting electrons spend more time spinning around the larger oxygen there is less magnetic cloud around the two hydrogen atoms, thus causing $^1_1$H it to create the most intense MR signal.

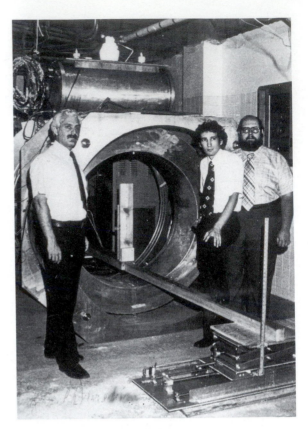

Figure 1-12. In 1977 Dr. Raymond Damadian and his associates, Dr. Larry Minkoff and Dr. Michael Goldsmith, successfully completed the construction of the world's first whole body MRI scanner. Named Indomitable to capture the spirit of its seven-year construction, it is now located at the Smithsonian Institute in Washington, D.C. (Courtesy Dr. Damadian and Fonar Corporation, Melville, New York.)

numerous setbacks and hardships: however, on July 3, 1977, they performed the first whole body transaxial proton density weighted slice image requiring 4 h 45 min [Figure 1-13]. During the scanning procedure, the patient had to be physically moved 106 times on a trambler to accomplish spatial excitation. Dr. Damadian states that only his inner religious faith and strength sustained him through those seven tumultuous years.

Dr. Damadian named his whole body scanner Indomitable, which portrays their dauntlessness, resolve, and determination in building it. The Indomitable is now located at the Smithsonian Institute of Technology in Washington, D.C.

PAUL LAUTERBUR, Ph.D.

Irrespective of his great success and fame in the field of test tube spectroscopy, Dr. Lauterbur [Figure 1-14] was not content with the fact that a substance had to be pure to obtain a spectroanalysis. He knew there must be some scientific approach utilizing the principles of NMR where selective excitation could be achieved. He agonized and deliberated over this dilemma for months.

The solution came to him one day while he sat eating at a fast-food restaurant. He theorized that by superimposing a controlled weaker magnetic gradient field onto a stronger static

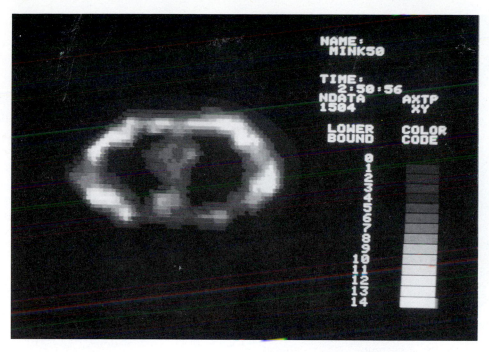

Figure 1-13. The first whole body transaxial image took 4 h 45 min to produce. Made on July 3, 1977, it shows the thoracic spine (nipple line) of Larry Minkoff, who built the Indomitable scanner with Damadian and Goldsmith. (Courtesy of Dr. Damadian and Fonar Corporation, Melville, New York.)

magnetic field going through the specimen, a magnetic tomographic region of the same frequency value could be isolated and its signals detected and transformed into an image.

Once the idea was conceived, it required many weeks of painstaking research and experimentation before Dr. Lauterbur was convinced of the following.

1. Selected NMR signals could produce a magnetic tomographic region.
2. These signals would be of sufficient magnitude for the implementation of the principles of Fourier transformation (FT) to produce a spatial image.
3. Magnets could possess sufficient magnetic homogeneity for selective image quality.

As part of the Herculean task of integrating and perfecting these three theoretical conditions,

in 1973 Dr. Lauterbur astounded his peers by designing and implementing the use of G_x, G_y, and G_z gradients for selective excitation imaging of various animal and plant matter [Figure 1-15].

In 1988 President Ronald Reagan bestowed this nation's most prestigious award, the National Medal of Technology, upon Doctors Damadian and Lauterbur for their outstanding contribution to improving the well-being of the nation through the promotion of technology.

Scientists and physicists throughout the world continuously researched and expanded on the foundation and knowledge set heretofore by their predecessors. The MRI world owes considerable recognition to many. The list is long, but the most eminent certainly would include the following.

1950s **Erwin L. Hahn, Ph.D.:** currently at the University of Berkeley, for his

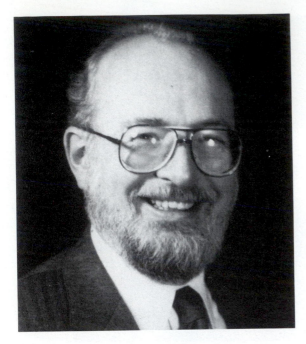

Figure 1-14.   Dr. Paul Lauterbur.

discovery of the Hahn spin echo pulse sequence. At the time, his discovery (1949) was so revolutionary he could share it with no one.

1960s **Prof. Dr. R.R. Ernst:** currently at Eidgenossische Technische Hochschule, Zurich, Switzerland, for enormously increasing MRI detection sensitivity by creating the phase vs. frequency coordinates on the MR (grid) matrix and implementation of the Fourier transformation (FT) spatial imaging process. In addition, he maximized the sensitivity and balance between the flip (Ernst) angle – the essence of fast scanning imaging.

1980s **Sir Peter Mansfield:** Nottingham, England, is primarily known for his discovery of gradient echo relative to multiecho train imaging – the inevitable prelude to real-time MRI scanning. Sir Peter was knighted by Queen Elizabeth II

for his considerable contribution to diagnostic MR imaging.

TODAY

Damadian and Lauterbur made believers of the previous skeptics as MRI units were being designed and manufactured at an unprecedented rate. There are close to 10,000 MR systems worldwide. Initially MRI units were only manufactured in the United States, but it did not take long for the MRI industry to expand overseas.

International MRI competition became fierce as each exporter strove to obtain the competitive edge over the others. As a result, new and confusing terms invaded the technical arena, and it was with great difficulty that the MRI operator began to immobilize the MRI language. Eventually the educational gap between industry and MRI sites widened as MRI production increased as sites were scattered throughout the United States. At best the training given to the rapidly immobilized MRI personnel, some of whom never were health career oriented, generally consisted of a 1 to 2 week crash program usually given by the manufacturer. Problems related to protocol and safety were usually answered by making a telephone call to the closest manufacturer's headquarters. Even the most adept operators had great difficulty knowing how, when, and where to override the computer during a patient's claustrophobic anxiety attack or how, when, and where to enhance image contrast for a particular lesion.

During this interim, three basic system strengths were being used: low, mid, and high; each with their own advantages and disadvantages. With the advent of FDA-approved invasive contrast media in 1988, the superconductive, high-field MRI system became the preferred method for neurological, low contrast, pathologically oriented images. Significant gains in hardware improvements at all field strengths today eliminate this preference. Newer, open architecture mid-field systems using superconductive

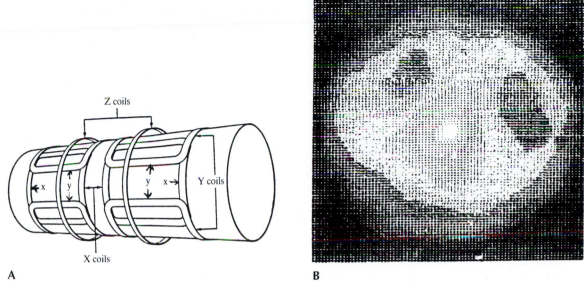

A   **B**

Figure 1-15. **A** Gradient coils G_x, G_y, and G_z interact upon the magnetized patient and collectively create a preselected spatial excitation. **B** Oil distribution in a pecan nut, Lauterbur's 1973 prototype selective excitation image (graphically enhanced) taken using NMR.

technology may now have a competitive edge over the more expensive high-field, close-bore systems.

Additionally, advances in MRI computer software and electronics have led to improved imaging applications, particularly with vascular imaging, known as magnetic resonance angiography or MRA. Upgrades to non-invasively image the body's vascular network – specifically the brain's anatomy and corresponding quantitative blood flow rate – have been made. Several vascular imaging options are presently being employed, such as time-of-flight and phase contrast. The selective application of gradient echoes, presaturation, fast scanning, spoiler reminder pulses, and preparatory pulses has significantly improved image quality.

A spin-off from MRA is the ongoing research of MRI for selectively mapping the brain's neuronal pattern. Since civilization began, mind readers have made a lucrative living by amusing and beguiling the general public, allegedly forecasting their future. This myth and trickery has now yielded to (MRI) technology where specific blood ingredients and flow dynamics cause the cognitive thinking areas of the brain to literally "light up" on the monitor during appropriate stimulation.

For instance, the patient is placed in the scanner and stimulated by watching a videotape, until one or more segments of the brain's audio, visual, and/or sensory cortex get excited. The excited neuronal target area(s) will subsequently demand more energy and the blood volume/flow is increased specifically to supply the deprived neural tissues of the energy-bearing glucose.

Concurrently, the site will also receive arterial-enriched oxygenated hemoglobin. It is this juncture, where the oxygen is removed from the red blood cells (erythrocytes) and the deoxygenated blood returns to the heart, that causes a significant dipole–dipole intensity alteration. These magnetically excited centers are becoming readily MR detectable and will "light up." Intense signal areas indicate where thinking is located, where it is going, how long it will stay, and whether it is a normal or an abnormal reaction.

MRI researchers are intensely focused in using MRI for imaging cognitive centers specifically to determine whether a condition is completely neurologically rooted, whether a condition is short-circuited, or whether specific segments of the brain are diseased. MRI and PET scanning are continuously being researched for more definitive cognitive-related diagnoses and for the means to more effective treatment planning. Among the research areas, by no means all, are epilepsy, learning disabilities, compulsive disorders, schizophrenia, Parkinson's disease, and Alzheimer's disease.

In perspective, it is apparent that MRI is today where X-ray was at the turn of the century. Just what lies ahead for MRI/MRA/MRS, neurological brain mapping, etc., is sheer conjecture.

CHAPTER 2

Magnetic Resonance: A Technical Overview

Gary M. Schwartz and Yanmin Huang

BASIC PRINCIPLES OF MAGNETIC RESONANCE

Magnetic resonance imaging (MRI) is founded on the principle of nuclear magnetic resonance (NMR). NMR has been an important branch of physics and chemistry since the 1940s, when it was discovered independently by Bloch[1] and Purcell[2].

Initially a tool used by chemists to better understand the properties of materials, NMR came to be thought of as having applications for biological systems as early as 1971[3]. Over the time since then, techniques have evolved to the point at which NMR has become indispensable in the diagnosis of disease.

In this chapter we will discuss the fundamental principles of MRI. We'll take a look at the properties of atomic nuclei that allow magnetic resonance: magnetic moments and proton precession in a magnetic field. Then we'll examine the properties of magnets that allow a large object to be imaged, as well as the types of magnets that are typically used in commercial MRI systems. We'll discuss the properties of spin relaxation that allow us to discriminate between protons that live in various environments, and we'll take a look at the radio frequency pulses that produce the information used to create MR images.

PROTON PRECESSION AND RESONANCE

The principles of NMR are based on the fact that the nuclei of certain elements have a magnetic moment. This means that if a sample of atoms of one of these elements was placed in a magnetic field, its nuclei would tend to line up with the field.

The nuclei don't actually line up exactly in the direction of the magnetic field, however. The laws of quantum mechanics dictate that they align at an angle to the direction of the field.

Each type of nucleus has a quality known as angular momentum associated with it. The idea

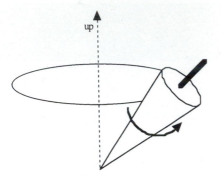

Figure 2-1.   A spinning top precessing about the vertical axis.

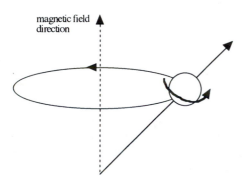

Figure 2-2.   A spinning nucleus precessing about the magnetic field.

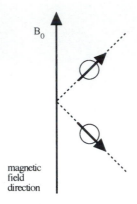

Figure 2-3.   A proton has two orientations in which it can align with respect to the magnetic field.

the nuclei are commonly referred to as *spins* that are manipulated to generate images.

In quantum mechanics the angular momentum is represented by a number called the spin of the nucleus. Depending on the value of the spin number of a particular nucleus, there will be several different orientations in which the nuclei may line up in a magnetic field. Each orientation is represented by a different angle from the direction of the magnetic field about which the nucleus will precess [Figure 2-3].

MRI takes advantage of the fact that the nucleus of a hydrogen atom (a single proton) has a magnetic moment. The spin of the proton is such that the proton has exactly two possible ways to line up with the applied magnetic field. Because of its abundance in the body, hydrogen is a wonderful candidate for use in magnetic resonance imaging.

The frequency at which the nucleus precesses is a function of both the strength of the magnetic field and the particular nucleus. This frequency, called the *Larmor frequency*, is equal to the product of the strength of the magnetic field and a constant called the *gyromagnetic ratio*. The gyromagnetic ratio is unique for each nucleus that has a magnetic moment.

The Larmor frequency is important because it is the frequency at which the nucleus will absorb

of an intrinsic angular momentum of the nucleus is fundamental to magnetic resonance imaging. It can be likened to the example of a spinning top. When a top is spun at an angle to the vertical, it will precess about the vertical axis [Figure 2-1]. That is, the top will rotate about its own axis, and the axis of the top's rotation will revolve about the vertical axis.

This precession is due to the angular momentum of the top, which is in turn due to the spinning of the top. In the same way, a nucleus that is aligned at an angle to the direction of the magnetic field will precess about the axis of the field [Figure 2-2]. The analogy is so exact that energy that will cause it to change its alignment. In proton imaging, this energy is in the radio frequency (RF) range, meaning that the frequency typically varies from 1 to 100 MHz.

If an RF pulse at the Larmor frequency is applied to a proton, the proton will change its alignment so that rather than being aligned with the main magnetic field, it will be aligned opposite the field. Over a period of time the proton will flip back to align with the field. In doing so, it will emit energy whose frequency is also exactly the Larmor frequency. It is this emission of energy that makes NMR such a useful means to locate and image protons.

The term *resonance* refers to that property of the precessing nucleus in which it absorbs energy only at the Larmor frequency. If the frequency is off even by a small amount, the nucleus will not absorb any energy, nor will it change state.

Later we will see how the property of nuclear magnetic resonance is used to generate information about the distribution of protons.

MAGNETS AND STATIC MAGNETIC FIELDS

As we have seen from the above discussion, placing a sample in a magnetic field is a fundamental requirement of magnetic resonance imaging. However, it's not sufficient merely to place an object in any type of field. In order to have confidence in our imaging experiment it is critical for the field to be extremely uniform. That is, the strength of the magnetic field must be nearly the same at all points within our sample.

This importance is a result of the dependence of the resonant frequency on the strength of the magnetic field. As we saw earlier, the Larmor frequency is directly proportional to the strength of the field; the proportionality constant is called the gyromagnetic ratio. Therefore, if the strength of the magnetic field is the same for all points in the sample, then all points in the sample will resonate at the same frequency.

In our imaging experiments we apply a radio frequency pulse to the anatomy being imaged. In order to have confidence in the spatial dependence of the image, we must therefore begin with confidence that all the protons at all the points in the imaged anatomy resonate at the same frequency.

First we discuss the magnets that have been designed to produce these highly uniform fields. Next we examine how it is possible to shape the magnetic field in order to create a large homogeneous volume.

Magnets

Three types of magnet are used in commercially available MRI systems: superconducting, resistive, and permanent. All have in common that they can generate large, uniform magnetic fields. They differ in the cost to produce the magnet, the strength that can be produced, energy requirements to support the magnet, and the direction of the main magnetic field.

Superconducting Magnets By far the most commonly used magnet is the superconducting magnet. This type of magnet is notable in that the magnetic field can be maintained for a very long period of time without requiring a constant source of energy. This allows the use of this type of magnet in systems that require extremely strong magnetic fields (above 0.5 T).

A superconducting magnet is based on the principle that a moving electric charge induces a magnetic field. Further, if the charge moves in a circle, the magnetic field is generated along a line orthogonal to the circle [Figure 2-4]. An easy way to picture this is to curl the fingers of your right hand, then stretch out your thumb (as if you were trying to hitch a ride along the side of the road). Imagine that the fingers of your hand represent the direction of the electric current. Your thumb then points in the direction of the magnetic field generated by the current in your fingers.

A superconducting magnet consists of many windings of wire that carry an electric current. The magnetic field generated by this cylinder of

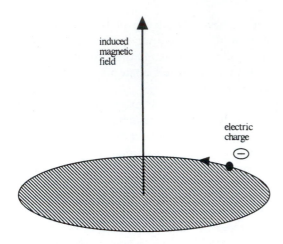

induced
magnetic
field

electric
charge

⊖

Figure 2-4. An electric charge moving in a circle induces a magnetic field in a line orthogonal to the plane of the circle.

wires runs in the direction along the long axis of the cylinder.

Because of the requirement that the cylinder be wide enough to accommodate a human for imaging (typically 55 to 70 cm in diameter), the magnet is generally very long in order to provide a uniform field large enough for imaging.

As you might expect, the current required to generate very large magnetic fields (as large as 2 T) is quite great. Therefore the energy required to maintain this current must be quite great as well, since the resistance in the wires of the magnet will cause the current to decay over time.

We are able to reduce the energy requirement by taking advantage of a principle called *superconductivity*. This phenomenon, discovered in 1911[4], is a state in which the resistance in a conductor goes to zero at very low temperatures. The temperature is in fact typically very close to absolute zero. Therefore the wires of the magnet are bathed in liquid helium at 4 K to maintain the superconductive properties of the magnet.

The liquid helium can be insulated by a Dewar filled with liquid nitrogen. This layer of insulation keeps the liquid helium from boiling

off quickly. A magnet equipped with both helium and nitrogen tanks will require that those liquids be refilled periodically.

It has become common recently for magnets to be equipped with only a liquid helium tank and a refrigeration unit that keeps the helium cold. This reduces operating costs by eliminating the requirement for liquid nitrogen, but this reduction is balanced by the cost of the electricity required to run the refrigeration unit.

Resistive Magnets Resistive magnets are similar to superconducting magnets in that they are typically coils of wire through which a magnetic field is induced. However, the wires are not cooled to a superconductive state. Therefore, the wires are resistive, and if a current were applied and the power supply disconnected, the current would eventually die out.

The major difference, therefore, is one of trade-offs in operating cost. A resistive magnet does not require liquefied gases (cryogens), but it does require a power supply to keep the magnet at a stable field. As a result of the increase in cost, these magnets are not seen in commercial systems at field strengths over 0.4 T.

Permanent Magnets The permanent magnet is gaining in popularity for systems that operate at magnetic fields up to about 0.4 T. A large part of this popularity is due to the fact that a permanent magnet has few requirements to maintain it. While a superconducting magnet requires cryogens, and a resistive magnet requires a power supply to maintain its current, a permanent magnet requires neither.

The direction of the magnetic field of a permanent magnet is along a line connecting the two poles of the magnet [Figure 2-5]. The distance between the pole faces of the magnet is generally a trade-off between the weight of the magnet, the desired strength of the field, and the minimum distance necessary to fit a human for imaging. A smaller gap allows for a stronger field, and therefore, a lighter magnet to create the field. Because of the small gap required to create

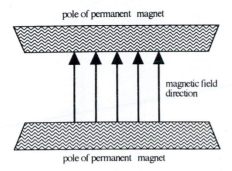

pole of permanent magnet

magnetic field direction

pole of permanent magnet

Figure 2-5. The direction of magnetic field lines between the poles of a permanent magnet.

a strong field, the distance between the poles is typically very small (just enough to image a human). This means that the direction of the magnetic field is no longer along the long axis of the human body.

The alignment of the magnetic field in a permanent magnet system therefore requires RF coils whose axis is along a different axis (since the axis of the RF coils must be in a plane orthogonal to the direction of the main magnetic field). This manifests itself in the difficulty in designing comfortable quadrature coils for systems whose field is along the vertical axis.

In the mid-1990s, magnets whose gap is large enough to image extremities, but not large enough for whole-body imaging, became available commercially. Because of the reduced size (and cost) of the magnets, these systems were priced less than whole-body imagers. For imaging centers whose needs do not include whole-body imaging, these systems might be a viable alternative.

The disadvantages of using a permanent magnet are its weight and the cost of the magnet and supporting structures. In addition, permanent magnets are susceptible to hysteresis (a time-varying change in the field). They are commonly used now for low cost systems; the cost (and weight) of the magnets has precluded their use at higher field strengths.

Field Homogeneity

As we discussed earlier, it is critical to have a very uniform magnetic field in order to generate high quality MR images. The uniformity, or homogeneity, of a magnetic field is defined by the difference in the strength of the field at various points on the surface of the imaging volume. For most commercial MR imagers the volume is a sphere.

The homogeneity is measured by measuring points along the surface of the sphere. The requirements of MRI are such that the homogeneity is measured in parts per million (ppm) of deviation from the mean value of the field. For example, for a 1.5-T magnet, one part per million is equal to 1.5×10^{-6} T. Typical magnet specifications require that the system be uniform to ± 2.5 ppm over a 40-cm sphere.

While the magnet may meet the homogeneity specifications in the factory, once it is placed in the imaging environment it is subject to the effects of materials in the surrounding area, including magnetic shielding. Magnets have been placed under surgical suites and above parking lots, and in order to shield those rooms from the effects of the magnet it is necessary to place magnetic shielding near the magnet. This shielding will affect the homogeneity of the magnet; this effect must be compensated.

So how do we shape (or shim) the magnetic field in order to achieve the desired homogeneity? Let's look at the example of shimming a superconductive magnet.

In many systems it is common to place pieces of steel inside the bore of the magnet in order to shim it. Figure 2-4 shows how the magnetic field is generated by a circle of current. In Figure 2-6 we can see a cross-section of the magnet, showing the walls of the magnet and the magnetic field. The arrows on the field lines indicate the direction of the magnetic field.

If we place a piece of iron inside the walls of the magnet, the iron acts like a magnet itself; therefore, it generates its own magnetic field. Figure 2-7 shows the field of a bar magnet.

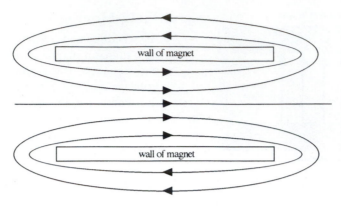

Figure 2-6.   A cross-section of a superconductive magnet showing magnetic field lines within the magnet. Note the return of the field (in the opposite direction) outside the walls of the magnet.

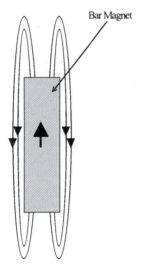

Figure 2-7.   Magnetic field lines of a bar magnet.

Notice in the figure the lines showing the direction of the field in the two magnets. The poles of the bar magnet are aligned with those of the main magnet. At the center of the magnet, the field lines of the bar magnet (which wrap from one pole to the other) run in the opposite direction to the lines of the main magnet. This has the effect of lowering the strength of the overall field.

Similarly, if we were to place the bar magnet outside the walls of the main magnet, we would see the opposite effect at the center of the main magnet. This is because the poles of the bar magnet are now opposed to the field at the center of the main magnet, and the field lines from the bar magnet will now add to the strength of the main magnet rather than subtract from it; this is shown in Figure 2-9.

LONGITUDINAL AND TRANSVERSE MAGNETIZATION

Net Magnetization and its Components

When a collection of protons (a person, an imaging phantom, a fruit, or a slab of meat) is placed into the magnet, the protons line up with the field. Recall from our earlier discussion that there

Notice how the field lines wrap along the sides of the magnet to reach from one pole to the other. This is similar to the situation with the superconducting magnet, in which the lines also wrap from one end of the magnet to the other end.

When the iron bar magnet is placed along the wall on the inside of the superconducting magnet, the bar magnet's field interacts with the main magnet's field; this is shown in Figure 2-8.

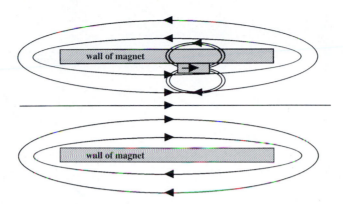

Figure 2-8. When a bar magnet (a piece of iron) is placed inside the wall of a superconductive magnet a field is induced in the bar magnet. The field within the iron is in the same direction as that of the superconductive magnet. The field lines connecting the poles of the bar magnet therefore run in a direction opposite to that of the superconductive magnet. The result is a reduction in strength of the field inside the superconductive magnet.

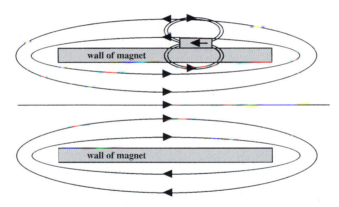

Figure 2-9. When the iron bar is placed outside the wall of the magnet it lines up with the field outside the magnet. Its field lines, therefore, add to the field inside the magnet, causing it to increase in strength.

are two possible orientations in which the protons may line up. Ideally all of the protons would want to line up in the same orientation: in the direction of the field. Quantum mechanic principles and the thermal motion of the molecules and atoms, however, dictate that not all do. Some of the protons will line up with the field, some will line up opposed to the field; most will therefore cancel each other out. The distribution is dependent on the temperature and on the field strength. At room temperature, approximately one proton in every million protons will be aligned with the magnetic field, the rest cancel each other out. The excess protons that line up along the magnetic field contribute to our ability to generate a signal and, therefore, an image.

That more protons align in one direction than in the other creates a *net magnetization*, which can be easily understood as the sum of the contributions of all the magnetic moments of the individual protons [Figure 2-10]. It is common among MR physicists to discuss manipulations of

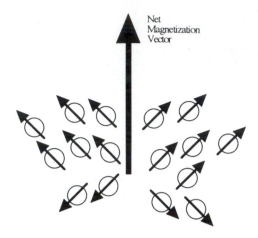

Figure 2-10. The magnetic moments of individual spins add up to create a net magnetization vector.

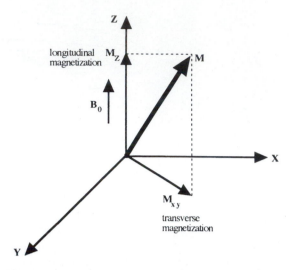

Figure 2-11. The net magnetization vector can be broken down into two components: the longitudinal magnetization (M_z), aligned in the direction of the magnetic field, and the transverse magnetization (M_{xy}), in the plane orthogonal to the field.

the net magnetization, rather than to discuss the effects on individual spins.

The net magnetization need not be aligned with the direction of the magnetic field. We take advantage of our ability to manipulate this vector in order to create an image. As we can see in Figure 2-11, the net magnetization may be aligned in any direction in the plane. It can be broken down into two components: the *longitudinal magnetization* and the *transverse magnetization*.

The longitudinal component is the projection of the net magnetization along the direction of the static magnetic field. The transverse component is the projection of the net magnetization onto the plane orthogonal to the direction of the static magnetic field. Note that it is not necessary for the net magnetization to have *both* a longitudinal and a transverse component.

Initially, the net magnetization is aligned with the direction of the static magnetic field. When an RF pulse at the Larmor frequency is applied, the protons begin to change states, or flip to the other alignment. The flipping of individual protons causes the net magnetization to move away from the longitudinal axis. If the RF pulse is of sufficient strength or duration, the net magnetization is moved completely onto the

transverse plane [Figure 2-12]. Since the effect of this pulse is to have rotated the net magnetization vector 90 degrees from one axis to the other, the pulse is commonly referred to as a *90-degree RF pulse*.

Relaxation of the Magnetization

Once the net magnetization is rotated onto the transverse plane, the protons begin to flip back to their original alignment, and the net magnetization vector eventually returns to its initial state along the longitudinal axis. Although one could follow the net vector in space as it relaxes back, it is common to decompose the net magnetization vector into two components, each of which gives specific information about the protons in the sample.

Relaxation of the Longitudinal Component Referring to Figure 2-13A, the first component that we look at is the longitudinal

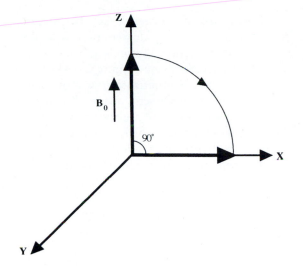

component, which grows as the net magnetization vector returns to its original state. The relaxation of this component is referred to as *T1 relaxation*. T1 is a measure of the time in which the longitudinal component has grown to 63 percent of its initial value.

T1 is commonly referred to as spin–lattice relaxation. This means that the interactions that are involved in this relaxation mechanism are between the spins and their environment. T1 relaxation is the regrowth of the magnetization along the longitudinal axis, which is along the direction of the magnetic field. We are therefore seeing the spins as they become realigned with the magnetic field.

We saw above that it requires energy to move the spins from one alignment to the other. Therefore, as the spins realign themselves with

Figure 2-12. Depiction of the rotation of the net magnetization vector away from the longitudinal axis and completely onto the transverse plane – a 90-degree rotation.

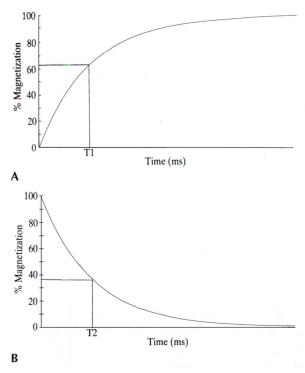

Figure 2-13. **A** Curve showing relaxation of the longitudinal magnetization. At time T1 the magnetization has relaxed to 63 percent of its initial value. **B** Curve showing decay of the transverse magnetization. At time T2 the magnetization has decayed to 37 percent of its initial value.

the magnetic field, they must be able to give up some energy. This energy is given up to the environment in which the spins reside. This could be other nearby electrons or nuclei.

You will see in a later chapter that the T1 of protons is different in different tissues in the body. This is a result of the different environment in different tissues at the molecular level, primarily the proportion of water that is *bound* in macromolecules and that which is *free* (in solution)[5]. Tissues with a high proportion of bound water, like liver, will have a shorter T1. That is, they will relax to equilibrium more quickly than those that have more free water, like fluids which have a much longer T1.

Relaxation of the Transverse Component

The other component that we examine is the transverse component [Figure 2-13B]. While the longitudinal component is growing, the transverse component is decaying back to its initial state, which is zero (since at the initial state, all of the net magnetization is along the longitudinal axis). However, the two do not necessarily relax at the same rate. The relaxation of the transverse magnetization is referred to as *T2 relaxation*. The term T2 is similarly a measure of the time in which the transverse component has decayed to 37 percent of its initial value.

Note that it is possible for the transverse component to decay to zero before the longitudinal component reaches its initial state. However, it is not possible for the transverse magnetization to exist after the longitudinal component has relaxed back to its initial state. This means that T2 must always be less than or equal to T1. It can never be greater than T1.

T2 relaxation is commonly referred to as spin–spin relaxation. The mechanism that causes the decay of the transverse magnetization is the dephasing of the spins over time. This is due to contributions from T1 relaxation, a dipolar interaction between the spins, inhomogeneities in the static magnetic field, and local inhomogeneities caused by magnetic susceptibility effects.

Dephasing of Transverse Magnetization

At the time a 90-degree pulse is applied, the net magnetization vector is moved entirely onto the transverse plane [Figure 2-14]. At this instant the net magnetization vector begins precessing in the transverse plane. Initially the individual spins can be thought of as all being in phase, as all of their individual components add up to create the net magnetization vector.

Over time the spins begin to lose their phase coherence, as a result of the spin–spin interaction. As they lose their phase coherence, the sum of their individual vectors begins to cancel out and the net magnetization vector becomes smaller.

There are several ways to visualize this process. What does it mean that the spins precess at different frequencies? The classic example is that of runners on a racetrack [Figure 2-15A]. At the start of a race, all of the runners are lined up at the same point along the track (let's assume there's no staggered start). This is analogous to all of the individual spins lined up together in the transverse plane [Figure 2-15B].

A few seconds or minutes into the race, the faster runners pull ahead, and the slower runners fall behind. The runners are now spread out along the track [Figure 2-15C]. Similarly, after a short time, some of the spins that are precessing more quickly are ahead of those that are precessing less quickly [Figure 2-15D]. So even though

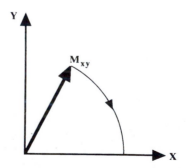

Figure 2-14. Precession of the net magnetization vector in the xy plane.

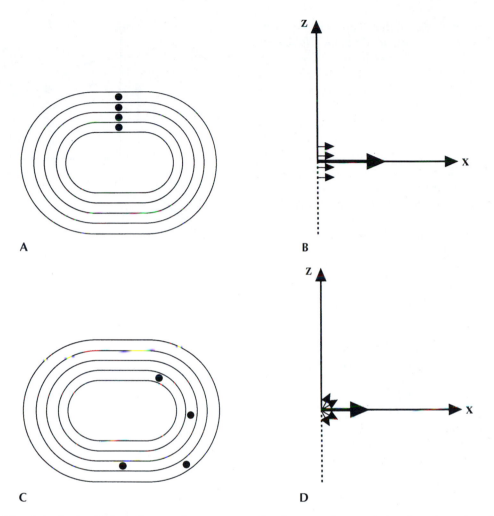

Figure 2-15. **A** At the beginning of a race the runners are lined up together on the track and are therefore *in phase*. **B** The spins lined up together in the *xy* plane create a net magnetization vector pointing in the *x*-direction. **C** As the race progresses the runners move at different speeds, no longer lining up together on the track; they have lost their phase coherence. **D** As the spins precess at different frequencies, they no longer line up together in the plane. When added together they create a net magnetization vector that is smaller than the initial vector; they have lost their phase coherence.

the spins are still precessing in the transverse plane, their contribution to the net magnetization vector does not add completely in the direction of the net magnetization vector. Some of their contributions cancels out, and the part that doesn't cancel contributes to a smaller net vector.

RADIO FREQUENCY WAVES: GENERATION AND APPLICATION

Free Induction Decay

Now that we have an understanding of the mechanism of spin relaxation, we can discuss how we apply RF energy to generate a signal in an

MRI experiment[6]. Recall that there is a frequency at which protons in a magnetic field will absorb energy and change their orientation with respect to the magnetic field. This Larmor frequency is dependent on the strength of the magnetic field and the nucleus we want to image.

Imagine a net magnetization vector (magnetization) precessing in a magnetic field (we'll refer to the main field as the static magnetic field since it doesn't change over time). The goal of the imaging experiment is to move the magnetization away from the direction of the static field so that we can observe its relaxation.

The way to change the orientation of the magnetization is to cause it to precess about another magnetic field that we introduce into the system. If we apply a magnetic field with the RF coil at the appropriate frequency, we can cause the magnetization to precess about it. In Figure 2-16A we see an example of a magnetization that is pointing in the direction of the static field, which we'll call the z-axis. We want to rotate the magnetization onto the xy plane (the transverse plane) so that we can watch the T2 decay and the T1 relaxation.

We apply an RF field whose frequency is also the Larmor frequency. The field is applied in a

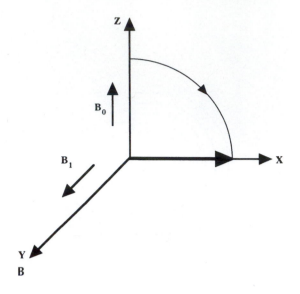

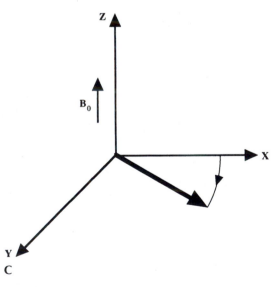

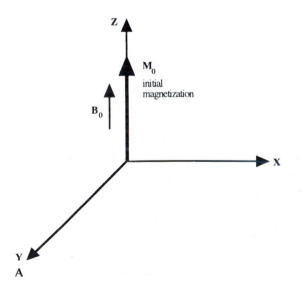

Figure 2-16.   **A** At the beginning of the imaging experiment the net magnetization vector points in the direction of the magnetic field (B_0). Its initial value is M_0. **B** An RF field (B_1) whose frequency is the Larmor frequency has been applied. The net magnetization vector processes about B_1 and is rotated 90 degrees into the xy plane. **C** When B_1 is turned off, the net magnetization vector precesses once again about B_0.

direction perpendicular to that of the static field. When this field is turned on, the magnetization begins to precess about the new field [Figure 2-16B]. When the RF field is turned off, the magnetization will stop precessing about it. Therefore, we can control the rotation of the magnetization by controlling the intensity and duration of the applied RF field.

Once the applied RF field is turned off the magnetization precesses about the static field [Figure 2-16C]. It induces a current in an RF coil, which could either be the same coil used to transmit the RF pulse or a separate receiver coil. As we saw above, the component of the magnetization in the transverse plane will dephase and therefore decay. Because of the decay of the signal strength it is called a *free induction decay*, or FID.

It is the manipulation of the FID that gives us the signal we use to create MR images. One could either image the FID, or use the FID to create refocused *echoes* that may be imaged. In spin echo pulse sequences we use RF pulses to refocus the FID and create an echo. In gradient echo sequences we use the magnetic field gradients to refocus the FID and create an echo. These sequences are described in Chap. 8.

RF Coils

RF coils are the radio antennas that transmit the energy with which we manipulate the spins and receive the signals generated by the spins as they precess about the static field. They are similar to the coils of a superconductive or resistive magnet in that a current is passed through the coil to induce a magnetic field. In addition a current is generated in the coil by the precessing magnetization.

Geometry is a tremendously important consideration for the coil. For human imaging experiments the coil must be large enough to comfortably hold a person, yet the larger the coil the less sensitive a receiver it will be. Similarly, the larger the transmit coil, the more power is required for the same effect inside the subject.

We saw above that in order to rotate the net magnetization vector off the axis of the main magnetic field the axis of the RF pulse must be orthogonal to that of the main magnetic field. For magnets whose axis is vertical (e.g., permanent magnets) it is convenient to produce solenoid coils. These coils generally consist of turns of wire that wrap around the imaging subject. The RF field generated by this coil is in the horizontal plane and can therefore both rotate the net magnetization vector and receive a signal as the magnetization precesses [Figure 2-17].

For magnets whose field is along the long axis of the human body (e.g., superconducting magnets), coil construction is made somewhat more complicated. The RF field cannot be in the same direction of the main magnetic field. It must be either vertical or along the patient's left to right direction. Coils such as saddle coils and birdcage coils have been developed to obtain the appropriate field direction.

In 1985 quadrature RF reception was introduced in order to increase the signal to noise ratio. Signals from both axes orthogonal to the main magnetic field are received using coils and added together. Theoretically this increases the signal to noise ratio by over 40 percent. In

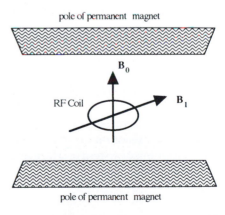

Figure 2-17. In a permanent magnet system B_0 is a vertical field. A solenoid coil creates B_1, a horizontal field that rotates the net magnetization vector.

practice isolating the two coils and geometry reduces this somewhat.

Surface coils were introduced to image body parts in which it was not necessary to have a symmetric, homogeneous field for imaging. For example, it is convenient to image the brain with a coil that surrounds the brain, since we're interested in imaging the entire head. This lends itself to the design of a circular or oval coil, in which the RF field is nearly homogeneous (that is, it doesn't vary much over the imaging volume).

For other body parts (e.g., the spine) we're more interested in anatomy closer to the posterior surface rather than anterior. Here we can design a coil whose field is very intense close to the surface, but which dies out as we move further away from the coil. This surface coil will produce a good signal at depths through the vertebral bodies, but we won't see much signal further away.

Surface coil technology has enabled us to image body parts (such as the spine, shoulder, orbits, etc.) at very high resolution without having to worry about receiving signal from anatomy that's not of interest.

One last consideration is the difference between transmit and receive coils. For some applications it is convenient to use the same coil to transmit and receive the RF signal. This is generally the case for brain, knee, and body imaging, where the RF coils tend to have nice geometries that lend themselves to creating homogeneous transmit fields. For other applications, especially surface coil imaging, one wants to have separate transmit and receive coils.

The transmit and receive coils must both be orthogonal to the axis of the main magnetic field. In order to optimize system performance it is critical that the transmit and receive coils are well isolated from one another. If the coils couple (interact with one another) the signal to noise performance will decrease.

CONCLUSION

In this chapter we've taken a look at the hardware that makes up an MR imaging system, and compared and contrasted the benefits and trade-offs of the various types of magnets available in commercial systems. In addition we've introduced the concept of magnetization and the manipulation of magnetic spins. We've examined the relaxation properties of spins that give rise to our ability to discriminate their environments. In the next chapter you'll build upon this knowledge and learn about the characteristics of tissue in the human body that make MR imaging feasible. Afterwards you'll see how RF pulses are combined with *gradient* magnetic fields to provide spatial information that gives us a meaningful image. This material will then be pulled together in the discussion on imaging pulse sequences.

REFERENCES

1. Bloch F, Hansen WW, Packard ME. *Phys Rev* 69:127, 1946.
2. Purcell EM, Torrey HC, Pound RV. Resonant absorption by nuclear magnetic moments in a solid. *Phys Rev* 69:37, 1946.
3. Damadian R. Tumor detection by nuclear magnetic resonance. *Science* 171:1151, 1971.
4. Kamerlingh Onnes H. *Akad. van Wetenschappen* (*Amsterdam*) 14:113, 1911.
5. Mansfield P, Morris PG. *NMR Imaging in Biomedicine.* New York: Academic Press, 16, 1982.
6. Fukushima E, Roeder SBW. *Experimental Pulse NMR: A Nuts and Bolts Approach.* Reading MA: Addison-Wesley, 7–12, 1981.

CHAPTER 3

Magnetic Resonance Tissue Contrast Characteristics: Proton (Spin) Density, T1, and T2

Roger D. Freimarck

One of the outstanding diagnostic aspects of MR imaging is its ability to allow us to "see" various types of normal and abnormal tissues. By using the right parameters, MR imaging allows us to create desirable tissue contrast. *Dorland's Illustrated Medical Dictionary* defines the term contrast as "comparison in order to distinguish differences." For accurate diagnosis, MR images must be able to distinguish differences in tissues. Equally important, the operator must understand the underlying principles that produce this aspect of tissue contrast. In most imaging facilities, the bulk of clinical day-to-day MR imaging still centers on the use of spin echo imaging. The purpose of this chapter is to describe the building blocks of tissue contrast as they relate to spin echo imaging. We will take a close look at tissue signal characteristics using spin density, T1, and T2 weighted imaging parameters. The term *weighted* simply means that image parameters have been chosen to produce a desired type of tissue contrast in the final image.

LONGITUDINAL AND TRANSVERSE MAGNETIZATION

Before tackling the issue of how to create a spin density, T1, or T2 weighted image, it is necessary to remind ourselves that, in a typical MR imager, one can only measure transverse magnetization. In a strong static magnetic field (produced by the main magnet), the majority of hydrogen protons at rest (equilibrium) will be precessing ever so slightly around the vector of that main magnetic field. The longitudinal magnetization produced by these resting protons will not be measurable simply because their precessional magnetic vectors are not in phase and are not slicing through a receiving coil. Remember, for an electric current or signal to be induced into an imaging coil, the coil must have a moving magnetic field to slice through.

A simple analogy of this is the following scenario. Consider a small darkened room with

27

light detectors built along each sidewall at approximately shoulder height. These devices measure the intensity or amount of light and are most sensitive when the light is pointed directly into their sensor. In this scenario, these detectors represent your imaging coil. Now, with a flashlight in your hand, enter the room and stand in the very middle. Turn on the flashlight and extend your arm above your head, aiming the beam of light at a mark on the ceiling directly above you. Looking at this mark, begin to rotate the beam of light around it in a circular fashion. Your extended arm and the beam of light coming from the flashlight now represent a precessing proton in a strong magnetic field [Figure 3-1]. The beam of light represents the magnetization vector of the proton and your body position (foot to head) represents the magnetization vector of the main magnet. The light sensors in the wall (your coil) cannot efficiently detect the full intensity of the light beam because it is pointed 90 degrees away from them.

Now begin to rotate your body as you slowly lower your arm holding the flashlight. As you rotate and lower your arm, you represent what happens to a proton exposed to a burst or pulse of properly tuned radio frequency (RF) energy

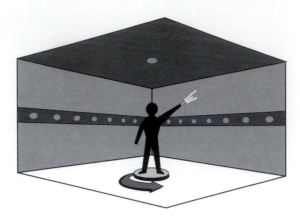

Figure 3-2. Following a 90-degree RF pulse, the proton magnetization begins to spiral downward (light sensors begin to sense light, or signal).

(in spin echo imaging, we begin the imaging process by utilizing a 90-degree RF pulse). Continue to rotate while lowering your arm [Figure 3-2] until it is pointing straight out (90 degrees) from your body. With your arm and the flashlight at a 90-degree position to your body (and the walls), each of the shoulder high light sensors in the wall can now efficiently detect the light (or signal) as you rotate in a circle [Figure 3-3]. As you rotate, the beam of light points directly into each sensor, and the light is at its highest level. In this model, you have taken undetectable longitudinal magnetization (light beam pointed at the ceiling) and made it detectable by tipping it 90 degrees into the transverse plane (light beam pointed at the walls).

If longitudinal magnetization is not measurable, why is it so important to know about it? Because the strength or amount of magnetization a tissue has in the longitudinal plane will convert on a one to one basis when tipped into the measurable transverse plane [Figure 3-4]. In our model, if your flashlight beam has an intensity of 10 W while it is pointed at the ceiling (not measurable by the sensors), it will have a measurable intensity of 10 W when it is pointed 90 degrees at the light sensors in the walls, no

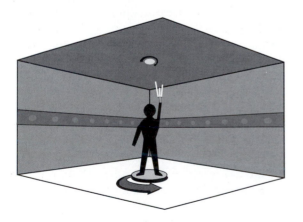

Figure 3-1. An arm with flashlight represents a precessing proton magnetization in a strong magnetic field with no measurable signal. Light sensors in the walls represent a coil (cannot sense light).

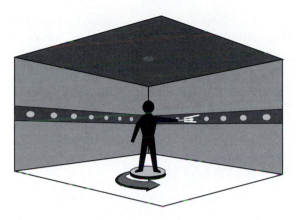

Figure 3-3. As the proton magnetization vector precesses at a 90-degree angle, the light sensor (coil) detects a full light beam (signal).

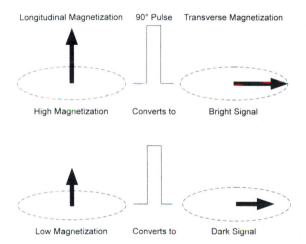

Figure 3-4. Two tissues with different amounts of longitudinal magnetization. The amount of magnetization attained in the nonmeasurable longitudinal plane converts directly to the same amount of magnetization (signal) in the measurable transverse plane.

more, no less. From this model, one might think it would always be desirable to have an intense longitudinal signal (light beam pointed at the ceiling) so that one has an intense signal when tipped into the transverse plane (light beam pointed at the walls). However, this is not always the case.

LONGITUDINAL (T1) AND TRANSVERSE (T2) RELAXATION

It is equally important to review the basic fundamentals of longitudinal and transverse relaxation before discussing our three main image weighting techniques. To keep things simple, we will use the same arm and flashlight model to demonstrate proton magnetization relaxation aspects. We left that scenario with you rotating and holding the flashlight at a 90-degree angle to your body and to the walls containing the light sensors. After the RF pulse (which tipped the precessing proton magnetization vector through 90 degrees) is turned off, two distinctive *and* independent things begin to happen: longitudinal and transverse relaxation.

First, we examine *longitudinal* relaxation. After the RF pulse is turned off, the arm holding the flashlight begins to rise until once again the beam of light is making small circles around the original ceiling mark (Figs. 3-1, 3-2, and 3-3 in reverse). This process of returning the magnetization vector to the original longitudinal direction, or equilibrium, is termed spin–lattice or T1 relaxation. It is easiest to remember this "T one" relaxation strategy by thinking of *one* hydrogen proton magnetic vector and how it behaves following a 90-degree RF pulse. When at rest, the single proton precesses around the static magnetic field. A 90-degree RF pulse causes it to tip (and precess) 90 degrees into the transverse (measurable) plane. When the RF is turned off, the single proton magnetic vector begins to spiral back up to its original precessional position around the static magnetic field. Longitudinal relaxation occurs simply because each individual proton (itself a tiny magnet) is attempting to realign with the main magnetic field after having been knocked off its axis by a 90-degree RF pulse.

To examine the mechanism of *transverse* relaxation, we must add a second proton, or flashlight, to our scenario. Holding a second flashlight in your other hand, you aim its beam of light at the mark on the ceiling. To be accurate, you should move the two flashlight beams around the ceiling mark so they never point to the same place at the same time. In reality, individual magnetic vectors of precessing protons do *not* all point to the same place. However, that changes when the RF pulse is turned on. The 90-degree RF pulse causes the two flashlight protons to tip 90 degrees into the transverse plane *and* causes them to converge the two separate light beams into a single light beam. The two beams of light are now precessing *in phase* with each other and point to the same spot on the wall light sensors. Why is this fact important? If each of our individual beams of light has a signal intensity of 10 W, adding the two beams together (and pointing them at the same spot) will double the measurable signal intensity to 20 W. In reality, we have an extremely large number of proton vectors precessing in phase, which allows us to add together the sum of all the tiny individual amounts of signal into one large amount of measurable signal. However, this in phase process begins to rapidly break down. In the flashlight model, very soon after the 90-degree RF pulse is turned off, one of your beams of light begins to move slightly faster than the other. As a result, your precessing beams of light begin to separate once again into two individual beams of light. They become *out of phase* with each other. This relaxation process, which occurs in the transverse plane, is termed spin–spin or T2 relaxation. It is easiest to remember this "T two" relaxation process by thinking of *two* proton vectors and how they interact with each other following the 90-degree RF pulse. In reality, the motion of individual hydrogen nuclei at room temperature is so rapid and chaotic that they often come into contact with each other, causing some to lose energy to other nuclei. This constant state of interaction simply allows some protons to be lost from the MR imaging process. As this transverse relaxation process takes place, we lose measurable signal by having fewer and fewer protons (flashlights) in phase with each other.

It is imperative we remember that these two relaxation processes occur at the same time but are *independent functions*. Individual proton magnetization vectors are trying to return to their original longitudinal precessional positions at the same time as multiple proton magnetization vectors are becoming out of phase with each other.

T2* RELAXATION

A second and very important type of transverse relaxation, often glossed over in many MR publications, T2* (T2 star) relaxation is not a tissue specific entity but one which mainly occurs due to the static magnetic field used in all MR imaging. One should know that before true T2 transverse tissue relaxation has a chance to occur, total T2* relaxation (loss of all signal) just kind of happens. Why? As mentioned earlier, following the 90-degree RF pulse all proton magnetic vectors begin to precess in phase. The rate of individual hydrogen proton precession is *always* proportional to the magnetic field strength they reside in (Larmor equation and gyromagnetic ratio). At *precisely* 1.0 T, the precessional frequency for hydrogen protons is 42.6 MHz, which is 42,600,000 cycles/s. In reality, there is no such thing as a perfectly even, or homogeneous magnetic field. For example, the field strength of a 1.0 T system will vary ever so slightly throughout the patient imaging area. It will be slightly higher in some areas and lower in others. As our volume of protons is tipped 90 degrees and the protons begin to spin in phase, individual protons are very quick to realize that they may be in a slightly stronger or weaker magnetic field than their neighbors. As a result of this slight difference in field strength, they begin to precess faster or slower than their neighbors, which puts them out of phase, creating transverse relaxation (and loss of measurable signal). Manufacturers spend a great deal of time, effort, and money to make their magnets as homogeneous as possible in order to lessen the impact of T2* loss of signal.

SPIN DENSITY VALUES

Most clinical MR imaging exploits the use of hydrogen protons as its source of signal. The simple reason for this is the abundance of hydrogen atoms in the human body. Approximately 90 percent of the average human is composed of water tissue which in turn is composed of mobile hydrogen nuclei. These mobile hydrogen nuclei are MR visible. As it turns out, the concentration of hydrogen protons or spin density differs by only a few percent between tissue types [Table 3-1]. However, this slight difference in proton concentration is enough to give reasonable tissue contrast when the MR imaging parameters are adjusted to give a spin density type of image. Each tissue acquires a high, intermediate, or low level of longitudinal magnetization based on its value of spin density, or hydrogen proton concentration. Although we cannot measure precessing longitudinal magnetization, its value converts directly to the same amount of measurable signal when tipped 90 degrees into the transverse rotating plane. As a result of this 1:1 aspect ratio, high levels of longitudinal magnetization convert to high levels of measured signal in the transverse plane (and end up being bright areas on the final image). Conversely, lower levels of longitudinal magnetization convert to lower levels of measured signal in the transverse plane (and end up as dark areas on the final image). To summarize, spin density imaging produces tissue contrast (bright to dark areas) based on a difference in the concentrations of hydrogen protons within the tissues.

T1 AND T2 TIME VALUES

What are the values of T1 and T2 relaxation times for various types of tissues and what do they mean? These values, as it turns out, were the driving force behind the initial diagnostic success of spin echo MR imaging. Unlike proton density (concentration) which may vary by just a few percent between various tissues [Table 3-1], T1 and T2 relaxation times can vary as much as several hundred percent [Tables 3-2 and 3-3]. With such profound variation in these imaging values, it is relatively easy to take advantage of

Table 3-1

Spin Density Values: Relative Values of Mobile Hydrogen Concentrations in Various Tissues

Muscle	100
White matter	100
Fat	98
Cerebrospinal fluid	96
Kidney	95
Gray matter	94
Spleen	92
Liver	91
Blood	90
Pancreas	86
Cortical bone	1–10
Lung	1–5
Air	< 1

Table 3-2

T1 Time Values: Approximate T1 Relaxation Times for Various Tissues (Measured at 1.0 T)

Fat	180 ms
Liver	270 ms
White matter	390 ms
Spleen	480 ms
Gray matter	520 ms
Muscle	600 ms
Blood	800 ms
Cerebrospinal fluid	2000 ms
Water	2500 ms

Table 3-3

T2 Time Values: Approximate T2 Relaxation Times for Various Tissues (Measured at 1.0 T)

Muscle	40 ms
Liver	50 ms
Spleen	80 ms
Fat	90 ms
White matter	90 ms
Gray matter	100 ms
Blood	180 ms
Cerebrospinal fluid	300 ms
Water	2500 ms

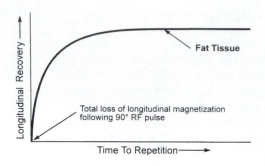

Figure 3-5. A typical T1 relaxation curve for fat tissue.

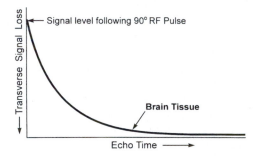

Figure 3-6. A typical T2 relaxation curve for brain tissue.

this and adjust the imaging sequence to produce great separation in the area of tissue contrast. Each tissue type responds to T1 and T2 relaxation at a different rate. Relaxation times are generally expressed in values of milliseconds (ms); 1000 ms is equal to 1 s. In Tables 3-2 and 3-3 the T2 value of a given tissue is *always* shorter than the T1 value for the same tissue. This is a very important aspect of MR imaging to remember and will be discussed later in this chapter.

One cannot draw a simple linear graph to illustrate a tissue's T1 or T2 relaxation rate. These relaxation rates *never* occur in a simple linear fashion. Both processes occur exponentially, which indicates they take place at varying, nonlinear rates. Both processes start relatively quickly, then subsequently slow down [Figures 3-5 and 3-6]. You need to become familiar with what I term the 63 percent rule of tissue relaxation. A T1 value indicates how long it takes a tissue to regain 63 percent of its original longitudinal magnetization (after having been tipped 90 degrees by an RF pulse). As each additional T1 time value elapses, the tissue regains an additional 63 percent of the original level of longitudinal magnetization. For all practical purposes, it takes *five* T1 time values to elapse before a

tissue has regained almost all (99 percent) of its original level of longitudinal magnetization [Figure 3-7].

This same 63 percent rule holds true for T2 relaxation. A single T2 value indicates how long it takes for that tissue to lose 63 percent of its transverse magnetization (after it has been tipped 90 degrees by a burst of RF energy). As each additional T2 time value elapses, the tissue loses an additional 63 percent of the original level of transverse magnetization. Again, for practical purposes, it takes *five* T2 time values to elapse before a tissue has lost almost all (99 percent) of its transverse magnetization [Figure 3-8].

Earlier, we mentioned that transverse magnetization fades faster due to T2* relaxation than due to genuine T2 relaxation. The T2* process of signal loss (due principally to main field

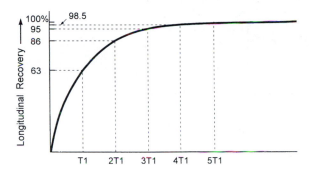

Figure 3-7. A typical T1 relaxation curve.

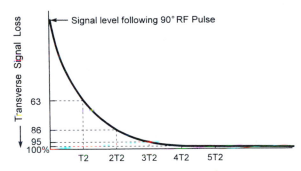

Figure 3-8. A typical T2 relaxation curve.

inhomogeneity) occurs much more rapidly than genuine T2 decay. One can see the effects of genuine T2 decay when measuring how much transverse signal can be rephased (or how much signal is lost) using spin echo imaging.

SPIN ECHO IMAGING

Up to now, we have utilized simple 90-degree RF pulses in our imaging scenarios. In reality, this is a very inefficient way to produce MR images. When protons are tipped 90 degrees, the resultant transverse signal pattern, termed *free induction decay* (FID) fades away very rapidly due to T2*. This FID rapidly fades away because the spins have become completely dephased

and all measurable signal is lost (remember the flashlight analogy). As it turns out, we can actually cause these spins to rephase by the introduction of a 180-degree RF pulse. Using the flashlight analogy again, as you rotate with flashlights in both hands, one beam of light starts to rotate a bit faster causing it to get ahead of the other beam (T2* dephasing). As the 180-degree RF burst is introduced, you reverse your rotational direction. At some point, the faster beam of light (proton) catches up to the slower beam of light (proton) and, for just an instant, the two beams of light are again in phase with each other, producing a strong signal. When you compare our two proton (flashlight) example to the billions of protons that actually participate in this dephasing and rephasing process, one interesting difference becomes apparent. The amount of signal which is rephased by the 180-degree RF pulse is never as much as the original FID [Figure 3-9]. *The loss of signal between the original FID and the 180-degree rephased echo is due to true T2 relaxation.*

The term *echo* simply refers to a process by which we can rephase spins that have become dephased. Spin echo imaging utilizes at least one 180-degree RF pulse to produce this so-called echo and may in fact utilize multiple 180-degree RF pulses producing a multiple spin echo sequence [Figure 3-10]. However, as each 180-degree RF pulse is given (rephasing the spins), there is a loss of measurable echo signal due to the ongoing effects of true T2 relaxation.

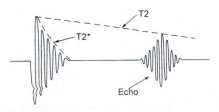

Figure 3-9. Simple spin echo.

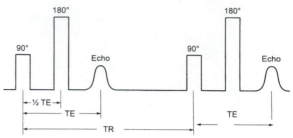

Figure 3-11. A spin echo sequence demonstrating TR and TE placement.

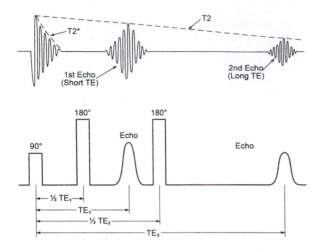

Figure 3-10. Multiple spin echo.

TISSUE CONTRAST IMAGING PARAMETERS

Which standard spin echo pulse sequence parameters directly control this process of spin density, T1, and T2 tissue contrast? In spin echo imaging, only two parameters determine tissue contrast, TR and TE.

TR or time of repetition is the amount of time that elapses between 90-degree RF pulses on a given slice [Figure 3-11]. TR is usually expressed in milliseconds and for standard spin echo imaging is generally set in the range 350 to 3000 ms. TR is the amount of time we allow individual proton vectors to realign with the main magnetic field. Although a long TR, such as 3000 ms (3 s), is not sufficient to allow long T1 tissues, such as CSF, to fully recover longitudinal magnetization between 90-degree RF pulses, it is considered to be adequate. TR affects tissue contrast by defining how much magnetization or signal each tissue recovers in the longitudinal plane, which in turn converts to the same level of measurable signal (bright to dark) in the transverse plane.

TE or time to echo is the amount of time between the 90-degree RF pulse and the measurement of the signal echo [Figure 3-11]. TE is also expressed in milliseconds and for standard spin echo imaging is generally set in the range 10 to 120 ms. TE affects tissue contrast by defining how much measurable signal is maintained or lost by allowing a little or a lot of dephasing to occur.

IMAGE WEIGHTING

As mentioned earlier, one weights a spin echo image by choosing the proper imaging parameters to produce the tissue contrast of choice in the final image. Keep in mind that all spin echo images actually have some amount of spin density, T1, *and* T2 image contrast. Initial longitudinal magnetization is always affected by a tissue's spin density and no matter what TR and TE choices one makes, some amount of T1 and T2 relaxation occurs before the signal can be measured. However, by selecting intelligent values of TR and TE, one can increase the tissue contrast of choice and minimize the others.

Spin Density Weighted Imaging

In spin density weighted imaging, desired tissue contrast is produced as a result of variations in the concentration of mobile hydrogen nuclei. Tissues should be fully realigned along the main magnetic field for these concentration variations to be seen. This is done by using a *long TR/short TE* sequence [Figure 3-12]. The long TR allows

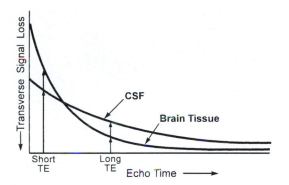

Figure 3-12. Multiple spin echo tissue contrast.

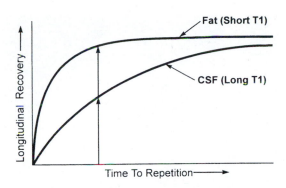

Figure 3-14. Tissue contrast with short TR and short TE.

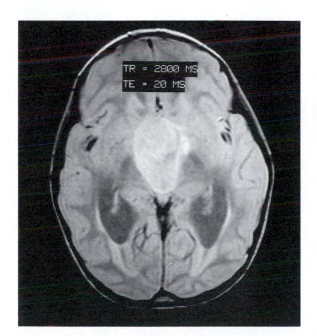

Figure 3-13. A spin density weighted brain image showing bright subcutaneous scalp fat and relatively dark CSF (note the relatively high pathological tissue signal).

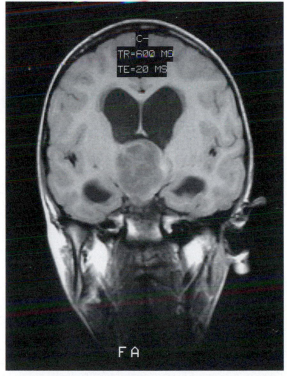

Figure 3-15. A noncontrast T1 weighted brain image showing bright fat, dark CSF, and an intermediate pathological tissue signal.

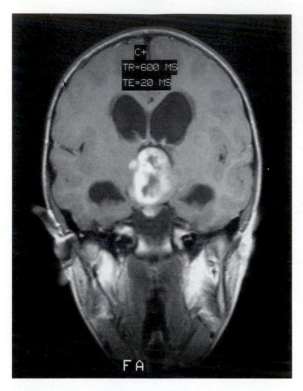

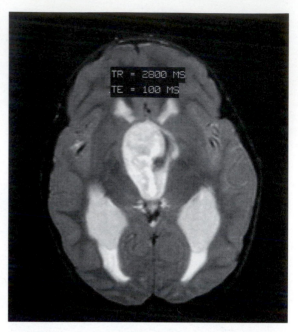

Figure 3-17. A T2 weighted brain image showing intermediate fat, bright CSF, and a bright pathological tissue signal.

Figure 3-16. A contrast enhanced T1 weighted brain image showing a bright pathological tissue signal (due to the T1 shortening effect of contrast agent).

tissues to reach full longitudinal magnetization. The short TE allows minimal loss of transverse signal due to T2 relaxation. In this sequence, the long TR reduces T1 effects and the short TE reduces T2 effects [Figure 3-13].

T1 Weighted Imaging

In T1 weighted imaging, desired tissue contrast is produced by looking at the variations in longitudinal relaxation rates. This is done by using a *short TR/short TE* sequence [Figure 3-14].

The short TR allows tissues with a short T1 value (such as fat) to fully recover along the longitudinal direction and tissues with a long T1 value (such as CSF) to only partially recover. The short TE allows minimal loss of transverse signal due to T2 relaxation. The short TR increases T1

effects and the short TE reduces T2 effects [Figures 3-15 and 3-16].

T2 Weighted Imaging

In T2 weighted imaging, desired tissue contrast is produced by looking at the variations in transverse relaxation rates. This is done by using a *long TR/ long TE* sequence [Figure 3-12]. The long TR allows tissues to reach full longitudinal magnetization. The long TE allows controlled loss of transverse signal due to T2 relaxation. The long TR reduces T1 effects [Figure 3-17]. The long TE highlights tissues with long transverse relaxation rates (such as fluid). It is extremely important to note that many pathological processes involve an abnormally high level of fluid in or around the area of interest. T2 weighted imaging is excellent for producing very bright signal from pathological fluids.

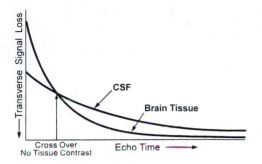

Figure 3-18. Tissue contrast reversal.

CROSSOVER

Tissue T2 relaxation curves can produce a very interesting imaging phenomenon. When examining a multi echo (short and long TE) imaging sequence utilizing a long TR, one can follow the T2 relaxation curves of two different tissues and discover that they can actually cross over one another at some point, resulting in reversal of tissue contrast (Figure 3-18). For example, brain will appear brighter than CSF on the short TE (spin density) image and darker than CSF on the long TE (T2) image. If the signal could be measured at the precise instant of crossover, these two tissues would become isodense, that is they would look identical.

SUMMARY

MR is in a constant state of change and development. It seems that technologists barely have time to attempt to understand or comprehend a newly designed imaging technique before another comes along to take its place. Without a working knowledge of the intrinsic factors responsible for the production of spin density, T1, and T2 tissue contrast, it is very difficult if not impossible to move forward and understand more complicated imaging techniques.

CHAPTER 4

Relating Frequency to Space: The Fourier Transform and Gradient Fields

Gary M. Schwartz and Yanmin Huang

INTRODUCTION

We've seen earlier how a radio frequency pulse can be used to create a signal in a sample of spins. The RF signal received depends on the T1, T2, and spin density within the sample. However, in a homogeneous magnetic field all of the spins will resonate at the same frequency. This means that in a homogeneous field there is no information about the spins at particular positions within the volume. In order to create a meaningful image, spatial information must be generated.

A convenient method to generate this information is to use that quality of magnetic resonance which allows us to image in the first place: a specific frequency RF pulse dependent on the magnetic field is required to generate the signal. Recall that the resonant frequency of the protons in our sample is determined by the strength of the magnetic field. If we could change the magnetic field at various positions within our sample in a predictable way, then we could also change the resonant frequencies of the protons at various positions within our sample in a predictable way. This would allow us to derive information about the properties of the spins at different positions in our sample.

The method that has been adopted is to change the static magnetic field by adding gradients to it. These gradients cause the field to vary by position in the field. RF pulses that excite protons of several frequencies are created so that we can image a volume of spins. This is done using Fourier transform technology.

Use of magnetic field gradients, coupled with appropriate RF pulses, has given rise to a tremendous number of methods to generate images. Different sequences of RF and gradient pulses, known as *pulse sequences*, have been invented to create images that look at different properties of the body. Not only can static anatomy be imaged, but flow can also be imaged. Sequences have been designed to take advantage of different relaxation mechanisms, generating images with different contrast.

In this chapter we introduce the concepts of the Fourier transform and magnetic field gradients, we discuss how gradients are applied in different directions to generate an image (slice select, phase encoding, and frequency encoding), and we look at a more advanced idea, gradient moment nulling and how it applies to image quality.

THE FOURIER TRANSFORM AND ITS APPLICATION

We've seen how critical it is to transmit RF power at the Larmor frequency. It is this frequency at which the spins resonate and return signal. However, if the spins are in a uniform magnetic field, all of them will resonate at that frequency. This means that no spatial information is generated in the sample.

To obtain an idea of the position and relaxation properties of the spins at different points in the volume, we must be able to change the Larmor frequency of the spins at different points. Magnetic field gradients allow us to change the frequency of the spins so that in lines across the sample the spins will absorb RF power in a continuous range of frequencies.

The power of this technique is that it is possible to tailor RF pulses in such a way that a continuous range of frequencies is excited. This is performed with Fourier transform MRI.

The Fourier transform is a mathematical method that allows us to "decompose" a complicated waveform into the sum of waveforms of different frequencies. For example, consider the function $\cos(f_0 t)$. This function is shown in Figure 4-1A. It consists of a single frequency, f_0, and is graphed with respect to time, t. Figure 4-1B shows the function $\cos(2f_0 t)$, also a single frequency, but twice the frequency of the function in Figure 4-1A. If we add the two functions together, we obtain $\cos(f_0 t) + \cos(2f_0 t)$, shown in Figure 4-1C. We see how a

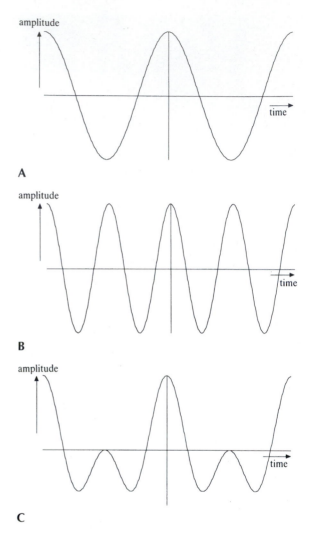

A

B

C

Figure 4-1.   Graphs of cosine function: **A** $\cos(2f_0 t)$, **B** $\cos(2f_0 t)$, and **C** $\cos(f_0 t) + \cos(2f_0 t)$. The frequency of the curve in **B** is twice the frequency of the curve in **A**. Notice how a complex curve may be created easily from simpler curves.

complex curve may be generated by simply adding cosine functions of different frequencies.

The curves in Figure 4-1 are graphed as functions of time. We could also graph these as functions of the frequencies used to compose them. For example, Figure 4-1A is composed of a single frequency, f_0. We could graph this as shown in Figure 4-2A. Note that the curve is now a single line whose frequency is f_0. This represents a transformation of the cosine curve from the time domain into the frequency domain. The two curves are equivalent.

Similarly, Figure 4-1B can be shown in the frequency domain as in Figure 4-2B. The single line is now depicted at frequency $2f_0$. Once again, the two curves are equivalent. One is simply a representation of the curve with respect to time, one with respect to frequency.

The complex curve shown in Figure 4-1C may be decomposed into a more straightforward-looking curve as shown in Figure 4-2C. The curve now consists of two lines, one with frequency f_0, and one with frequency $2f_0$.

The Fourier transform is essentially a representation of the frequencies and amplitudes of the cosine curves required to create a particular function.

Note that the common convention is to show the curves as the sum of two frequency components, each with half the amplitude of the original curve. The frequency components are f_0 and $-f_0$. These are shown in Figure 4-3. They are equivalent (in the frequency domain) to the curves in Figure 4-1 (in the time domain).

Using the same technique, we could compose a different function, this time a square pulse. A square pulse can be decomposed into a series of cosine curves. The greater the number of different frequencies we include in the series of cosine curves, the better the representation of the square wave. Figure 4-4A[1] shows an approximation of a square wave formed by the sum of two cosine curves: $\cos(2t)$ and $-(1/3)\cos(6t)$. Figure 4-4B, C, D show better and better approximations of the square wave by adding more cosine curves to the series: (B) $(1/5)\cos(10t)$, (C) $-(1/7)\cos(14t)$, (D) $(1/9)\cos(18t)$.

Note that the left half of Figure 4-4 shows the square wave in the time domain, and the right half of Figure 4-4 shows the square in the frequency domain. As more cosine curves are added we see that more frequencies are added to the frequency domain.

Finally, in Figure 4-5 we show the time and frequency domain curves as if we had an infinite number of frequencies with which to compose the square wave. The frequency domain curve now appears as a continuous curve. This curve also defines a function; its value at any point on that curve is $(\sin x)/x$.

Therefore, the Fourier transform of a square wave is the curve $(\sin x)/x$. This transformation works in both directions. If we were to graph the curve $(\sin x)/x$ in the time domain and decompose it into its component frequencies, the result would be a square wave in the frequency domain.

The importance of this is that in order to excite spins with a continuous range of frequencies we must transmit an RF pulse whose shape in the time domain is the waveform. In the frequency domain, we will be exciting spins whose frequencies combine to make up the waveform $(\sin x)/x$.

MAGNETIC FIELD GRADIENTS

In Chapter 2 we saw how a coil of wire could be used to induce a magnetic field. In particular we looked at the generation of a high intensity, stable magnetic field in which we perform MR imaging. While the coils of wire in the main magnet have a stable current through them, it is possible to build separate coils through which we will pulse a current in order to create time-varying magnetic fields. These gradient fields are superimposed on top of the main, static field, and they allow us to manipulate the strength of the static field in a very predictable way.

In this discussion we'll concern ourselves with linear gradient fields. The purpose of a linear gradient is to alter the environment of the protons so they resonate at a different frequency at different locations in the magnet. Since we'll know how we've altered the field, this is the first step in gaining information about spins at particular in the magnet.

In Figure 4-6 we see a depiction of a static, homogeneous magnetic field. The field strength

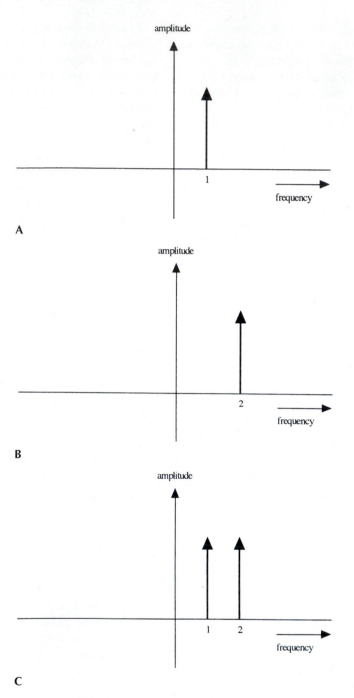

Figure 4-2. Representation of the curves from Figure 4-1 as functions of frequency. This is a representation of a Fourier transform of the cosine functions. **A** Since Figure 4-1**A** consists of a single frequency, it is shown as a single line at frequency 1. **B** Since Figure 4-1**B** consists of a single frequency (twice that of Figure 4-1**A**), the curve is shown as a single line with frequency 2. **C** The sum of the curves in Figure 4-1**A,B**; this is equivalent to the curve in Figure 4-1**C**.

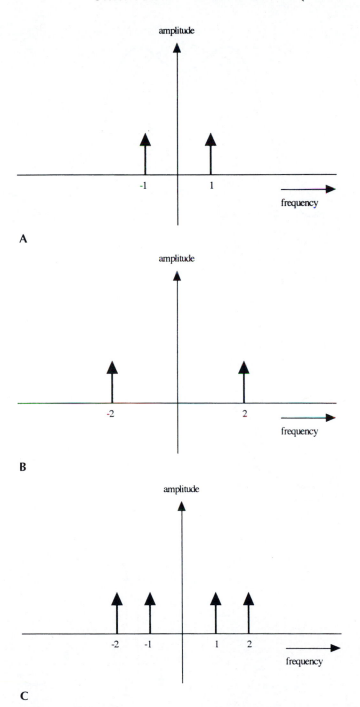

Figure 4-3.   The convention is to draw the Fourier transform as the sum of two curves whose frequencies are positive and negative. Each curve has half the amplitude of the original curve. Figure 4-3**A** is equivalent to Figure 4-2**A** and similarly for parts **B** and **C**.

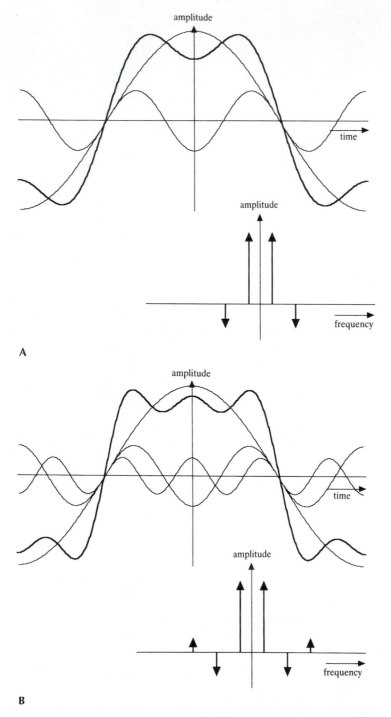

Figure 4-4. Representation of how to add cosine curves of different frequencies to create a square wave: **A** sum of the curves $\cos(2f_0t)$ and $-(1/3)\cos(6f_0t)$, **B** sum of curve **A** and $(1/5)\cos(10f_0t)$.

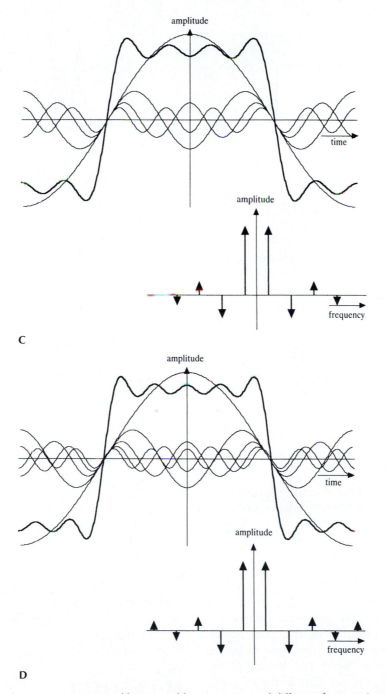

Figure 4-4 (*continued*).   Representation of how to add cosine curves of different frequencies to create a square wave: **C** sum of curve **B** and $-(1/7)\cos(14f_0t)$, and **D** sum of curve **C** and $(1/9)\cos(18f_0t)$. Notice how the profile of the square wave improves with each new cosine curve added. Note the Fourier transform plotted with each curve.

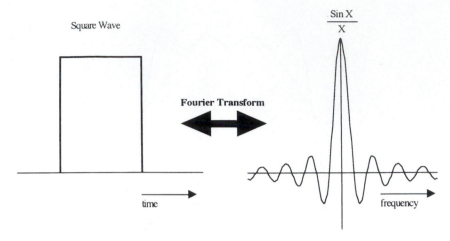

Figure 4-5. A perfect square wave requires an infinite number of cosine curves to create it. The Fourier transform of the square wave, plotted here, is the function $(\sin x)/x$.

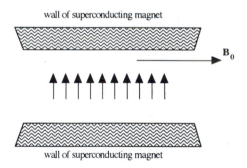

Figure 4-6. Representation of the strength of the B_0 field at 10 points in the magnet. Note that the direction of the field is horizontal. The vertical arrows simply indicate that the strength of the field is the same at all ten points.

at each point in the field is represented by a vertical arrow. Note that the vertical arrow *does not* represent the direction of the field. Merely the strength of the field is represented by the length of the arrow. Since the length of the arrows is the same, the strength of the magnetic field is the same at each point.

In Figure 4-7 we see a depiction of the gradient that we will apply to the main field. Again the length of the arrows shows the strength of

the gradient field. The direction of the arrows shows that we are either adding to or subtracting from the main field. Note that at the center of the gradient field there is no arrow, and therefore, no effect on the main field.

The effect of the gradient on the main magnetic field is shown in Figure 4-8. Here we see that the strength of the main field is different at each of the points shown in the figure. Note that the strength changes in a predictable, linear way. The result of changing the field strength is that the Larmor frequency of the spins at each point is also changing in a predictable, linear way.

Gradient coils are built so that the field can be manipulated in each of the three axes independently. One could also pulse the gradients in such a way that they add up to rotate the three axes so that we can image in phases other than the original frame. This is the idea behind oblique imaging.

SLICE SELECT

The slice select gradient starts the process of providing the information for an image. The purpose of this gradient is to divide the volume

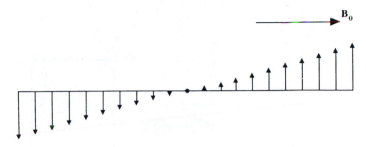

Figure 4-7. Representation of a linear gradient field. Note that at the center the strength of the gradient is zero. The direction of the gradient field is the same as that of the B_0 field. The arrows indicate the strength of the gradient field. The arrows pointing down will subtract from the B_0 field while those pointing up will add to it.

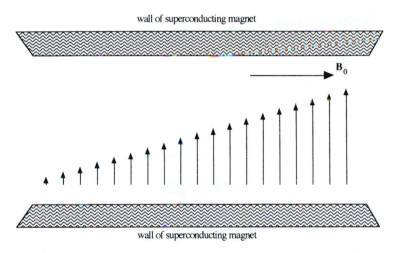

Figure 4-8. Representation of the effect of the gradient field on the B_0 field. Here Figures 4-6 and 4-7 have been added together. Note that the strength of the B_0 field is different at each of the points. This means that the Larmor frequency is also different at each point.

of interest into discrete slices. The theme that repeats itself throughout the application of gradient fields is that we are using the gradients to create a distribution of frequencies, and we use an RF pulse to excite a range of frequencies.

In the case of the slice select gradient, we turn on the RF pulse while the gradient is being applied. As we saw earlier, one may tailor the RF pulse for particular purposes. For example, one could obtain a square slice profile by using a sinc pulse, sinc $x = (\sin x)/x$. The sinc pulse excites a discrete range of frequencies with equal amplitude at each frequency [Figure 4-9].

Recall from the discussion of magnetic field gradients that the gradient creates a range of frequencies in the volume. The sinc pulse excites spins whose position in space corresponds to the frequencies determined by the gradient. Therefore, the slice profile is square. This RF pulse shape takes a relatively long time to

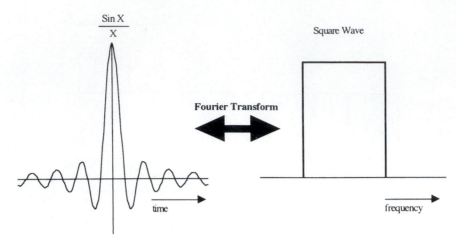

Figure 4-9. A (sin x)/x pulse transforms into a square pulse, therefore it excites a range of frequencies with the same amplitude at each frequency in the range. A square slice profile is the result.

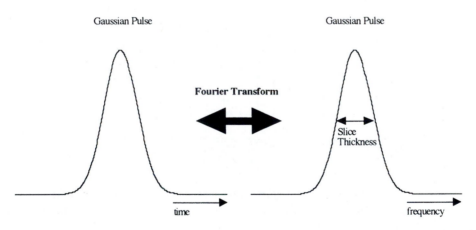

Figure 4-10. A Gaussian pulse transforms into a Gaussian pulse, therefore the amplitude of the signal generated within the slice is dependent on position within the slice. Spins at the center of the slice contribute more to the signal than spins at the edges of the slice. The slice thickness is defined as the width of the slice at half the maximum amplitude.

produce, so it is less desirable for fast sequences, as well as those with a short TE.

Alternatively, one could use a Gaussian pulse to save time, and excite a slice whose profile is itself a Gaussian distribution [Figure 4-10]. The drawback with this RF pulse is that the slice thickness, defined as the full width at half maximum (FWHM) of the slice profile, is such that slices whose centers exactly lined up would have some overlap in the slices, causing a degradation of signal to noise [Figure 4-11]. This is sometimes referred to as *crosstalk*. The solution is to increase the gap between the slice centers so there is no interference.

Let's assume that we use a sinc pulse to excite the slice. As we saw earlier, the Fourier transform of a sinc pulse is a square wave. This square wave represents a discrete range of frequencies, and, as we change the frequency range of the square wave, we change the position in space of the pulse excitation. This is how we're able to image slices at different positions in the volume.

The slice thickness can be changed by either changing the width of the range of frequencies

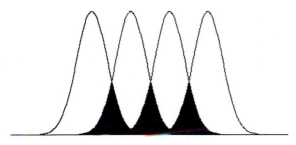

Figure 4-11. Overlap of closely spaced Gaussian pulses. If these slices are imaged consecutively the spins in the shaded area do not have time to relax, therefore they contribute less signal than if they had relaxed completely. This can alter the contrast of the image. One must increase the gap between the slices to eliminate this crosstalk.

excited by the sinc pulse, or by changing the strength of the gradient field. Changing the width of the range of frequencies generally means changing the length of time the sinc pulse is applied. Since that can change the timing of the pulse sequence (and may change TE as well as other parameters), it is not commonly done.

It is more common to change the slice thickness by changing the strength of the gradient. Figure 4-12 shows examples of slices whose thickness is changed by changing the gradient strength. As the gradient is made stronger, the frequency distribution across the same distance increases. Another way to look at changing the gradient strength is that for the same range of frequencies, a higher gradient defines a narrower distance. We see in Figure 4-12 that for the same RF pulse (and therefore the same frequency spread), different gradient strengths produce different slice thicknesses.

One important consequence of this discussion is that the minimum slice thickness for a given RF pulse is dependent upon the maximum gradient strength of the system. This desire for thinner slices and better spatial resolution is why manufacturers are always looking at ways to increase the capabilities of their gradient systems.

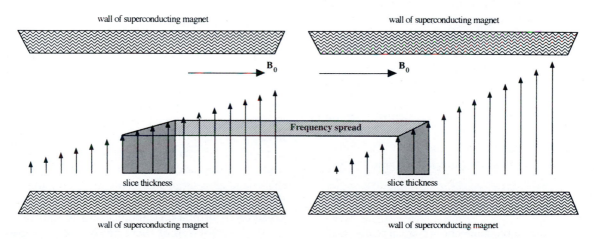

Figure 4-12. Representation of how gradient strength can be changed to change slice thickness. The horizontal shaded area represents the selected frequency range. Note that the selected slice thickness is larger in the magnet on the left than in the magnet on the right. This is a result of the stronger gradient being applied on the right-hand side.

FREQUENCY ENCODING

Having excited a slice using a selective RF pulse with an appropriate slice select gradient, we apply another gradient to read the echo. The gradient is applied in a direction along the plane of the slice, rather than through the slice. It produces a spread of frequencies along the slice in the direction of the gradient, the same way a spread is produced by the slice gradient.

The frequency range of interest is selected by the bandwidth of the readout sampling window. The bandwidth is inversely proportional to the amount of time spent listening to each data point. Since the convention is to call the center of the echo zero frequency, the quoted bandwidth is half the total width (so a 6 kHz total window width is actually a 3 kHz bandwidth, from −3 kHz to +3 kHz).

Once the desired frequency range is set, the gradient strength is adjusted to provide the desired field of view (FOV). Since a stronger gradient produces a larger frequency spread over a given physical space, for a given frequency spread (set by the sequence designer) a stronger gradient produces a smaller FOV. This is exactly the same as the situation shown in Figure 4-12. In fact you could replace the words "slice thickness" with the words "field of view" in Figure 4-12 to describe how gradients affect FOV in the frequency encoding direction. Once again we see that the search for better resolution lies in stronger (and faster) gradients. It is also why the gradient strength determines a system's maximum resolution.

As we will see later, the demand of more complicated and strenuous sequences combined with the need for high resolution also creates a demand for stronger (and faster) gradient fields.

PHASE ENCODING

Each time we read an echo we are actually reading the information in the entire slice. This provides information about two of the three dimensions of the slice. We know we've excited a slice of a specified thickness (first dimension). By reading the echo with a frequency encoding gradient we've determined the distribution of spins at specific frequencies in that direction (second dimension). How then can we generate information about the third dimension in the slice?

The solution is to read the echo many times, but to slightly change the conditions under which we read the echo each time. We do this by applying a gradient in the third direction, called the phase encoding gradient.

We saw earlier that every gradient applied introduces a frequency shift. A gradient applied along the phase encoding direction will similarly produce a spread of frequencies of the spins along the gradient. Recall from the discussion in Chapter 2 that when spins are precessing at different frequencies they tend to lose their phase coherence. This is analogous to the example of runners on a track.

The way we encode the data is the change the strength of the phase encoding gradient for each line of data we acquire. Since the frequency spread is different for each line of data we acquire, the phase coherence is also different. That is, our runners have changed speeds relative to one another. Thus, the gradient affects the relative phase of the spins.

Figure 4-13 shows the effects of phase encoding gradients of different strengths. In Figure 4-13A no gradient is applied; all the spins are moving at the same frequency, therefore all the runners are aligned together on the track. In Figure 4-13B a low PE gradient is applied; the spins move at slightly different frequencies, and if we stop them at a given time we'll see that some have traveled further than others, like our runners on the track. The phase coherence is somewhat degraded. In Figure 14-13C we see the effect of a large PE gradient. Compared to the low PE gradient in Figure 4-13B there is a greater loss of phase coherence of the spins.

In the right half of these figures we see a grid that represents how we write the data onto the computer disk. Each horizontal line represents the data of a single echo. Each time we change

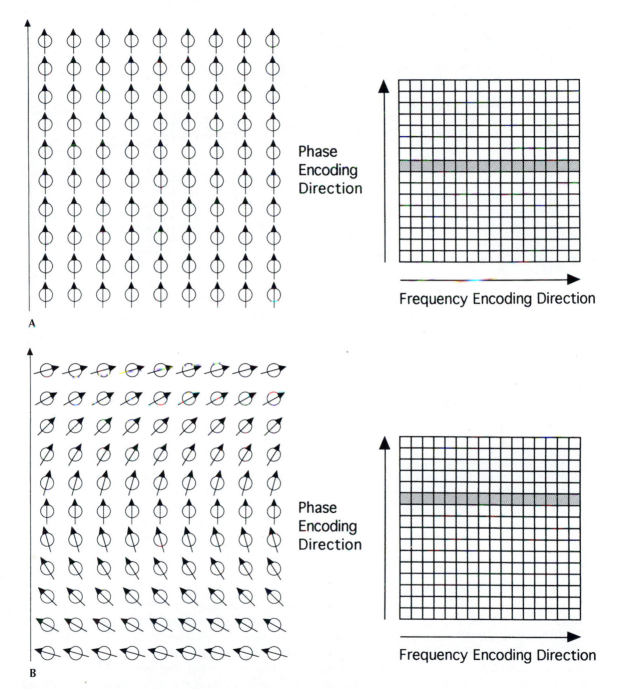

Figure 4-13. Representation of the effect of the phase encoding gradient on the spins at different positions in the magnet. **A** No gradient is applied, and the spins all have the same phase; the data collected with no gradient is placed at the center of the image data. **B** A small PE gradient is applied, and the phase of the spins varies with position.

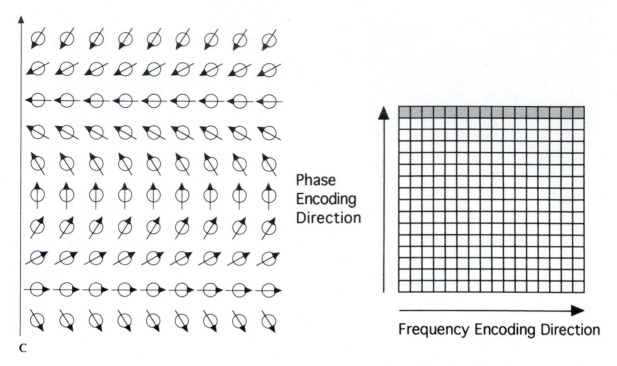

C

Phase Encoding Direction

Frequency Encoding Direction

Figure 4-13 (*continued*).   Representation of the effect of the phase encoding gradient on the spins at different positions in the magnet. **C** A large PE gradient is applied, and the variance in phase of the spins is increased.

the phase encoding gradient we acquire and write another line of data. Then a Fourier transform is applied in each direction (PE and Freq.) to create the image.

The low phase encoding lines are written in the center of the image, while the high phase encoding lines are written to the edges of the image. Because of the phase coherence of the lines with little phase encoding gradient applied, there is more signal in those lines.

Once we've collected all of the lines of data we have a whole set of information about the distribution of spins. This is a result of the addition or subtraction of signal from spins at different positions depending on their relative phase in each line of data. The data is decoded by performing a Fourier transform on it.

Just as for the frequency encoding gradient the maximum strength of the phase encoding

gradient determines the FOV of the imaging experiment. The number of lines of data acquired determines the resolution.

One very important concept with respect to phase encoding is *wraparound*. Look at Figure 4-13. Notice that as we increase the strength of the gradient (or move further away from the center of the magnet), the spins become more and more out of phase. Eventually, like runners who move at different speeds, the spins will "lap" one another. When they do this, it's impossible to tell whether they are on the same lap or on different laps.

The result is that the spins will be treated as if they actually have the same phase. The effect is that in the image, objects whose position with respect to one another is such that they have the same phase will appear in the same location on the image. This is an important source of image artifacts, and therefore you must carefully select the phase encoding direction when you set up a protocol.

GRADIENT MOMENT NULLING

Gradient moment nulling is a technique in which we are able to greatly reduce, if not eliminate, image artifacts due to moving spins. These artifacts are commonly caused by flows of blood or CSF. Not only does this technique improve image quality by reducing the artifact, it also improves image contrast by correctly placing the signal from the moving spins where they belong in the image.

When spins move while a gradient is on they accumulate a phase shift. This is why you see the flow artifact in the phase encoding direction. In sagittal imaging of the knee with the phase encoding direction in the A/P direction, for example, blood flow in the popliteal artery causes artifacts that can obliterate the anatomy in the joint. The reason for this artifact is that the moving blood acquires a different phase than stationary tissue at the same position. It then is mapped in the wrong location in the phase direction.

One of the common misperceptions of the gradient moment nulling technique is that we might be nulling out the signal. In fact, what we are nulling is the gradient moment. In order to understand how this works, we need to take a closer look at what is meant by a gradient moment.

Let's take a look at a moving spin. Its position at any time is directly related to its starting position, its velocity, and its acceleration. There are other things that contribute, such as pulsitility, but we won't be concerned with them at this time. If we were to look at this as a physics problem, we might write an equation as:

Position equals starting position plus
velocity plus acceleration

The spins acquire a phase shift when they're under the influence of a gradient field. In fact, this phase shift is directly proportional to the strength of the gradient. It's also directly proportional to the position of the spins in space. We might write this equation as:

Phase shift is proportional to
strength times position

Recalling that position is related to the starting position, the velocity, and the acceleration, we discover that the phase shift is also proportional to the gradient strength times the starting position, the gradient strength times the velocity, and the gradient strength times the acceleration.

Each of these represents what is called a *moment* of the gradient field. The goal of designing the sequence is to use the gradients to minimize the phase shift due to each moment, since we only have control over the gradients, not the position of the spins. If the phase shift can be reduced to zero (by choosing the appropriate gradient), then that gradient moment will have been *nulled*.

The moment related to the position is the zeroth moment, the velocity term is the first moment, and the acceleration term is the second moment. This means that a system that supports first and second order flow compensation is able to reduce the effect of constant flow (the velocity term), and flow whose velocity changes (the acceleration term).

CONCLUSION

In this chapter we've seen how we use RF pulses and magnetic field gradients to generate information about spins at different positions in the sample. We've looked at the Fourier transform, a powerful technique that allows us to include a tremendous amount of information in a single RF pulse. We've examined magnetic field gradients, especially with respect to how gradients are used to derive spatial information in three dimensions. Finally, we've seen how a more complex gradient sequence may be designed to remove flow artifacts. In the following chapters you will build on this and see how gradients and RF pulses may be combined to create MR imaging pulse sequences, and how to optimize those sequences for your clinical work.

REFERENCE

1. Brigham EO. *The Fast Fourier Transform*. New York: Prentice Hall, 5, 1974.

CHAPTER 5

Imaging Coil Technology

William Faulkner, Jr.

INTRODUCTION

MR is based on the interaction of magnetic fields and radiowaves. The MR signal is produced when the tissue magnetization moves through an antenna orientated in the transverse xy plane. The current induced in the antenna is used to create the final image. The RF coils are the antennas. Before discussing how we use coils, let's begin with a very basic explanation of how transmission and reception of a signal can be accomplished. Figure 5-1A shows a very simple dipole transmitter. The signal generator produces an alternating flow of electrons (current) along the axis of the dipole. A receiver is configured the same as a transmitter except that a receiver is positioned in place of the signal generator and the conductor (antenna) acts to receive the signal rather than transmit the signal. If we position our receiver along the same axis as the transmitter in what is known as a collinear fashion [Figure 5-1B], the signal generator causes current to flow along the axis of the dipole.

The current in the wire produces an electric field (E field) and a magnetic field (B field); in other words, an electromagnetic wave. The electromagnetic wave from the transmitter interacts with the electrons in the conductor of the receiver. This interaction has the effect of causing the electrons in the receiver to oscillate at the same frequency as the electromagnetic wave along the conductor producing a current in the conductor at that frequency.

In magnetic resonance imaging, the sample of tissue being imaged is the signal generator. The transverse magnetization vector rotates in the xy plane rather than oscillating in a linear orientation. When this magnetic vector rotates through our receiver coil, the electrons in the conductor (wire within the coil) move and produce a current in the receiver coil. This principle is known as *Faraday's Law of Induction*. When a magnetic field moves through a loop of wire, a current is induced in that wire. The strength of the current (amplitude of the signal) is related to the conductivity of the wire, and the strength of the magnetic field [Figure 5-2]. The higher the magnitude of the magnetization vector (amount of transverse magnetization), the greater the amplitude of the resultant signal. Because the rotating magnetic field passes in and out of plane with our receiver

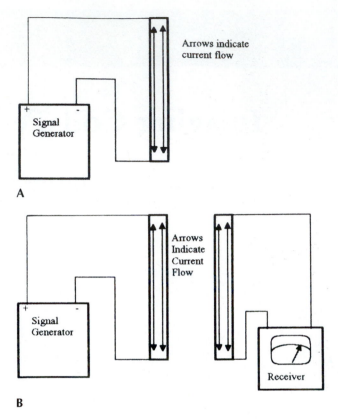

Figure 5-1.   A In a simple dipole transmitter a signal generator produces an alternating current flow in a transmitter (conductor). **B** A transmitter and receiver in a collinear orientation. Current flow in the transmitter causes current flow in the receiver, which produces a detectable signal.

coil, the signal in the coil oscillates at the frequency of the magnetic field precession.

In this chapter we will look at the overall applications of coils as well as their various configurations. We will also look at some strategies for their use.

COIL CONFIGURATIONS

Transmit and Receive Coils

Most MR systems have two main types of imaging coils, receive-only and transmit and receive (T/R); these will be the focus of this section, although other configurations may exist.

With high field systems, the two most common coils to be configured as transmit and receive are the body coil and the head coil. Coils used for extremity imaging can be either, depending on the manufacturer's preference. With low field systems, most coils are receive-only. The transmit coil is located within the enclosure on the magnet "face." Typically, transmit and receive coils are felt to be more efficient than receive-only. The closer a coil is to the area or part to be excited, the less RF energy is needed to create transverse magnetization. This directly reduces the specific absorption rate (SAR) to the patient. In addition, having a receive coil close to the excited volume will detect a larger signal, hence improving the signal-to-noise ratio (SNR). With low field systems, since less RF power is needed and thus SAR is of less concern, receive-only coils are likely sufficient.

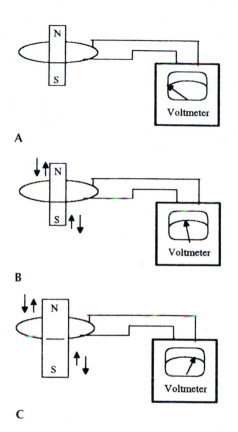

A

B

C

Figure 5-2. **A** When the magnet is not moving through the coil of wire no voltage is produced. **B** Moving the magnet back and forth through the coil of wire will produce a voltage. **C** Increasing the size of the magnet will increase the strength of the voltage produced.

Several types of smaller coils may be configured as T/R coils. They are typically used for imaging the head and/or extremities as shown in Figure 5-3. In a vertical field system where the *xy* plane is along the axis of the patient's body, the basic design of the coil is a solenoid, or wraparound configuration.

Receive-Only Coils

Coils that only receive MR signal are called receive-only coils. These coils may come in a variety of shapes, configurations, and sizes. Initially, coils that were designed to be placed around or on a

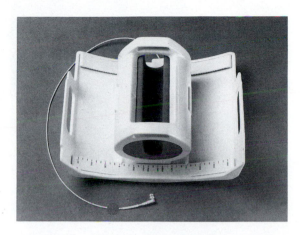

Figure 5-3. A T/R coil used for imaging extremities.

specific area were called *surface coils*. Now, some are designed to be placed internally within the body, such as the endorectal coil used to image the prostate. There are three different configurations of this particular coil. Each one is specifically designed to image the prostate, rectum, or uterus. An example of this type of coil and sample images are shown in Figure 5-4. Surface coils and other small-body-part-specific coils are now often referred to as *local coils*. It is now a standard practice to use some type of local coil specific to whatever area of the body we are imaging.

Surface Coils

One of the big battles in MRI is to produce images with high SNR. Noise can be defined as *unwanted signal*. The advent of surface coil imaging was a big help in that battle. A surface coil is a receiving antenna which can be placed close to the source of our signal. Surface coils help improve our SNR by "listening" to a more limited area than a larger coil, such as the body coil, thereby reducing signal we don't want or need. In other words, surface coils increase signal. Getting an antenna close to the source of the MR signal enables more efficient reception of the MR signal. The major advantage of using a surface coil is related to this increase in SNR.

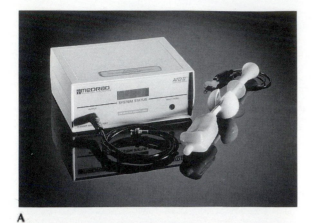

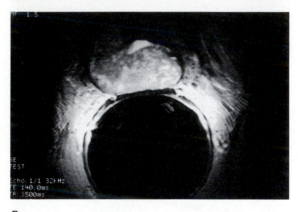

Figure 5-4.   A Prostate coil, **B** Sample image.

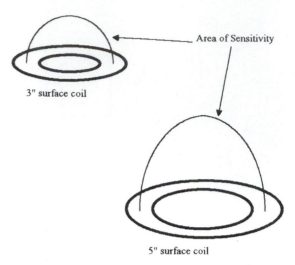

Figure 5-5.   By increasing the size of a planar surface coil we increase the area from which we receive MR signal, the area of sensitivity.

is important to remember that the basic idea behind surface coils is to improve SNR, and that increasing the size of the coil we use actually decreases the SNR. Increasing the area of coverage without decreasing the SNR can be done and will be addressed later. But as a general rule *increasing the size of the coil will increase the area of coverage* and decrease the SNR.

We can often use an increased SNR to compensate for a smaller voxel volume in order to improve our spatial resolution or we can acquire less signal averages to reduce our overall scan time.

Just as a coil transmitting radio frequency has a certain distance over which it radiates its signal, a receiver coil has a certain *area of sensitivity* over which it receives signal. Outside this area, minimal signal is received. The area of sensitivity is related to the diameter of the coil [Figure 5-5]. Increasing the size of the coil increases the area of sensitivity; almost everything in MR is gained at a price. Increasing the area over which we receive MR signal increases not only the amount of MR signal, but also the amount of noise we receive. It

GENERAL RULES FOR SURFACE COIL USE

I use some basic rules of thumb to select a surface coil. First, *match the coil to the anatomy or the area you desire to image.* There is no need to use a coil larger than the area of interest because of the negative impact on SNR. Secondly, *match the field of view (FOV) to the size of the coil.* If this is done, the resolution can be optimized and the need for anti-aliasing techniques can be eliminated. The images in Figure 5-6 are from a study of the temporomandibular joint (TMJ). Figure 5-6A was acquired using a 5-in. circular coil and a 12-cm FOV. Not only is the SNR low, but since the

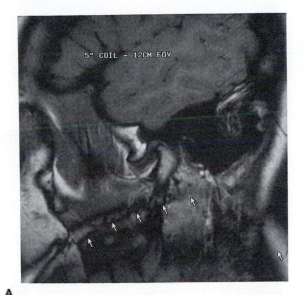

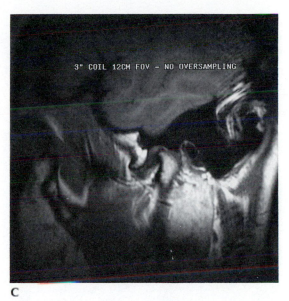

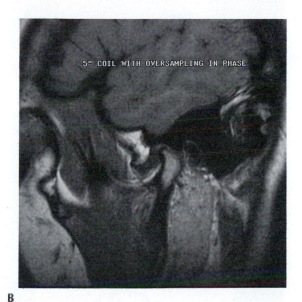

Figure 5-6. Images of the temporomandibular joint (TMJ) acquired using **A** a 5-in. coil and a 12-cm field of view (FOV), **B** a 5-in. coil and a 12-cm FOV with anti-aliasing, and **C** a 3-in. coil and a 12-cm FOV, no anti-aliasing because it isn't necessary.

however, an anti-aliasing option was used that oversampled in the phase direction. Although this removed the aliased signal, the overall SNR was not improved. Oversampling option used in the phase direction will increase the scan time in proportion to the amount of oversampling but can be compensated for by reducing the number of signal averages used. This however reduces the motion reduction effect of multiple averages, but since there is less "noise" from aliasing, the SNR may remain unchanged. Maintaining the original average parameter will result in improvements in SNR. Figure 5-6C was acquired with a 12-cm FOV, no anti-aliasing option, and a 3-in. coil. Notice the absence of aliased signal since the FOV is roughly the same size as the receiver coil. In addition, the overall SNR is greatly improved.

Increasing the length of the coil along the lumbar spine does allow us to image more of the structures along the axis of the spine [Figure 5-7A and B]. While the superior to inferior coverage

receiver coil is larger than our FOV, signal from tissue outside the FOV is aliased into the FOV (indicated by arrows). Figure 5-6B was acquired using the same 5-in. coil and 12-cm FOV, is better in Figure 5-7A when compared with Figure 5-7B, the SNR is not as high as in Figure 5-7B, which was acquired using a smaller surface coil. Figure 5-7C and D shows the main reason for the noise increase in the image acquired with the larger coil. Using a narrow window width allows us to get an idea of the area of sensitivity of each type of coil. The larger coil's increased area of sensitivity allows more signal to be detected from the bowel and even the anterior abdominal

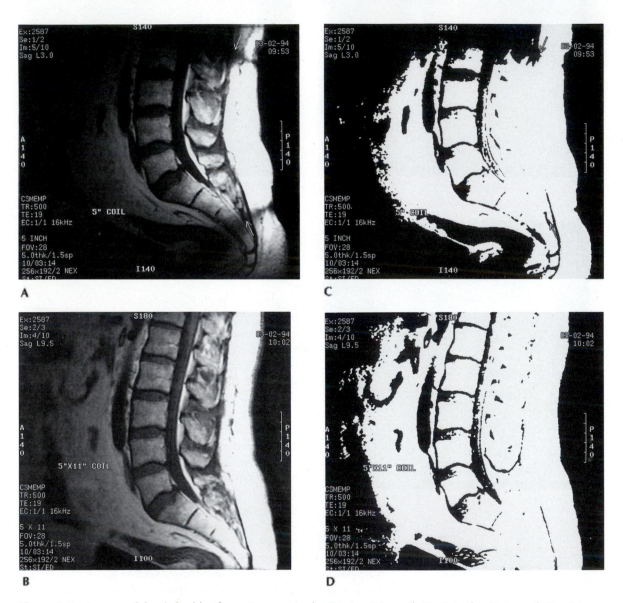

Figure 5-7.   Images of the sagittal lumbar spine acquired using **A** a 5-in. coil, **B** a 5-in. by 11-in. coil, **C** a 5-in. coil with a narrow window showing the area of sensitivity, and **D** a 5-in. by 11-in. coil with a narrow window showing the area of sensitivity.

wall. Both of these structures are moving, therefore contribute even more to the reduction in image quality by causing motion artifacts. This can be minimized by the use of multiple signal averages. The obvious penalty, however, for increasing averages is a direct increase in scan time. Among other remedies are respiratory compensation techniques and the use of spatial presaturation pulses within the imaging FOV. Using a coil matched to the area of interest allows us to optimize the SNR for the desired scan time. Smaller coils reduce the area of coverage, yet increase the inherent SNR of images and therefore less signal averages are needed, as demonstrated by the TMJ example.

It is often desirable to obtain the best spatial resolution possible, given the SNR dictated by other parameter choices. Using a coil specific to the size of the area being imaged will help by giving us more SNR than if we had chosen a coil larger than needed. We can use the extra SNR to acquire images with smaller voxels, thereby increasing spatial resolution. Increasing the SNR also improves the ability to see small differences in tissue contrasts by improving the contrast-to-noise of our image [Figure 5-8].

There is a continual effort to balance time, SNR, and spatial resolution using MRI. The use of surface coils gives us more flexibility by improving the SNR of our images.

LINEAR AND QUADRATURE DESIGN

In constructing both transmit and receive coils and surface coils, two basic designs are generally employed, linear and quadrature. Going back to the initial explanation of a dipole transmit and receive configuration, it may seem fairly clear regarding signal production and reception. In the world of MRI, however, that description is not really accurate. The transmitter, you will recall, is really the sample of tissue. More specifically, the rotating magnetic field within the sample transmits the signal. You may also recall from the initial explanation that maximum signal occurs when the direction or polarization of the receiver is collinear or aligned with the direction or polarization of the transmitter. Since our transmitter is rotating, we say that our transmitter is circularly polarized. We could get optimum reception if we rotated the receiver in phase along with the transmitter. At 1.5 T, that means someone would have to circle the coil around the patient at approximately 63 MHz. Since this is not practical, we adopt the configuration of Figure 5-9A. In this case the coil is linear; it is linearly polarized. As the rotating transverse magnetization becomes aligned with the coil (360 degrees and 180 degrees) the signal will be at its strongest. When the magnetization vector is orientated at 90 degrees and 270 degrees, the signal will be at its weakest.

In the situation just described, we have magnetization in the x-direction and the y-direction but we receive only in the x-direction. In other words, our transmitter is circularly polarized but our receiver is linearly polarized. A quadrature

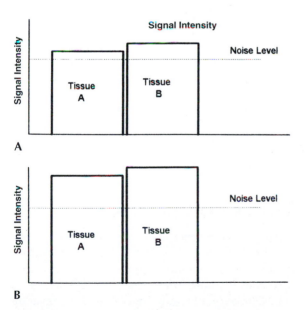

Figure 5-8. A graphic representation of the results of increasing the SNR in an image. By increasing the SNR, that is raising the amount of signal, we improve our ability to differentiate tissues with lower contrasts. **A** Lower SNR, **B** higher SNR.

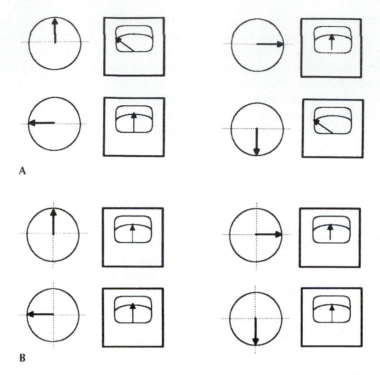

Figure 5-9. **A** A linear coil aligned along the 90–270-degree axis (dotted line). As the transverse magnetization rotates through the coil, the signal is strongest when the magnetization vector is aligned with the polarization direction of the coil (collinear). **B** A quadrature coil is also known as a circularly polarized or CP coil. In the CP design the magnetization vector is collinear more often than in the linear design and this improves the overall signal strength.

coil is configured so that we receive in the y-direction as well as the x-direction. This situation is illustrated in Figure 5-9B. When the rotating magnetization is aligned with the coil component at 90 degrees and 270 degrees (horizontal dotted line), the signal will be at its strongest. The signal will become weaker as it rotates away from the horizontal dotted line. With the quadrature design, however, the signal starts to become stronger as it approaches the vertical dotted line and will be strongest again as it becomes aligned with the vertical dotted line. In the linear coil configuration, the signal would be weakest at this point. The two coils receive the signals which are offset in their phase by 90 degrees. These two signals are added electronically and have the effect of improving the SNR by 41 percent (a factor of the square root of 2).

In summary, since our signal generator (the voxel) is circularly polarized due to its rotation, we get improved signal detection when we use a coil that is also circularly polarized, a quadrature coil, for example.

OTHER COIL CONFIGURATIONS

There are two other styles or configurations we need to mention. The first is a Helmholtz configuration. A Helmholtz pair can be described as two coils working in tandem. Figure 5-10 shows an example of a Helmholtz coil used for imaging the anterior neck and/or the cervical spine. This is sometimes referred to as a volume coil. The Helmholtz pair differs from the quadrature coil in that it is actually two linear coils. The purpose is to improve the signal through a volume of tissue.

A more recent configuration is called phased array or multicoil. In the first type of phased array to be commercially available, each coil in the array is wired to its own receiver board or channel. In this type of configuration, each single coil does not see any other coils in the array. Usually if two coils are placed close together, they will interact with each other reducing the overall SNR of the image because each coil detects noise from the other (coupling). With phased array coils, each coil is independent of the other; each has its own separate receiver channel. This yields the SNR of an individual coil and the coverage of the entire array. If coils are linked together in a linear fashion, longer areas of anatomy can be imaged without the penalty of signal being received from deeper in the anatomy. This has great benefit when imaging larger areas of the spine. It is not uncommon to have requests to image multiple levels of the spinal cord for various reasons, such as multilevel metastatic disease to the vertebral bodies. These patients are often in extreme pain and lengthy exams are not possible without considerable compromise in image quality (increased motion artifacts) and patient discomfort. For the sake of time, decreasing the number of signal averages

benefits the patient, but also decreases SNR. The use of a linear coil array greatly improves the success rate of imaging such patients. Figure 5-11 shows an example of a linear array coil and a sample image.

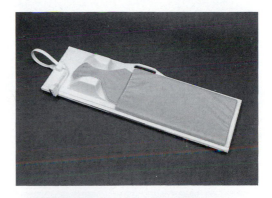

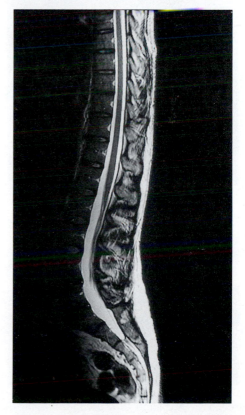

Figure 5-10. A volume neck coil.

Figure 5-11. A spine array (above) and sample image.

Another variation of the multicoil array can be termed the *volume array*; an example is shown in Figure 5-12. This array is used for imaging of the pelvis. Two coils are in the posterior component and two coils are in the anterior component. As with the linear spine array, the area of sensitivity is that of each small coil. In this type of array, however, the total depth of tissue that can be imaged is actually the sum of the posterior and interior components. And as with the linear array, the SNR is that of the small, individual coils. This type of array could have application in extremities, abdomen, and chest.

Phased array technology has been a tremendous aid in the development of specialty coils. Figure 5-13 shows an example of an array used

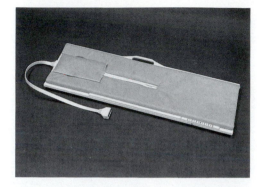

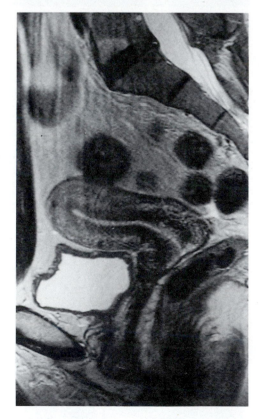

Figure 5-12. A volume array used for imaging the pelvis (above) and sample image.

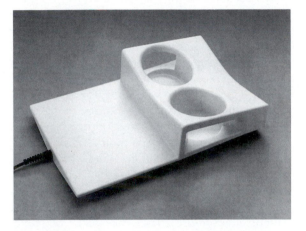

Figure 5-13. An array used for breast imaging.

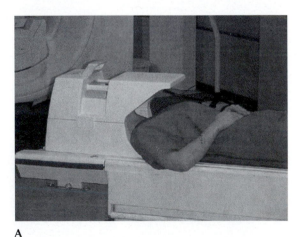

A

Figure 5-14. A Multicoil array for imaging the head and neck. (Courtesy Erlanger Medical Center, Chattanooga, TN.)

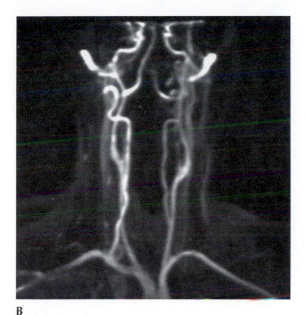

B

Figure 5-14. **B** Large field-of-view coronal image shows vessels from superior aorta to inferior circle of Willis using a multicoil head/neck array.

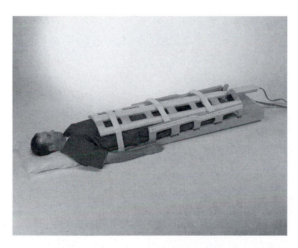

Figure 5-15. Phased array peripheral vascular coil for imaging the peripheral vascular system. (Courtesy USA Instruments, Inc.)

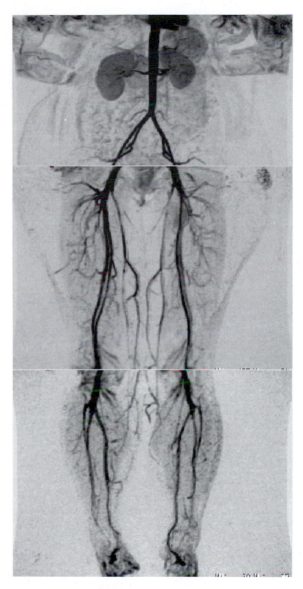

Figure 5-16. Continuous image of the peripheral vascular system from the renal vessels to the lower legs using a multicoil peripheral vascular array. (Courtesy USA Instruments, Inc.)

for breast imaging. The advent of contrast enhanced MR angiography techniques have spawned the need for specially designed coils. Phased array designs lend themselves well to this type of application due to the ability to cover a large volume without a penalty in SNR. Figure 5-14A shows an example of a multicoil array for imaging the head and neck *along with a sample of the type of study one can perform* with this type of coil [Figure 5-14B]. A multicoil array for imaging the aorta and peripheral vasculature is shown in Figure 5-15. Software can be written to advance the scanning table and simultaneously switch to the appropriate coils to produce the images shown in Figure 5-16.

There have been tremendous improvements in coil technology in the past decade. The advent of surface coil imaging has been instrumental in the improvement of MR image quality. Advances such as quadrature design, transmit and receive coils, dedicated local coils, and phased array (multicoil) technology prove that imaging coils are, and will be, an intricate part of magnetic resonance imaging now and in the future.

CHAPTER 6

Assessing the Interaction of Image Sequence Parameters

Peggy Woodward

Since the first successful brain scan was performed less than two decades ago, we have known that the viability of this diagnostic imaging procedure is directly related to our ability consistently to produce high-quality diagnostic images. The selection of image sequence parameters is paramount to producing image quality that separates excellent from good from bad. It is the radiologist and the MR technologist who are ultimately responsible for this selection. Therefore, emphasis must be placed on educating these groups to understand how the selection of scan parameters affects the final image. It can make or break an imaging center.

WHAT IS IMAGE QUALITY?

Image quality in MRI is a measure of the diagnostic accuracy and appearance of an image. It is defined by the contrast of the images, the ability to resolve detail spatially, and the signal-to-noise ratio (SNR).

CONTRAST

In MRI, contrast is the difference in relative brightness between pixels: the result of the signal intensity received from each voxel during the NMR experiment. Signal intensities vary, predominantly due to variations in the spin relaxation rates. Hydrogen density of the tissues also varies and plays an important role in contrast discrimination. Since contrast is inherent in tissues, it is the goal of MR imaging to enhance that contrast without misrepresentation.

The MRI system produces visual contrast by means of the graphics processor. The primary calculation performed during a Fourier transform separates the encoded signal into its individual frequency components. These signals are translated into gray scale ranges between 1 and 256 shades of gray. The pixel with the most intense signal is assigned the brightest value and the pixel with the least intensity is assigned the darkest value. The perception of contrast depends on how many of the pixel intensities are represented by each of the 256 shades of gray. If a limited

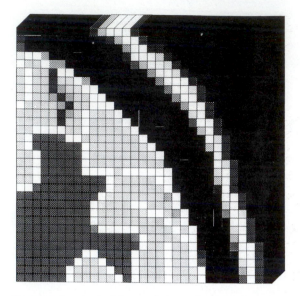

Figure 6-1. A pixel interpolation of gray scale assignment to a transaxial MRI of the head.

number of pixel intensity values are included in each of the 256 steps, the image will appear to have high contrast, that is, fewer shades of gray between the brightest and the darkest pixel. Figure 6-1 represents a pixel interpolation of gray scale assignment of a transaxial MRI of the head.

Factors Which Affect Contrast

Contrast depends on the relationship of signal intensities among the tissues that appear in the image. As the signals are received, the appropriate pixel intensity represents the signal of each voxel within the tissue.

Contrast discrimination is affected by many factors: pulse sequence types, repetition time (TR), echo time (TE), inversion time (TI), flip angle (FA), relaxation rates (T1 and T2), hydrogen density, flow, contrast media; and in fast scan imaging, echo train length (ETL), and effective echo time (ETE).

TR, TE, FA, TI, ETL, and ETE are all controlled by the imaging sequence selected. They can affect greatly the perceived contrast of an image and must be chosen with care according to clinical criteria and expected results.

Pulse Sequence The pulse sequence selected is chosen to intensify tissue contrast based on diagnostic needs. Each pulse sequence has a unique application and benefit for a desired result. In general, spin echo pulse sequences give us information about T1, T2, and the proton density of tissues. Field or gradient echo sequences use gradient reversal techniques to give us T1- and T2-like contrast in a shorter scan time than for a spin echo sequence. Inversion recovery sequences are predominantly T1-weighted sequences and require the use of a 180-degree inverting RF pulse to initiate the sequence. Let's take a closer look.

A spin echo (SE) pulse sequence may be manipulated via explicit imaging parameters to yield T1 contrast, T2 contrast, or proton density images. Table 6-1 identifies relative scan TR and TE parameters used for weighting images. Figure 6-2 represents the contrast associated with the selection of scan parameters to produce T1, T2, or hydrogen proton density images when using spin echo techniques.

Field (gradient) echo sequences can be devised to provide images with contrast that is very similar to the traditional spin echo pulse sequence. However, the selection of an additional imaging parameter, the flip angle, is necessary to implement a field echo sequence. The flip angle ultimately controls image contrast by flipping only a portion of the spins into the transverse plane.

Table 6-1

TR and TE Parameters used for Weighting Conventional Spin Echo Pulse Sequences

TE	TR	Weighting
Short	Short	T1
Long	Long	T2
Short	Long	Hydrogen density

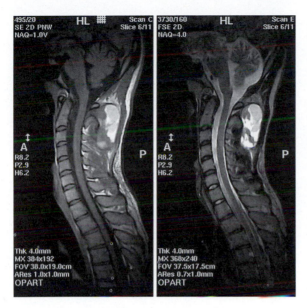

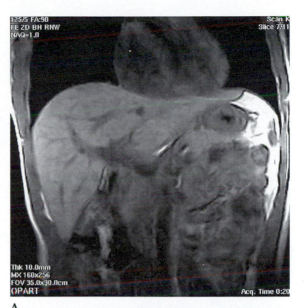

Figure 6-2. Spin echo T1 weighted sagittal cervical spine on the left; T2 weighted image fast spin echo of the same patient on the right.

The result is a much quicker T1 recovery period for those spins, necessitating a concomitant decrease in the TR selection.

In addition, gradient reversal techniques do not compensate for all magnetic field inhomogeneities, therefore T2 dephasing occurs more quickly than when imaging with a conventional spin echo pulse sequence. Much shorter echo times are typically used for even heavily T2-weighted images. Figure 6-3 shows the contrast differentiations of field or gradient echo imaging when varying the flip angle.

Inversion recovery (IR) sequences are predominately T1 weighted. TI (inversion time) is the main controlling factor of contrast. When fat suppression is the objective, a short TI (approximately 69 percent of the T1 relaxation time of fat) is used; the sequence is commonly known as a STIR sequence (short TI recovery). IR sequences can also be used to differentiate, for example, periventricular fluid from CSF in the lateral ventricles by attenuating the signal from fluids based on molecular structure of the fluids.

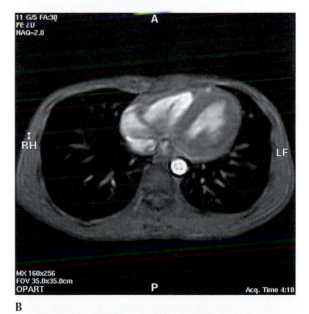

Figure 6-3. **A** Field echo image using a high flip angle (FA = 90 degrees) and breath-hold technique to produce a T1 weighted image of the abdomen; **B** Field echo cardiac gated image using a low flip angle (FA = 30 degrees) to produce a T2-like image of the heart. Note the contrast difference between the two images of the heart.

This sequence is known as FLAIR for fluid attenuated IR. Figure 6-4 shows examples of IR sequences in the pelvis.

Repetition Time (TR) This is the time interval necessary for longitudinal magnetization to occur after RF perturbation as represented by Figure 6-5. The longer the tissue vector is allowed to recover its longitudinal magnetization, the more signal will be available to be flipped into the transverse plane during the next excitation. However, tissue contrast discrimination is less apparent as all tissues will have recovered a sufficient amount of signal. Therefore, the best T1 contrast is obtained when TR is short enough to allow longitudinal recovery of few tissues. The remaining tissues within the imaging volume will have varying recovery rates, hence a variation in contrast. When repetition time is short, it has the net effect on image contrast of increasing signal dependence on tissues with short T1 values, directly controlling T1 contrast. When T2 contrast is desired, long TRs will minimize any T1 contrast so that T2 effects predominate. Figure 6-6 shows a typical T1 contrast curve. A change in TR can vary the resultant contrast of the image, as shown in Figure 6-7.

Echo Time (TE) This is the time from the original RF pulse to the peak of its reemitted echo, see Figure 6-8. The selection of a particular TE controls the amount of spin dephasing (T2 effects) allowed to occur before the signal is collected. The longer the echo time, the more dephasing has occurred for most tissues, resulting in a significant loss of signal but a higher degree of T2 contrast. When the voxel sees less signal due to significant dephasing, it assigns a lower gray scale value. The smaller the dephasing effects seen by the computer, the greater the gray scale value corresponding to higher signal per voxel. Figure 6-9 shows a typical T2 contrast curve.

From our knowledge about T2 relaxation times, we know that tissues with loosely bound

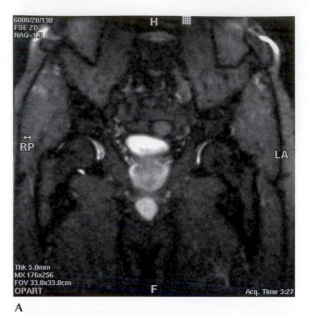

Figure 6-4. **A** Inversion recovery (IR) FastSTIR; TR = 6000 ms, TE = 20 ms, TI = 130 ms. **B** FastIR image: TR = 6000 ms, TE = 20 ms, TI = 550 ms.

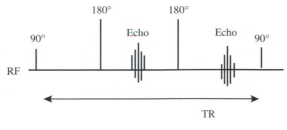

Figure 6-5. Repetition time (TR).

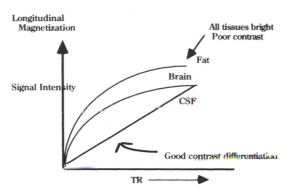

Figure 6-6. A typical T1 contrast curve.

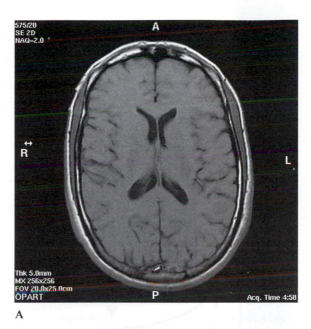

A

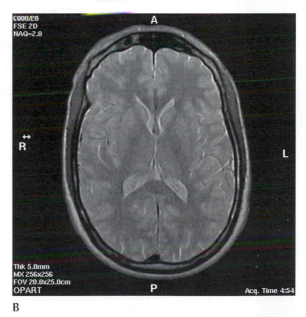

B

Figure 6-7.   **A** SE image; TR = 575 ms, TE = 20 ms.
B Fast SE image; TR = 6000 ms, TE = 20 ms.

hydrogen protons will take a longer time to dephase, therefore they will remain brighter for a longer period of time. Examples of long T2 tissues are fluid-filled structures such as the ventricular system, urinary bladder, simple cysts, and most pathologic structures. Short T2 tissues have a more tightly bound molecular structure, which contributes to shorter T2 relaxation times. Tissues such as brain, liver, spleen, muscle, ligaments, and tendons are examples of short T2 tissues. They have a dark appearance on a sequence with a long TE due to considerable dephasing effects. Figure 6-10 represents T2 contrast variations when the TE is manipulated. T2 contrast is maximized between short and long T2 tissues when using a long echo time. The long echo times allows for sufficient dephasing while a long TR minimizes T1 contrast.

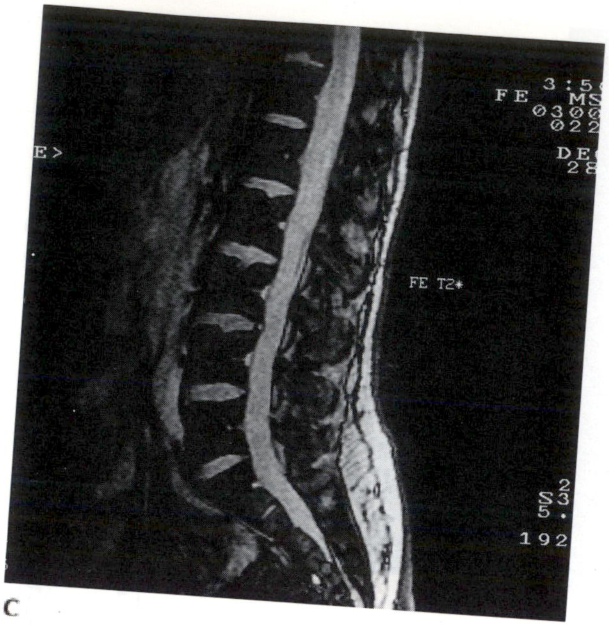

Figure 6-15 (continued). **C** FE 2DFT image; TR = 300 ms, TE = 22 ms, flip angle = 28 degrees.

a brief fluctuation of the nuclear magnetic fields to which the nuclei respond. This response determines the rate of energy loss corresponding to T1 relaxation and the rate of dephasing measured by T2. Any process, naturally occurring or externally stimulated, that affects thermal motion will have an influence on the relaxation rates. These processes include temperature, static field strength, and macromolecular content of the tissue.

The T1 relaxation times are contingent in part on the field strength of the magnet as well as on general tissue characteristics (solids versus liquids). Therefore, tissue contrast will be dependent on these factors as well as the imaging sequence parameters chosen for a particular pulse sequence. TR, TE, TI, and flip angles are selected to enhance the tissue contrast at a unique field strength. The graphs in Figure 6-16 represent T1 contrast curves associated with mid- and high-field MR imaging systems.

As field strength decreases, solids have a shorter T1 value. There will be more signal at any

one TR with a result of improved lesion detectability and better contrast discrimination between gray and white matter, and CSF. The T1 value of liquids such as CSF is relatively constant with field strength and will appear darker than solids. As field strength increases, TRs must be long enough to produce brighter signal from CSF so that lesion detectability improves. At shorter T1 values, such as seen with low-field MRI, there is a wider range in the choice of TR that will permit better contrast discrimination.

T2 relaxation times are primarily based on magnetic field inhomogeneities at the level of the cell and in the static external field. The spin phases of different nuclei drift out of phase rapidly due to T2 relaxation and static field inhomogeneity. Even though field strength has a small influence on T2 relaxation, the effects of inhomogeneity can be reversed by a 180-degree RF pulse. But T2 relaxation cannot be reversed.

T2 contrast is determined by the dephasing properties of liquids and solids. Local inhomogeneities around the protons in solids (e.g., cortical bone where molecular bonds are relatively fixed) are significant so there is easy and rapid spin–spin interaction leading to dephasing. T2 for solids is therefore very short. Liquids on the other hand (e.g., soft tissue with freely bound molecules) have weak spin–spin interactions because their local magnetic fields have rapidly averaged to a small value. Dephasing for liquids then takes a long period of time resulting in longer T2 values.

Hydrogen Density This is the concentration of resonating hydrogen atoms in a given anatomical region. The MR signal from a tissue is determined in large part by its hydrogen concentration. The molecular structure of the tissues will determine the T1 and T2 relaxation rates or to what degree molecular interaction will occur, this in turn will contribute to contrast.

Flow This refers to hydrogen in motion during the time of acquisition. Examples of flow

Table 6-2
Clinical Imaging Guidelines

Parameter	Action	Effect Image Quality
TR	Increase	Increases signal-to-noise
		Increases no. of allowable slices
		Decreases T1 contrast
		Increases scan time
		May allow decrease in no. of acquisitions
	Decrease	Decreases proton density
		Increases T1 contrast
		Shortens scan time
		Decreases motion artifacts
		Decreases signal-to-noise
		Decreases no. of allowable slices
TE	Increase	Increases T2 contrast
		Decreases signal-to-noise
		Decreases T1 contrast
	Decrease	Increases signal-to-noise
		Decreases T2 contrast
		Increases proton density and T1 contrast
Flip angle	Increase	Increases total spins directed to transverse magnetization
		Increases T1 dependence
		Increases T1 contrast
	Decrease	Increases T2* contrast
		Decreases spins flipped into transverse plane
		Decreases signal-to-noise
Matrix	Increase	Increases spatial resolution
		Increases signal-to-noise for entire image (by $\sqrt{2}$)
		Decreases signal-to-noise/voxel volume
		Decreases truncation artifacts
		Increases scan time
	Decrease	Decreases spatial resolution
		Decreases signal-to-noise for entire image
		Increases signal-to-noise/voxel volume
		Increases truncation artifacts
		Decreases scan time
Field of view	Increase	Increases total area imaged
		Increases signal-to-noise/voxel
		Decreases spatial resolution
Number of acquisitions	Increase	Increases signal-to-noise (by $\sqrt{2}$)
		Increases scan time
		May decrease FID artifacts

(continued)

Table 6-2 (*continued*)
Clinical Imaging Guidelines

Parameter	Action	Effect Image Quality
	Decrease	Decreases signal-to-noise
		Decreases scan time
		May increase appearance of FID artifacts
Slice thickness	Increase	Increases signal-to-noise
		Increases total imaged area
		Decreases spatial resolution
		Increases partial volume effect
	Decrease	Decreases signal-to-noise
		Decreases total imaged area
		Increases spatial resolution
		Decreases partial volume effect
ETL (Echo train length)	Increase	Decreases scan time
		Increases contrast mix
		Decreases no. of allowable slices
		May increase blurring artifact
ETS (Echo train spacing)	Increase	Increases contrast mix
		May increase blurring artifacts
		Decreases coverage
ETE (Effective TE)	Increase	Increases T2 contrast
		Decreases signal-to-noise

include blood, CSF, bile, and other body fluids. Hydrogen density and flow are considered to be constant for the imaging period of any one image, no matter what imaging sequence we use. For example, moving spins, such as blood flow, predictably dephase when in the presence of a gradient. If sufficient dephasing has occurred due to varying magnetic fields as well as turbulence and laminar flow, the vessel will appear as a signal void. We can manipulate the contrast of blood by selecting a pulse sequence which uses gradient reversals to refocus spin phases, such as gradient moment pulling techniques (flow compensation) or field echo sequences. These methods allow flowing spins to rephase so they produce a signal within the vessel. This is the objective of MR vascular imaging and other techniques. We can also select scan parameters that yield black blood (signal void within the vessel) and a relatively high signal intensity for all other tissues.

Contrast Media MR compatible contrast agents are commonly used to enhance diagnostic proficiency. Paramagnetic materials are used as contrast media in MR imaging to shorten T1 relaxation time, thus influencing the perceived contrast of the resultant image. Examples of paramagnetic substances are transition metals, such as gadolinium and manganese, whose atoms are magnetic due to the structure of their outer electron shell. These substances are injected before the MRI in traces that will concentrate in blood vessels or tissues where the blood–brain barrier is defective. The resultant increase in contrast is based on the paramagnetic response to the magnetic field of nuclear species within the

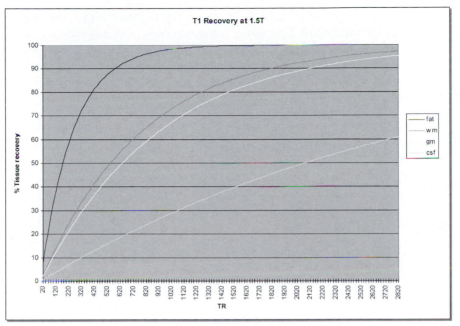

A

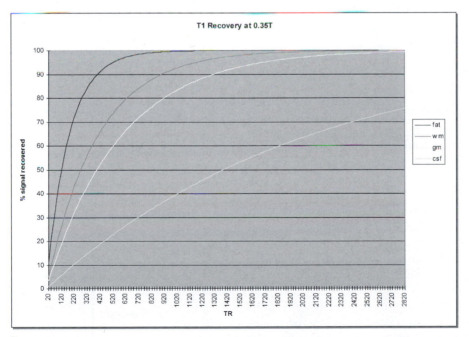

B

Figure 6-16. **A** and **B** T1 contrast curves related to high- and mid-field MR imagers.

tissues. Paramagnetics are also being used to enhance vascular signal for use in MR angiography, commonly known as contrast enhanced MRA (CE MRA).

Iron-based MR contrast agents may increase tissue contrast differentiation by causing a signal void in the area of uptake. Refer to Chapter 10 on MR contrast media for a more in depth description of the affect of contrast on signal or tissue intensity.

SPATIAL RESOLUTION

Spatial resolution is the sharpness of an image, or its ability to identify small objects and to define clearly edges and boundaries between tissues. The best spatial resolution obtainable on an MR image is when dimensional elements are very small. But we pay a price in SNR when the resolving power is high. The trick is to select parameters which yield a balance between the ability to define edge detail and to collect sufficient signal.

Factors Which Affect Spatial Resolution

Spatial resolution is controlled by those parameters that directly influence the volume units of our data collection. An image has three dimensions: the length and width are represented by the pixel size (resolution); the depth of the volume is controlled by the thickness of the slice. We can say then that the following factors affect spatial resolution: voxel size (pixel size or resolution and slice thickness), slice thickness, matrix size, and field of view (FOV).

Voxels These are three dimensional units from which signal is obtained during the reconstruction process. Voxels also directly affect the spatial resolution of an image by representing the intersections of hundreds of data lines during spatial encoding. The smaller the voxel volume,

the more highly defined the region of interest. Voxel volume is manipulated by selections of slice thickness and matrix dimensions so that a change in one of the three dimensions will have an influence on the resolving power. Figure 6-17 represents a simple voxel.

Pixels These are individual units that collectively comprise the dimensions of the matrix. They are the two-dimensional unit of the voxel whose signal has been averaged during Fourier transformation. They also represent the displayed image after reconstruction. If pixel size is extremely small, the matrix will essentially be sliced into thousands of tiny elements that produce a more well-defined area of interest with an increase in edge detail. Imaging areas which demand high resolving power include vascular tissue, brain structures, nerve roots, and extremities. Figure 6-18 shows a pixel.

Figure 6-19 was obtained using different resolution (pixel size) values from 0.95 mm-square pixels to 2.0 mm-square pixels. Except

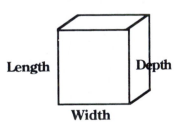

Figure 6-17.   Voxel dimensions.

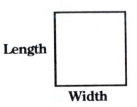

Figure 6-18.   Pixel dimensions.

for FOV, all other factors remain unchanged FOV changes according to the formula:

$$FOV = matrix \times resolution$$

Slice Thickness A change in the slice thickness, the third dimension of our voxel volume, will affect spatial resolution by increasing or decreasing the volume imaged in 2D FT imaging

techniques. When the volume increases, a loss in spatial resolution is noted because information is gathered from a larger area so that the region of interest is not sliced into the smallest units, all other factors being equal. In addition, the partial volume affect may be present when one slice contains information from overlapping tissues, especially those tissues which have contrary signal intensities at the interface, such as the pituitary and spheroid sinus. A signal misregistration then occurs during Fourier transformation (see Chapter 14 for details).

Gap The gap between slices also may affect spatial resolution. Slice selection during the spatial encoding process of MR imaging is accomplished by generating an RF pulse at the resonant frequency of the slice as specified by the Larmor equation. RF slice profiles on MR systems can be Gaussian profiles, square profiles or any variation thereof. Cross-contamination between slices can occur with a corresponding decrease

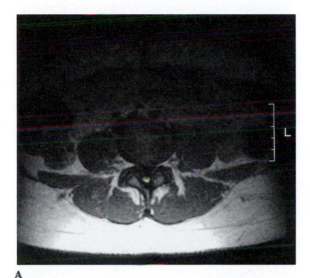

A

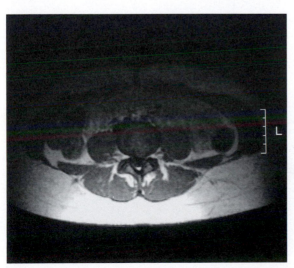

B

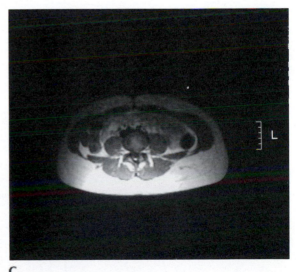

C

Figure 6-19. **A** Resolution 0.95 mm × 0.95 mm; matrix = 256. **B** Resolution 1.25 mm × 1.25 mm; matrix 256. **C** Resolution 2.0 mm × 2.0 mm; matrix 256. Note corresponding change in FOV if only resolution (not matrix) is adjusted.

in signal-to-noise ratio and variation in voxel contrast.

Contamination is a result of one RF slice profile overlapping another during slice selection of spatial encoding. During acquisition, the overlapped areas of the slice have received varying resonant frequencies which does not allow for accurate encoding. This can be significant when acquiring very thin slices, and is especially troublesome at higher field strengths. Figure 6-20 shows how cross-contamination occurs relative to slice profile overlapping. A gap is merely a space between consecutive slices controlled with the offset frequency of the RF pulses. This space is often operator selected and is usually a percentage of the slice thickness chosen as specified by the imaging system. When incorporated into the pulse sequence, cross-contamination can be decreased or eliminated. Figure 6-21 depicts gap insertion and its affect on slice profiles.

Matrix   This is the length and width of the entire imaged area and is comprised of a great number of individual pixels as depicted by Figure 6-22. We choose the matrix size by the number of phase encoding steps and the number of data sample points required to yield a desired spatial resolution. The more phase encoding steps per FOV the smaller the individual pixels and the better our definition. The number of frequency encoding steps (or samples) is normally fixed and also contributes to the size of the pixel, hence the spatial resolution. Figure 6-23A represents a matrix with x phase and frequency encoding steps. The matrix in Figure 6-23B shows the change in pixel size when the matrix is doubled. Figure 6-24A, B, C and D show how the spatial resolution of an image changes with a change in the matrix. Note that increasing the matrix by increasing the number of phase encoding steps also increases the scan time.

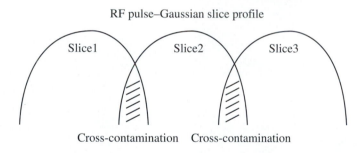

Figure 6-20.   Cross-contamination between slices.

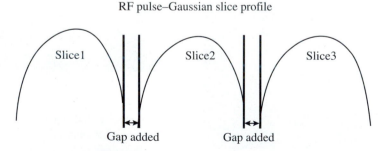

Figure 6-21.   Gap inserted between slices helps to eliminate cross-talk.

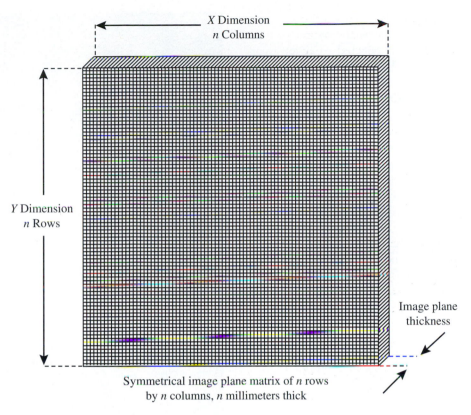

Figure 6-22. Matrix with *n* rows in *Y* dimension and *n* columns in *X* dimension.

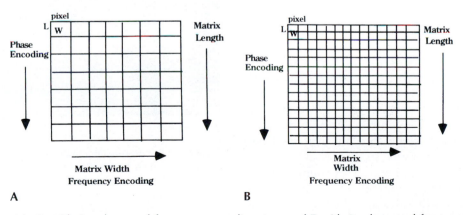

Figure 6-23. Matrix with **A** x phase and frequency encoding steps and **B** with 2x phase and frequency encoding steps.

Field of View (FOV)   This is the anatomic region of interest defined by the matrix and the resolution. Scan FOV is selected to cover a particular tissue volume. The larger the dimensions of the matrix and pixel size, the larger the FOV. For the same matrix size, a change in FOV will affect the pixel size and therefore the resolution. For example, if the FOV increases while the matrix remains the same, the pixel size will also increase, effectively increasing voxel volume. With phase encoding steps and data sampling points spread out in the enlarged FOV, definition of the area diminishes. Figure 6-25 represents an FOV with *x* and *2x* dimensions. The above changes will affect the spatial resolution of the resultant image, but will also contribute in a predictable manner to the SNR.

Fast Scan Techniques   When performing fast scan sequences such as fast spin echo imaging, the choice of echo train length (ETL) and echo train spacing (ETS) will affect spatial resolution.

Echo Train Length (ETL)   If the desire is to obtain ultrafast images, as well as to increase T2 contrast, the ETL is selected to be as long as possible. There are multiple echoes that will contribute to the overall contrast. The longest echo will contribute most to the resultant T2 contrast, due to its position in the echo train. A disadvantage of increasing ETL is a possible blurring artifact that may jeopardize edge detail. This occurs because of the abrupt differences in signal intensity from one TR to another.

Echo Train Spacing (ETS)   Echo train spacing determines the separation in milliseconds of the echoes in the echo train. Increasing ETS increases the contrast mix, thereby increasing the dependence on T2 contrast. And as there are larger jumps between each echo, there are larger jumps in signal intensity, so there is an increase in blurring. Edge blurring can be minimized by using the smallest echo train spacing possible. An added benefit is that this may allow a higher echo train to be used, thus decreasing scan time and possibly increasing T2 contrast.

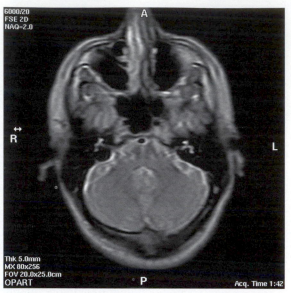

A

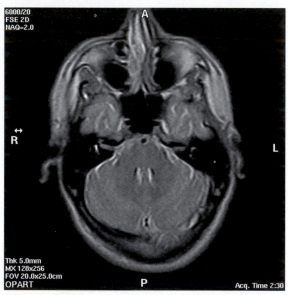

B

Figure 6-24.   Transaxial images through the internal auditory canal. **A** Matrix 80 × 256; **B** Matrix 128 × 256;

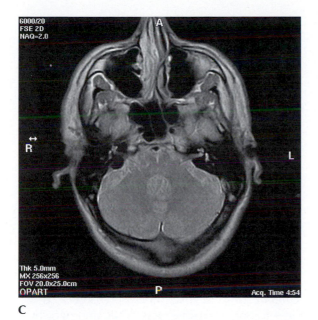

C

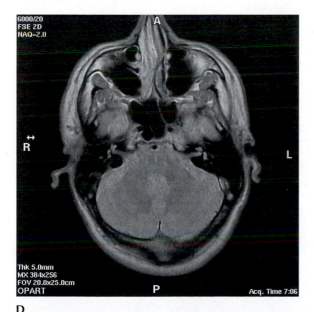

D

Figure 6-24 (*continued*).   Transaxial images through the internal auditory canal. **C** Matrix 256 × 256; **D** Matrix 384 × 256. Note also the increased scan time due to increased phase encoding steps.

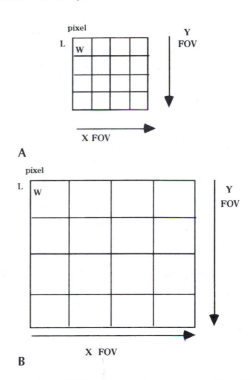

Figure 6-25.   FOV with **A** *x* dimensions and **B** with 2*x* dimensions.

SIGNAL-TO-NOISE RATIO

Signal-to-noise ratio (SNR) is a term used to describe the relative contributions to a detected signal made by the true signal and by random superimposed signals (noise). When the signal becomes relatively larger than the noise, SNR is improved and prettier images are obtained. But an improvement in SNR does not necessarily result in a more diagnostic image, since in 2DFT imaging detail is diminished. In fact, there is an inverse relationship between SNR and spatial resolution in 2DFT imaging. As technologists, we must recognize the benefits as well as the limitations of each scan variable selected and choose scan parameters accordingly.

Pixel values will fluctuate about a mean value when noise is superimposed on the signal. This means that on the image, sufficient noise will smear out the edges of the tissue interfaces. It impairs edge acuity so that small intensity differences that might be important may become impossible to see.

There are two types of noise. To some extent we can correct for noise that results from variations in the signal created by moving objects in the body. We can minimize this noise by selecting pulse sequences that incorporate artifact reduction techniques such as presaturation and flow compensation. The second type of noise is inherent in the system. We cannot correct for this noise with our imaging sequence parameters.

Factors Which Affect Signal-to-Noise Ratio

Imaging parameters include many factors that impact the signal-to-noise ratio (SNR). Remember there is an inverse relationship between SNR and spatial resolution in 2DFT imaging, so that by enhancing one we tend to diminish the other.

Hydrogen Proton Density This is the primary source of signal within our imaging volume. Depending on their chemical bonding properties, tissues will behave quite differently; this accounts for wide variations in resultant signal intensity. For example, CSF contains large quantities of loosely bound hydrogen atoms and yields a strong signal on T2-weighted imaging sequences. Ligaments and tendons contain a high concentration of tightly bound hydrogen protons and appear much darker. We cannot directly control proton density but we can manipulate imaging sequence parameters to bring out the available signal.

Field Homogeneity Field homogeneity is the product of the field strength of the system and the measured field homogeneity over a clinically useful imaging volume. Better absolute field homogeneity results in longer signal duration and a maximization of available signal.

Gap Depending on the type of RF pulse used in a particular pulse sequence, cross-contamination of slices may occur with a corresponding decrease in SNR. By adding a gap between the slices, this cross-contamination may be decreased or eliminated. Applied gaps also have a positive affect on spatial resolution and contrast.

Voxel Volume This is determined by slice thickness and pixel size or resolution. SNR may be improved by increasing the volume, because more protons will be available in the volume to contribute to the signal intensity. For example, if we double the length and width of the voxel (i.e., pixel size, directly or indirectly by a change in matrix or FOV), all other factors being equal, SNR increases by a factor of 4 (assuming the content of the voxel doesn't change). If we double only slice thickness, SNR improves by a factor of 2. However, a partial volume artifact may then be present.

Slice Thickness Increasing the slice thickness increases the signal volume per image, resulting in a higher SNR ratio. But a partial volume effect may degrade the image. A decrease in slice thickness when using 3DFT imaging methods does not affect signal adversely. 3DFT imaging is acquired by selectively exciting a "slab" of tissue then partitioning the slab into the desired slice thicknesses by using an additional phase encoding process. This means that signal is based on the entire volume being excited. In 3DFT imaging both detail and signal return are high. Figure 6-26 was acquired using different slice thicknesses as indicated, all other scan parameters remaining equal. They show how slice thickness affects the SNR of the resultant image on a 2DFT scan.

Repetition Time (TR) Lengthening the time between pulse repetitions improves SNR by increasing the time that longitudinal magnetization is allowed to recover for all tissues. More signal will then be available to be flipped to the transverse plane during subsequent RF pulses. A change in TR will affect the SNR of an image, as

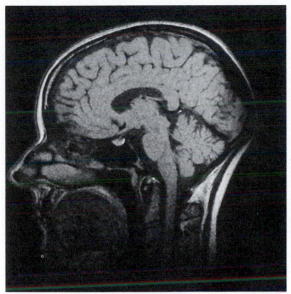

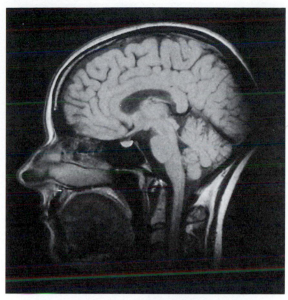

A

C

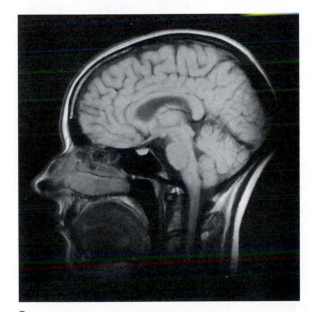

B

Figure 6-26. **A** Slice thickness 2.5 mm. **B** Slice thickness 5.0 mm. **C** Slice thickness 10.0 mm.

lose phase coherence. Dephasing effects are visualized as signal loss or void. Decreasing TE improves SNR by collecting the data before the signal has decayed. Figure 6-28 shows the SNR changes associated with manipulating the TE of the sequence. The longer we wait to collect the signal, the less signal will be available. A change in TE also affects the contrast of the image.

Number of Acquisitions Also referred to as the NEX (number of excitations) or averages, number of acquisitions represents the number of times we collect data for a given phase encode value and average the information to represent one image. Signal increases linearly but noise is random and adds incoherently. If we double the number of acquisitions, the signal will improve by $\sqrt{2}$. This calculates to an increase in signal of about 41 percent. But doubling the acquisitions also doubles scan time, which may result in more artifact noise due to the increase in allowable time

shown in Figure 6-27. Remember, TR also affects image contrast.

Echo Time (TE) Lengthening TE worsens SNR by allowing more time for tissue vectors to

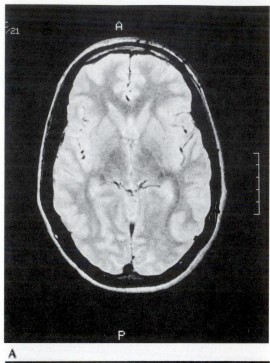

A

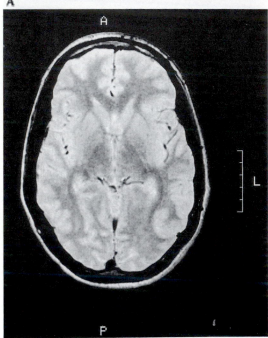

B

Figure 6-27. **A** SE at 0.35 T; TR = 500 ms, TE = 40 ms.
B SE at 0.35 T; TR = 3000 ms, TE = 40 ms.

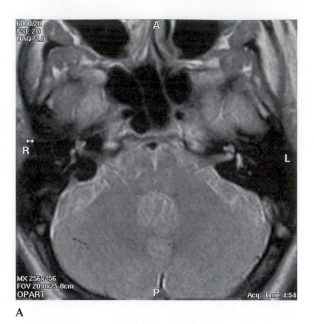

A

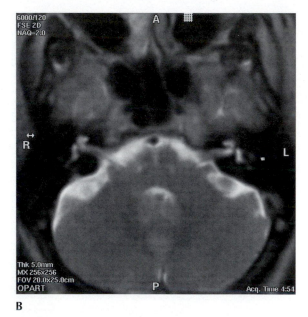

B

Figure 6-28. **A** FastSE; TR = 6000 ms, TE = 20 ms.
B FastSE; TR = 6000 ms, TE = 120 ms.

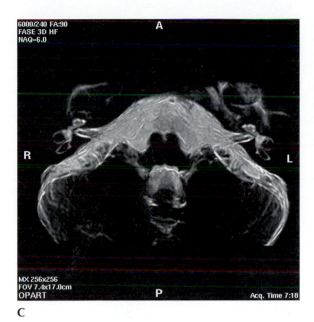

C

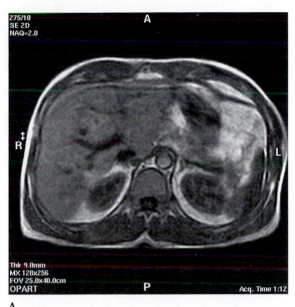

A

Figure 6-28 (*continued*).   **C** FastSE; TR = 6000 ms, TE = 240 ms.

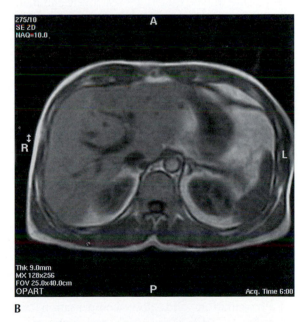

B

Figure 6-29.   **A** and **B** show a difference in SNR by almost a factor of 3 when increasing the number of acquisitions from 2 to 10 on an axial T1 abdomen. Note also the increase in scan time.

for physiologic motion or patient movement to occur. Obviously, the cost of doubling the scan time must be weighted against the potential benefit associated with an improvement in signal by less than 50 percent. Figure 6-29 represents SNR improvements when doubling the number of acquisitions.

Matrix Size   This refers to the number of rows and columns of pixels in our video image. Typically, our selection refers to the number of phase encode steps rather than frequency encode steps since the data sampling steps are commonly set by the manufacturer (often as oversampling). Increasing the matrix while maintaining the FOV decreases the pixel size, effectively decreasing voxel volume and therefore SNR per voxel. However, an overall improvement of signal may be realized by the fact that more lines of data are being averaged. Both factors contribute to the overall SNR and image quality.

Field of View (FOV)   The relationship between the matrix and the FOV has a definite effect on SNR by determining the size of the individual pixels within the matrix. When FOV is decreased while maintaining the matrix size, the pixels become very small. Therefore, there is less signal per unit volume. Remember, slice thickness is the third dimension of a voxel.

Artifact Reduction Techniques   There are several artifact reduction techniques that help to produce images with a competitive edge. Most artifacts are inappropriately encoded signals within an image, so their elimination or reduction will improve the image quality. Artifact reduction techniques are able to minimize flow (CSF and blood), breathing, swallowing, and other artifacts.

In the form of presaturation pulses, artifact reduction techniques are used to improve significantly image quality by selectively eliminating signal production in anatomic regions that are notorious for producing artifacts, such as the anterior cervical spine. The method uses repetitive RF pulses directed at regions adjacent to the imaging volume.

Flow compensation techniques use gradient reversals to refocus the phases of moving spins. Since moving spins (i.e., blood flow) and stationary spins (i.e., non-moving tissues) rephase differently during spatial encoding, an artifact will be generated such that the blood vessel will be seen as a variation of signals in a variety of locations on the resultant image. It is essentially being mismapped on the image. Flow compensation improves image quality by refocusing the phases of moving spins so that a signal is generated for the blood and is encoded in the proper location.

Presaturation and flow compensation are examples of artifact reduction techniques used to improve image quality by affecting the SNR of the resultant image. When used according to manufacturer's specifications they are very successful. Other techniques orient the artifact so it does not impede diagnosis (phase–frequency reorientation) or oversampling data during acquisition (no phase wrap or no frequency wrap).

CONCLUSIONS

Diagnostic accuracy in MR imaging is dependent on the selection of imaging sequence parameters that will enhance image quality. These parameters are manipulated in a balanced manner to improve the SNR, define the region of interest, and increase the image contrast. Each selection will affect the resultant image in a precise and well-defined manner. Teams of technologists and radiologists chain together these pulse sequence variables to produce images of the best diagnostic quality in the shortest possible scan time.

SUGGESTED READING

Hendrick RE. Signal-to-noise. *Magn Reson Imaging*, March 1990.
Kaufman L, Arakawa M, Hale J, et al. Accessible magnetic resonance imaging. *J Magn Res Q* 5:283–297, 1989.
Oldendorf W, Oldendorf W Jr. *Basics of Magnetic Resonance Imaging*. Boston: Martinus Nijhoff, 1988.
Schulz RA. *Resonant Ideas (Magnetic Resonance Newsletter of Diasonics MRI Division)* 2(7), Nov./Dec. 1998.
Wehrli FW. Parameters determining the appearance of the NMR image. In Newton TH, Potts DG, eds. *Advanced Imaging Techniques*, Vol. II. San Francisco: Clavadel Press, 1983.
Young SW. *Magnetic Resonance Imaging Basic Principles*, 2nd ed. New York: Raven Press, 1988.

CHAPTER 7

Standard MR Pulse Sequences: A Closer Look

Michael C. Sweitzer and David M. Kramer

INTRODUCTION

Few discussions of the basic physics of MRI bridge the gap between the basic physics concepts and the pulse sequence diagram – the tool employed by all MRI scanners to generate an image. The texts available focusing on this topic tend not to be written in a form understandable to the typical clinician, technologist, or MR user.

As a result, few users – operators or clinicians – have a working understanding of MRI necessary to predict sequence performance in terms of image contrast and lesion detectability. Current imaging techniques tend to be learned or memorized in an empirical fashion so as to generate the expected result. New techniques such as MR angiography or fast scanning, therefore, create a painful learning curve as advantages and disadvantages can only be revealed through slow, painstaking trial and error.

This chapter is intended to develop an understanding of how the physics of MR affect and shape pulse sequence techniques to generate a desired image. We hope it differs from other

texts available in that it provides the necessary connection between the basic physics of MRI to the implementation of pulse sequences. We assume the reader has already studied the conventional discussion of MR basic physics, including magnetic fields, radio frequency excitation, gradient spatial encoding, proton spin excitation and relaxation, and basic pulse sequence construction (Chapters 1 to 6).

While MR users on most systems generally do not have direct access to pulse sequence creation or modification, it is hoped that a more detailed understanding of this process will allow for better clinical decisions in sequence selection, as well as improve the feedback loop to the development process in the generation of more advanced techniques.

THE SPIN ECHO SEQUENCE

Our discussion begins with the basic spin echo pulse sequence – not because it is the simplest to construct, but because it represents the most widely used standard technique both at the early commercial introduction of MRI in the 1980s as well as today. Spin echo also is the most widely understood clinical technique for contrast generation, if only from an empirical perspective.

The basic sequence of events in spin echo is a 90-degree RF pulse excitation, spatial encoding, a 180-degree refocusing pulse, and signal readout. This is shown schematically in what is referred to as a pulse sequence diagram [Figure 7-1].

The pulse sequence diagram introduces several labeling conventions which shall be used throughout this chapter. Each horizontal line represents a primary component and/or function in the MRI system. In this case, radio frequency (RF) represents both the transmitted 90-degree and 180-degree radio frequency pulses (represented by single vertical lines for simplicity) and the received echo (represented by a sinc pulse shape).

Gss, Gro, and Gpe represent the gradient pulse timings for the slice select, readout, and phase encoding directions, respectively. Note that these could be – and often are – denoted as G_x, G_y, and G_z, though this can cause confusion in the arbitrary selection of the x-axis, the y-axis, and the z-axis. Using slice select, readout, and phase encoding serves to simplify matters by defining the gradients in relation to their function. The boxes along the gradient lines represent the gradient "on" times with the relative size, position, and shape of the boxes representing the gradient amplitude, polarity (positive or negative), and duration, respectively.

The diagram as shown is only an ideal depiction of the MR pulse sequence diagram. It is significant to note that in real life, RF pulses do not occur instantaneously nor do gradient pulses look like perfect boxes. Also, we do not always use perfect 90-degree or 180-degree pulses (we may use 89-degree or 181-degree pulses, for example) as the human body does not always react to the tools employed in MR as we would like. However, for the sake of simplicity, we will work with this idealized diagram as a starting point in the understanding of pulse sequences.

Excitation

Let's review the sequence shown in Figure 7-1 step by step. At the start of the sequence, it is assumed that the spins or protons within the body are aligned with the main magnetic field. We apply a 90-degree RF pulse in order to flip the spins from their longitudinal orientation into the $x - y$ or transverse plane. A gradient pulse in the slice select direction has been applied during this RF pulse in order to selectively excite the spins within a desired slice. That is, only the spins precessing at a frequency equivalent to that of the 90-degree RF pulse will be flipped into the transverse plane. By having applied a linear gradient in the slice select direction, only a plane or slice of spins perpendicular to this gradient is excited.

The effect of any gradient pulse is to momentarily speed up or slow down the precessional rate of the spins according to where they are located in the gradient field, as shown in Figure 7-2.

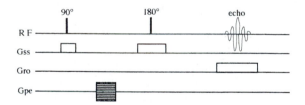

Figure 7-1.   Spin echo pulse sequence.

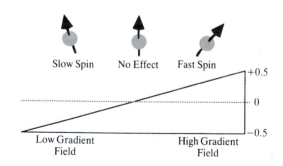

Figure 7-2.   Use of gradient magnetic fields for spatial encoding and the net effect on the precession rate of the protons.

The gradient effect is a direct result of the Larmor equation.

$$f_0 = \gamma B_0$$

where γ is the gyromagnetic ratio
f_0 is the precessional frequency of the spin
B_0 is the main magnetic field strength

It is from this equation that we determine the necessary operating frequency for our MRI system. For example

$$1.5\,T \sim 63\,MHz$$
$$1.0\,T \sim 42\,MHz$$
$$0.5\,T \sim 21\,MHz$$
$$0.2\,T \sim 8.3\,MHz$$

Applying a gradient of a specific amplitude means applying current to the gradient coil such that a small magnetic field is created in addition to the main magnetic field. Typically, gradients are measured in terms of gauss per centimeter (G/cm) or millitesla per meter (mT/m). Note that 1 G/cm equals 10 mT/m so that the terms may be used interchangeably. The gradient fields superimposed on the main magnetic field are therefore on the order of one to ten thousand times smaller than the magnetic strength of the main MRI magnet.

The term "gradient" refers to the fact that this small, applied magnetic field varies linearly from one end of the main magnet to the other (or from one side to the other). Typically, up to a 2 G/cm gradient is applied such that the zero gradient point is at the center of the bore of the magnet. This increases the local magnetic field by 100 G at one end of a 1-meter gradient coil, and decreases it by 100 G at the other.

From the Larmor equation, it also follows that applying a magnetic field gradient will effectively increase or decrease B_0, the magnetic field experienced by the proton. Since the gyromagnetic ratio is a constant for any given tissue, any change in B_0 directly affects f_0, the precessional frequency of the spin. Therefore, we can selectively change the precessional rate of a

spin by applying a gradient along a given direction. This change in frequency is what is employed to selectively excite a slice through the principle of resonance.

It is important to note at this point that we must flip the spins into the transverse plane in order to generate a signal. Due to the geometry of the receiving coil system, we cannot "see" any signal in the longitudinal direction aligned with the main magnetic field. Conversely, by applying a 90-degree RF pulse and flipping the spins into the transverse plane, we maximize the signal we can receive, as shown in Figure 7-3.

In our pulse sequence diagram [Figure 7-1], we have not shown any signal immediately following the 90-degree RF pulse. In fact, we should have drawn the signal as the decaying sinusoidal waveform in Figure 7-4. This waveform is known as free induction decay (FID). The signal decays in this fashion primarily due to T2* relaxation effects.

In summary, we apply a 90-degree RF pulse in order to flip the spins from their longitudinal orientation into the $x - y$ or transverse plane. A gradient pulse in the slice select direction is applied during this RF pulse in order to

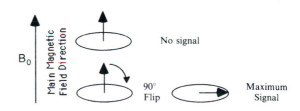

Figure 7-3.   Measurable MR signal.

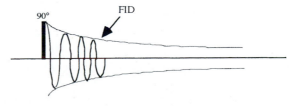

Figure 7-4.   Free induction decay (FID).

selectively excite the spins within a desired slice. By having applied a linear gradient in the slice select direction, only a plane or slice of spins perpendicular to this gradient is excited.

Encoding

Returning to the pulse sequence diagram, the next step following excitation of the slice with the 90-degree RF pulse is the application of the phase encoding gradient. In this case, the gradient pulse is turned on for a specific, finite period of time then turned off. Perhaps the simplest analogy is that of three clocks, all operating within the same time zone [Figure 7-5]. If we can apply a gradient to selectively make clock #1 run fast and clock #3 run slow, with no effect on clock #2, we can change the time of the clocks relative to each other.

Once we have altered the clocks to be exactly 15 min off with respect to each other, we turn the gradient off and each clock resumes its normal rate. The three clocks are now out of phase though they all operate at the same frequency. That is, one hour is still equal to one hour on all three clocks though they will each read 12:00 at different times.

Using a tactic similar to this, the phase encoding gradient distributes the rotation of the spins relative to their spatial location along the gradient axis. In the Fourier transform reconstruction process, the different phase rates

are assigned to spatial locations on the image (hence, the name phase encoding gradient).

In order to spatially encode using the phase encoding gradient, the gradient amplitude is varied as shown in Figure 7-6.

A different amplitude is employed with each repetition of the sequence. Hence, a 128 matrix requires 128 steps of phase encoding or 128 repetitions of the sequence. This is why the resolution in the phase encoding direction has a direct impact on the overall scan time in MR imaging and why the two factors become a direct trade-off in clinical imaging.

As a shorthand designation, the phase encoding gradient is generally shown as a large box with multiple horizontal bars representing the variations in amplitude [Figure 7-7]. In the strict sense, this designation implies multiple sequence repetitions.

So, in our pulse sequence diagram, we have now successfully obtained spatial information in two out of three directions. We have selectively excited only a slice of spins using the 90-degree RF pulse in combination with the slice select

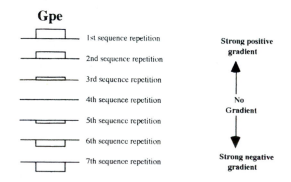

Figure 7-6. Phase encoding gradient amplitude designation.

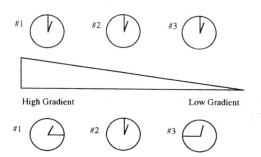

Figure 7-5. Phase encoding analogy of time.

Figure 7-7. Phase encoding gradient designation.

gradient. And, we now have created one-dimensional encoding within the slice by creating a phase distribution in that direction with the phase encoding gradient.

Refocusing

The next step in the pulse sequence is to generate the signal or echo. In the spin echo pulse sequence, this is accomplished using a 180-degree pulse. Recall that the spins undergo T2* relaxation, or dephasing, after they are flipped into the $x - y$ (or transverse) plane. This dephasing ultimately results in a net magnetization vector in the transverse plane of zero, as shown in Figure 7-8. Hence, no signal can be obtained.

At some period of time after the 90-degree RF pulse, the spins become evenly distributed in the transverse plane (pointing equally in all directions). This is the dephased condition. Complete dephasing results in the spins canceling each other out so that no vector remains in the transverse plane. This means no signal is available to be measured.

The 180-degree RF pulse serves to flip all spins about one axis within the $x - y$ plane. The spins are still traveling in the same direction, but now the faster spins are behind the slower spins, such that they will catch up at the time of the echo [Figure 7-9].

The refocusing pulse is a key element in virtually all MR imaging techniques. It should be noted, however, that a 180-degree pulse is not necessarily required to accomplish this as will be seen in the gradient echo techniques. However, the strategy to generate an echo by means of

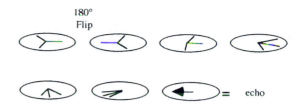

Figure 7-9. Refocusing of the signal (or echo).

some RF or gradient pulse is common to all MR imaging schemes.

One might note that in our sequence [Figure 7-1], the slice select gradient is once again turned on during the 180-degree RF pulse. In the ideal single-slice case, this would not be necessary as the original 90-degree RF pulse would flip only the spins from the desired slice into the transverse plane. Any spins not excited by the 90-degree pulse will remain aligned with the main magnetic field along the z-axis or longitudinal direction. A 180-degree RF pulse would then flip them into the negative z-direction where they would slowly relax in a straight line back to alignment with the main magnetic field. Since the spins are never flipped into the $x - y$ plane and we can only receive signal from spins in the transverse plane, we cannot see any of this undesirable signal.

The requirement for this Gss pulse becomes evident in the case of multislice spin echo sequences. In this case, spins from several slices will be in various stages of excitation and relaxation. It is critical in this situation that the spins see only the 180-degree RF pulse which corresponds to the appropriate slice. This will be discussed in greater detail in the section on multislice spin echo.

Signal Readout

The final step of the spin echo pulse sequence is readout of the echo. There are two key components of this phase: data acquisition and frequency encoding of the signal.

Data acquisition is almost trivial and is considered to happen in "the background" of the

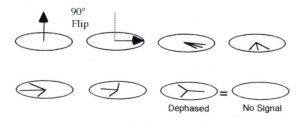

Figure 7-8. T2 relaxation in the transverse plane.

pulse sequence diagram. That is, there is generally no specific designation for the data acquisition process other than the sinc pulse to indicate the echo itself. The data acquisition process involves switching the RF coil into receive mode to "listen" for the RF signal returning from the tissue.

The data acquisition system (DAS) is then turned on and the signal is sampled multiple times corresponding to the desired resolution in the frequency encoding direction. Data acquisition is implicit in the basic spin echo sequence diagram, but becomes a significant consideration for fractional echo techniques and advanced pulse sequence timing.

The second component of signal readout, frequency encoding, is critical for proper spatial encoding of the data. We have already encoded the data in the slice and phase directions; the Fourier transform allows us to utilize frequency differences as a third dimension for spatial differentiation.

The goal here is to generate known variations in spin frequencies along a given data line. As we saw with the phase encoding gradient in Figure 7-2, application of a magnetic field gradient will speed up or slow down the spins precessing along that gradient direction. But unlike the phase encoding gradient, we do not want to turn off the frequency encoding gradient until we have completed readout of the signal. At the end of the readout period, all the spins will return to the frequency determined by the main magnetic field; they become indistinguishable from one another.

So, in essence, we create a variation in the precessional frequencies of the spins along the readout direction. This could be designated in a similar fashion to the phase encoding gradient with vertical rather than horizontal bars, as

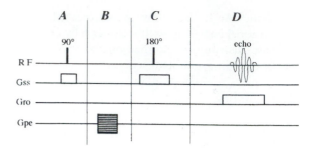

Figure 7-11. The four phases of the spin echo diagram. *A*, excitation; *B*, encoding; *C*, refocusing; *D*, readout.

shown in Figure 7-10. Since we do not vary the readout gradient amplitude from repetition to repetition of the sequence, we generally do not include this designation in our pulse sequence diagram.

As the gradient occurs during the readout period for the function of frequency encoding the signal, the terms readout gradient and frequency encode gradient are used interchangeably. The readout gradient pulse has a direct effect on the resultant image signal-to-noise since it is on during data acquisition – this is a key consideration in the understanding of low or narrow bandwidth techniques.

In summary, the spin echo pulse sequence progresses through four distinct phases: excitation, encoding, refocusing, and readout [Figure 7-11]. These four phases are actually common to all MR imaging techniques though different techniques will incorporate modifications to one or more of these phases.

GRADIENT PHASE EFFECTS

Now that we have created a spin echo pulse sequence from a general perspective, let's look at the effects of each gradient on the signal phase as well as strategies to compensate them. They are perhaps among the least understood of MR concepts and it may be because they are given inadequate attention in textbooks of basic MR physics.

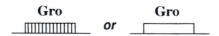

Figure 7-10. Readout gradient designation.

As you recall, magnetic field gradients in MRI have the net effect of momentarily speeding up or slowing down the precessional rates of spins within the main magnetic field. This creates a momentary dispersion of the spin phases used either to encode the data or for excitation of the appropriate spins. This effect is sometimes referred to as gradient phase dispersion.

It should be noted that gradient phase dispersion applies only to those spins in the transverse plane. Spins aligned with the z-direction, or main magnetic field, cannot become dephased, as shown in Figure 7-12.

If the applied gradient pulse is constant, the spins exhibit a linear dephasing response (assuming no additional external forces are applied). That is, the spins accelerate or decelerate in their precession at a constant rate proportional to the gradient field they experience. This is depicted graphically in Figure 7-13.

Note that the phase of the spins, ϕ, is zero before application of the gradient pulse. We can think of this as a sample of pure water in which all spins are in phase and precessing at the Larmor frequency as defined by the main magnetic field.

The moment the gradient pulse is turned on, the spins begin a steady and gradual dephasing process, either positive or negative depending upon the polarity of the gradient pulse applied. This continues until the gradient pulse is turned off, at which point the spin phase remains constant. Note that the phase in Figure 7-13*b* and *c* does not return to zero as we have done nothing in this simple example to cause this to happen.

Figure 7-13*d* does bring the phase dispersion back to zero provided the second (positive) gradient pulse is exactly equal in amplitude and duration to the first (negative) pulse. Also note that for the sake of this discussion, we are ignoring other T2 relaxation or dephasing effects (such as chemical shift, magnetic susceptibility, etc.). This is done for simplicity in order to examine the gradient-induced effects.

The phase dispersion diagrams in Figure 7-13 apply to the response of spins in the transverse plane to positive and/or negative gradient pulses. There are two other components of the spin echo sequence which must be considered – the 90-degree and 180-degree RF pulses. The effects of such pulses are shown in Figure 7-14.

In the case of the 90-degree RF pulse, we have drawn the gradient phase dispersion starting at the middle of the 90-degree pulse. Remember, with phase dispersion, we are looking only at the spins in the transverse plane. The intention of the 90-degree pulse in spin echo is to flip the desired spins from the longitudinal axis to the transverse plane. Hence, the gradient on-time prior to the 90-degree pulse has no effect on the phase

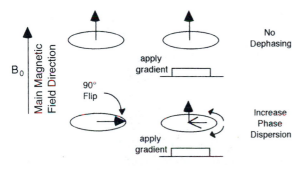

Figure 7-12.   Effect of gradients on phase dispersion.

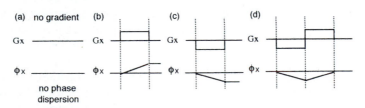

Figure 7-13.   Gradient phase dispersion diagrams, see text for explanation of parts (a) to (d).

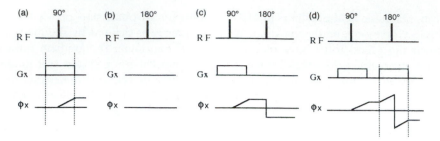

Figure 7-14.   Gradient phase dispersion diagrams, see text for explanation of parts (a) to (d).

dispersion. Therefore, we only create phase dispersion in the second half of the gradient pulse.

For the 180-degree RF pulse, we have three different cases to consider. In Figure 7-14b, we assume we have no phase dispersion prior to the 180-degree pulse (i.e., no gradient pulse applied). The 180-degree RF pulse flips all of the spins in the transverse plane. If our phase dispersion was zero before the 180-degree pulse, it will also be zero after the pulse. Conversely, if our phase dispersion is nonzero prior to the 180-degree pulse, it becomes flipped in polarity, or inverted, as shown in Figure 7-14c. Note that the amplitude of the phase dispersion is the same before and after the 180-degree pulse.

Finally, if a gradient is applied at the time of the 180-degree RF pulse as in Figure 7-14d, the dispersion increases prior to the 180-degree pulse, becomes inverted at the time of the RF pulse, and increases again after the 180-degree pulse in response to the positive polarity of the gradient pulse. It is important to note that the gradient phase dispersion continues in a positive, linear fashion regardless of the inversion by the 180-degree pulse.

This concept of phase dispersion will become the key to understanding more complex techniques in MRI. Let's look at how these diagrams work with our spin echo pulse sequence.

The Slice Select Gradient

Figure 7-15 represents an isolated view of the phase dispersion for the slice select gradient from

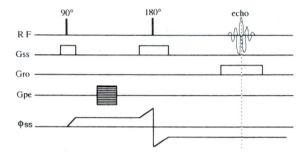

Figure 7-15.   Slice select gradient phase dispersion.

the spin echo pulse sequence diagram. In this case, we have added a line to represent the gradient phase dispersion induced by Gss and labeled as ϕ_{ss}.

In this example, ϕ_{ss} increases linearly during the applied gradient pulse for the 90-degree RF excitation. Following the gradient pulse, the phase remains constant at some nonzero value until the 180-degree RF pulse. At this second gradient pulse, the ϕ_{ss} again increases until the 180-degree RF pulse flips all the spins in the transverse plane such that the phase is inverted about the zero phase line. The phase continues to increase linearly through the second half of the gradient pulse, approaching zero phase dispersion, but not quite reaching zero phase.

Again, when the gradient is turned off, the phase remains constant through the echo, therefore at the time of the echo, the phase in the slice select direction is nonzero. That is, all the spins are not completely aligned in their rotation, as shown in Figure 7-16. This condition of nonzero phase dispersion leads to reduced signal due to cancellation between different spin vectors.

To avoid this situation, an additional gradient pulse is generally inserted into the pulse sequence diagram immediately following the 90-degree excitation pulse, as shown in Figure 7-17. This pulse is usually equal to one-half the area of the 90-degree slice select gradient pulse and is generally referred to as a balancing pulse.

Looking at the phase dispersion for the slice select gradient, we see that the pulse increases linearly as before during the latter half of the 90-degree RF pulse. The balancing pulse, however, brings the phase quickly back to zero immediately

following the excitation. This will happen as long as the amplitude and duration of the balancing pulse are such that the area defined equates to exactly one-half the area of the gradient during the 90-degree pulse (remember, the phase dispersion only occurs during the second half of the 90-degree pulse).

Now, at the time of the 180-degree RF pulse, the slice select gradient is once again turned on. The phase diagram follows the same path as we saw in Figure 7-14*d*, but now the resultant phase is zero through the echo. This results in maximum signal (or no reduction in signal due to slice select gradient effects) in the resultant image. So, now our general spin echo pulse sequence diagram can be redrawn to look like Figure 7-18.

The Readout Gradient

We can apply a similar analysis to the readout gradient design. Figure 7-19 demonstrates an isolated view of the phase diagram for the readout direction in our standard spin echo pulse sequence.

Once again, we see that the phase dispersion caused by the gradient pulse increases linearly during the gradient on-time. In this case, the phase remains zero through the sequence until the readout period begins. No dispersion in the readout direction occurs during the 90-degree or 180-degree RF pulses since we have not applied any readout gradient pulses.

Note that the phase at the center of the echo is again nonzero as was the case in the slice select direction. That is, all the spins are not completely aligned in their rotation. This again leads to

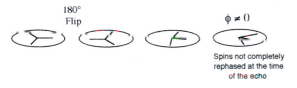

Figure 7-16. Incomplete rephasing due to gradient phase dispersion.

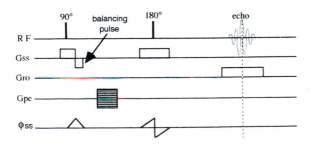

Figure 7-17. Modified slide select gradient phase dispersion.

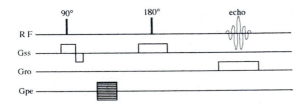

Figure 7-18. Spin echo pulse sequence diagram.

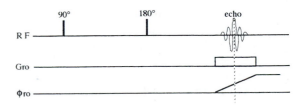

Figure 7-19. Readout gradient phase dispersion.

reduced signal due to cancellation between differing spin vectors.

To avoid this nonzero phase dispersion condition, an additional gradient pulse is generally inserted into the pulse sequence diagram immediately following the 90-degree excitation pulse and usually coincident with the phase encoding gradient, as shown in Figure 7-20. This pulse can also be thought of as a balancing pulse – this time for the readout gradient.

Reviewing the phase dispersion diagram for this modified readout gradient sequence, the phase increases linearly during the first gradient pulse on-time. Following this pulse, the phase remains constant at some nonzero value until the 180-degree RF pulse. At this second RF pulse, the phase in the readout direction is flipped (or inverted) about the zero phase line and is now negative due to the spin inversion in the transverse plane.

Phase dispersion remains constant at some nonzero value until the time of the readout pulse at the echo, where the phase increases linearly once more such that it crosses the zero phase line precisely at the center of the signal echo. This

results in maximum signal (or no reduction in signal due to readout gradient effects) in the resultant image. We can redraw our general spin echo pulse sequence diagram to look like Figure 7-21.

The Phase Encoding Gradient

We can repeat this process once more to analyze the phase diagram for the phase encoding gradient direction. Figure 7-22 demonstrates the phase diagram for the phase encoding direction in our standard spin echo pulse sequence.

Once again, we see that the phase dispersion caused by the gradient pulse increases linearly during the gradient on-time. In this case, the phase becomes nonzero fairly early in the pulse sequence. At the time of the 180-degree pulse, the phase is inverted about the zero phase line, but remains nonzero through the echo.

For the other two gradient directions, we balanced the pulse sequence in order to obtain zero phase at the time of the echo. But in the case of the phase encoding direction it is precisely this phase difference which provides us with the means to differentiate spins along one axis of the data set. Therefore, we do not want to balance or spoil the spins in the phase encoding direction.

In addition, the phase encoding gradient amplitude varies with each repetition of the sequence. Therefore, the phase dispersion diagram could be drawn as Figure 7-23.

Such a strategy will inevitably lead to a decrease in signal-to-noise, but it is exactly this effect which leads to signal-to-noise dependence on the phase encoding gradient amplitude.

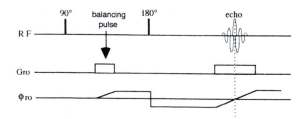

Figure 7-20. Modified readout gradient phase dispersion.

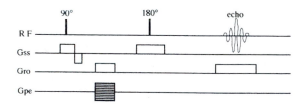

Figure 7-21. Spin echo pulse sequence diagram.

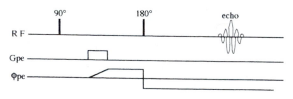

Figure 7-22. Phase encoding gradient phase dispersion.

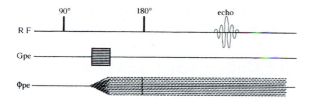

Figure 7-23. Phase encoding gradient phase dispersion.

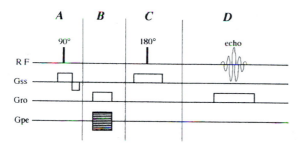

Figure 7-24. The four phases of the balanced spin echo diagram: *A*, excitation; *B*, encoding; *C*, refocusing; *D*, readout.

Hence, the center lines of our data file (or time domain) – where the phase encoding gradient amplitude is very low – typically exhibit higher signal, and therefore contribute the most to the resultant image signal-to-noise and contrast.

Standard Spin Echo Summary

To summarize what we have seen thus far, the standard spin echo pulse sequence diagram is actually more complex than we first thought. The signal at the time of the echo is dependent upon the gradient-induced phase dispersion created by each gradient applied. To correct for this effect, we have added extra gradient pulses in the slice select and readout directions. With appropriate timing, these balancing pulses provide maximum signal, and hence signal-to-noise, for the resultant data collection and image.

For most readers the phase diagrams introduced here in conjunction with the pulse sequence diagrams may be new, but they will become increasingly useful, if not critical, in understanding the physics and comparing the features of more complex techniques. Figure 7-24 shows the balanced spin echo sequence diagram labeled with the appropriate four stages of the pulse sequence diagram.

SEQUENCE MODIFICATIONS

Now that we have established the basic sequences used in MR imaging, we can discuss a variety of modifications employed to obtain better contrast or more clinical information. First, we will look at multiecho imaging which provides the acquisition of proton density in addition to T2 information on the long echo sequence without adding to the scan time. Next, we will look at multislice imaging, which uses the dead time of the spin echo pulse sequence to increase clinical coverage without sacrificing scan time.

The Multiecho Spin Echo Sequence

The spin echo diagrams drawn and discussed until now have involved a single echo. The extension to multiple echoes is straightforward and involves the simple addition of another 180-degree RF pulse and readout gradient, as shown in Figure 7-25.

The diagram shows an additional 180-degree RF pulse with a coincident Gss pulse – this is necessary in the instance where multislice acquisition is involved (to avoid the 180-degree pulse affecting any tissue other than the desired slice). Also, an additional readout gradient is applied for frequency encoding of the data during measurement. To ensure proper phase balancing of the

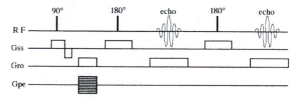

Figure 7-25. Double echo spin echo sequence.

signal, let's draw the phase dispersion diagram for each of the three gradient directions.

From Figure 7-26, we see that the addition of a second 180-degree RF pulse with a Gss gradient balances itself such that the phase in the slice select gradient direction is zero at the time of the second echo, as desired. The same holds true for the readout direction, thus maximizing the signal at the time of the echo.

In the phase encode direction, the phase is offset at the first and second echoes – a necessary condition for proper spatial encoding of the resultant data set. The reverse polarity of the gradient phase at the time of the second echo has no effect on the resultant images, as the phase encode variations will map out the raw data file in a symmetric fashion.

In summary, the multiecho spin echo technique is only limited by the additional time required for the extra RF and gradient pulse necessary to generate the second (or successive) echo. This may limit the number of slices available as it cuts into the dead time between multiple sequence repetitions during which the additional slices are acquired. It is also worthwhile to note that each echo in the multiecho technique is generally acquired at the same phase encoding gradient value. In this way, each echo is mapped as one line into separate raw data files in order to generate complete images from separate, but distinct echo times. Hence, we typically obtain one short echo (proton density) image and one long echo (T2 weighted) image from a single sequence.

The Multislice Spin Echo Sequence

In the clinical application of the spin echo sequence, the repetition time, TR, is generally much greater than the echo time, TE. The dead time between the end of echo collection and the next 90-degree pulse allows for excitation and acquisition of a data line of another slice. That is, the frequency of the 90-degree RF pulse is offset in order to excite spins precessing at a different frequency at a different location along the slice select gradient, as shown in Figure 7-27.

This sequence variation is essentially trivial in the phase dispersion diagrams due to the fact that adjacent slices are not excited simultaneously. The one possible interaction between slices occurs with the 180-degree RF pulse [Figure 7-28].

If the 180-degree pulse applied in slice #1 is a nonselective 180-degree – an RF pulse without a simultaneous slice select gradient – it is possible to create in slice #2 a contrast mechanism of the inversion recovery type. The spins in slice #2 are inverted 180-degrees into the negative z-direction; this situation is undesirable. As almost all sequences are used in multislice mode, it is generally correct to draw the spin echo pulse sequence with a slice select gradient pulse at each RF pulse; this avoids the undesirable effects of a nonselective 180-degree pulse on slice #2 spins.

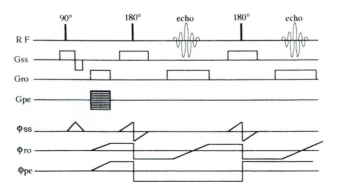

Figure 7-26.   Double echo phase dispersion diagram.

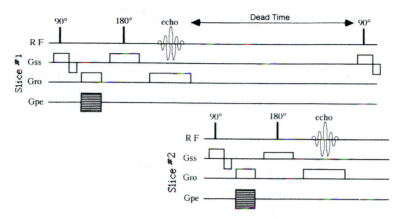

Figure 7-27.   Multislice spin echo diagram.

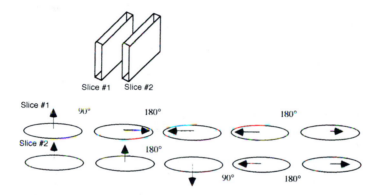

Figure 7-28.   Nonselective 180-degree pulse with multislice spin echo.

THE INVERSION RECOVERY SEQUENCE

The inversion recovery (IR) method, which provides heavily T1 weighted images, is often effective in defining small lesions or the internal structure of lesions where detectability may involve only subtle differences in T1 values.

In inversion recovery, the protons are pre-pulsed with a 180-degree inversion pulse prior to the standard spin echo pulse sequence. The sequence diagram is shown in Figure 7-29.

The preparation pulse serves to flip the spins 180 degrees into the negative longitudinal direction providing for a larger dynamic range in the relaxation process [Figure 7-30]. The receiver antennae (RF coils) can only detect magnetization perpendicular to the main magnetic field, therefore, a second RF pulse of 90 degrees is applied at a time, TI (the inversion time), after the 180-degree pulse. This 90-degree pulse flips the partially recovered spins into the transverse plane, so that a signal may be detected.

The effect of inverting the magnetization vector by the initial 180-degree RF pulse allows tissue to relax over twice the dynamic range possible with spin echo. Data is collected part way through the relaxation period by applying a 90-degree excitation pulse at a point when there is maximum (or desired) contrast. The magnitude

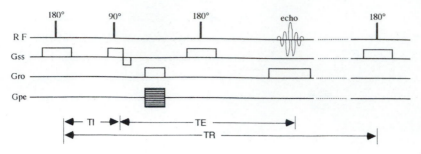

Figure 7-29.   Inversion recovery pulse sequence.

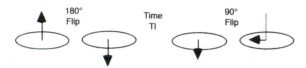

Figure 7-30.   Magnetization of inversion recovery.

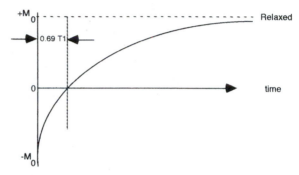

Figure 7-31.   T1 determination in inversion recovery.

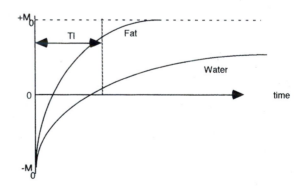

Figure 7-32.   Fat/water contrast curves in inversion recovery.

of magnetization is a function of time after a 180-degree pulse. The magnitude starts negative, passes through zero at $t = 0.69$ T1 [Figure 7-31], and recovers completely by $t = 5$ T1. Because of this expanded range in the longitudinal direction, excellent image contrast based on differences in tissue T1 values may be produced.

For example, since fat has a relatively short T1 relaxation and water has a relatively long T1; one can maximize the contrast difference between fat and water by initiating the spin echo portion of the sequence at approximately the average value of the two T1 values. Choosing the inversion time, TI, equal to the average T1 values of the two tissues produces optimum distinction between these tissues, as shown in Figure 7-32. The repetition time, TR, is usually chosen to be about three times longer than the inversion time (3 × TI) to optimize the signal-to-noise ratio.

It is significant to note that inversion recovery is designed to minimize T2 relaxation. In addition, this technique tends to have very long measurement times due to the incorporation of relatively long TR values plus the TI component into the scan time calculation.

The STIR Technique

Tissue signal suppression may be observed using STIR (short tau inversion recovery), a special case of the inversion recovery sequence. By using a very short TI, we can produce images with suppression of signals from specific tissue types, such as fat (Figure 7-33).

In STIR, the idea is to wait only until the fat signal crosses the null point ($0.69 \times$ T1), the time at which there is no fat signal available to be flipped 90 degrees into the transverse plane by the spin echo sequence. Remember, only signal in the transverse plane can contribute to the final image.

The T1 relaxation rates will vary with field strength, which will affect the recommended TI values to use with STIR. In addition, different systems may have variances in their calculation of TI values such that absolute values are difficult to provide. Consult with the vendor regarding recommended TI values for a specific system when attempting the STIR technique. As a general guideline, the parameters in Table 7-1 are offered as a starting point in defining the optimal inversion times.

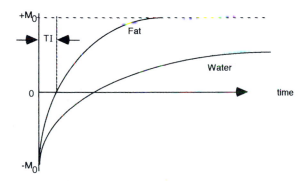

Figure 7-33. TI determination in STIR.

Table 7-1

Optimal Inversion Times for a Given Field Strength

Field (T)	TI (ms)
1.5	120–150
1.0	100–150
0.5	90–115
0.2	75–90

One of the advantages of STIR is that it is relatively reliable and system independent. As in spin echo, the contrast mechanism can be fairly easily reproduced from system to system and field strength to field strength, with appropriate correction of timing parameters.

The primary disadvantage lies with scan time. STIR scan time, as for inversion recovery sequences, can be computed as the product TR × NEX × Matrix. Since relatively long TR values are generally used, this results in scan times comparable to or even longer than standard T2-weighted spin echo sequences. NEX is the number of acquisitions.

In addition, we must be careful in the use of contrast agents in conjunction with STIR sequences. Gadolinium will shorten the T1 relaxation rates for vascularized tissues. Since fat generally has poor vascularity, its T1 value will not be affected. However, fatty lesions may experience some T1 shortening and therefore have reduced effectiveness in fat suppression. The combination of STIR with gadolinium enhancement has proven useful in the evaluation of breast lesions where sufficient suppression of the fat signal combined with enhancement of the lesion has been shown to increase detectability.

The FLAIR Technique

A variation on the STIR theme is the FLAIR technique (fluid attenuated inversion recovery). In this case, rather than using a short TI value to catch fat at the null point in longitudinal relaxation, we now use a very long TI to catch water at the null point [Figure 7-34]. This results in suppression of structures such as ventricles (CSF) and has been shown to help define even very small demyelinating lesions such as multiple sclerosis.

The drawback with the FLAIR technique lies in the fact that TR values of greater than 5000 ms are typically required with TI values of about 2000 ms. As should be immediately apparent, this technique has typical scan times of 20 min or more, even at high field strengths with reduced resolution.

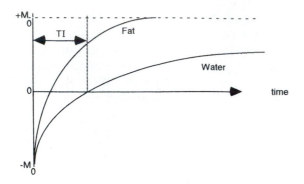

Figure 7-34. TI determination in FLAIR.

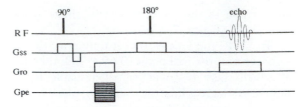

Figure 7-35. Spin echo pulse sequence.

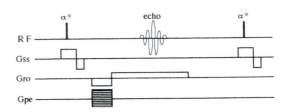

Figure 7-36. Gradient echo sequence.

Inversion Recovery Summary

In summary, the inversion recovery sequence is essentially the same as standard spin echo with the addition of a 180-degree preparation pulse for maximum contrast control. The technique involves relatively long scan times though provides exquisite T1 weighted contrast and a variety of tissue-specific signal suppression.

THE GRADIENT ECHO SEQUENCE

The spin echo pulse sequence has been the fundamental platform for MR imaging for more than a decade. While this sequence produces reliable and well-understood contrast, imaging times for spin echo tend to be fairly long (on the order of several minutes or more) in the clinical setting. With the inherent sensitivity of MRI to motion artifacts, this scan time becomes cumbersome for many patients.

In the mid-1980s, a new class of sequences began appearing which dramatically reduced the required scan time in MR imaging. These sequences are referred to as gradient echo sequences, and they vary from spin echo in two fundamental characteristics.

First, the spin echo sequence itself involves the use of a 180-degree RF pulse in order to accomplish refocusing of the echo, as shown in Figure 7-35. While this has proven to be reliable

for generating high quality T2 information in an image, the length of this pulse and associated gradient pulses significantly increases the minimum allowable echo time (TE).

Second, spin echo sequences generally involve relatively long repetition times (TRs) in order to allow sufficient time for longitudinal relaxation of the spins. Since the TR is directly involved in the calculation of scan time, spin echo sequences – particularly T2 weighted – tend to have relatively long scan times.

Gradient echo sequences overcome these two issues by utilizing a reduced (less than 90 degrees) flip angle for excitation, followed by a gradient reversal instead of the 180-degree RF pulse for echo formation [Figure 7-36]. Let's look at the advantages and disadvantages in more detail.

Gradient Reversal versus 180-degree RF Pulse

The essential feature of gradient echo sequences lies in the use of gradient reversal to create an echo rather than a 180-degree RF refocusing

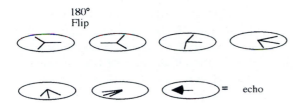

Figure 7-37.   180-degree RF pulse creation of a spin echo.

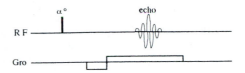

Figure 7-38.   Gradient echo gradient reversal.

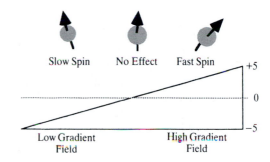

Figure 7-39.   Spin effects in gradient reversal.

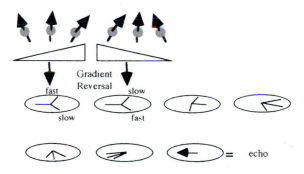

Figure 7-40.   Gradient reversal creation of a gradient echo.

pulse used in the spin echo pulse sequence. To review, the 180-degree RF pulse flips spins in the transverse plane, as shown in Figure 7-37.

All of the spins in the transverse plane are flipped by the 180-degree pulse such that the fast spins are now behind the slow spins in their precession. After a period of time, the faster spins will catch up and become aligned with the slower spins to create what we call an echo. In this case, the T2 effects controlling phase dispersion (spin–spin interactions, magnetic field inhomogeneities, magnetic susceptibility, etc.) are not affected and the spins continue their precession at the same rate and in the same direction. This is the fundamental mechanism in the creation of a spin echo.

In gradient echo sequences, a gradient reversal in the readout direction is employed to create the echo, as shown in Figure 7-38.

Spins which were "slowed down" by the first negative gradient pulse will now be "sped up" by the second readout gradient pulse, as shown in Figure 7-39.

It is important to note the result of T2 field effects in this scenario. T2* dephasing effects include items such as magnetic susceptibility, caused by the interface of adjacent differing tissues. At this interface, the protons of one tissue will precess faster than adjacent spins of the second tissue. These spins will affect each other such that the first spins will precess slightly slower than expected, and the second set of spins will precess slightly faster. The gradient reversal affects the rate at which the spins precess within the gradient field. The effect of this reversal on the transverse magnetization is depicted in Figure 7-40.

When the gradient is reversed, the spins which originally saw a high positive gradient amplitude now see a high negative gradient. The variation in precessional frequency of the spins through the application of the readout gradient pulse causes the spins to reform an echo – they are not flipped in the transverse plane as occurs with a 180-degree refocusing pulse for spin echo sequences.

Because the spins in one tissue are not precessing as quickly as they should (and the spins in another tissue are not precessing as slowly as they should), the spins at the tissue interface are not quite rephased at the time of the echo. This leads to a signal dropout and is the fundamental mechanism behind the magnetic susceptibility artifact seen in gradient echo images.

Gradient echo sequences will create an echo though this signal does not include information from regions where the magnetic field has been altered, such as by main magnetic field inhomogeneities or tissue interfaces. This modified T2 dependence is generally referred to as T2* contrast and is a fundamental property of gradient echo sequences.

The original goal behind the use of the gradient reversal was to eliminate the 180-degree RF pulse. The echo created by gradient reversal is limited only by the system's ability to rapidly switch the polarity of the gradient pulses. Therefore, the echo times attainable with standard gradient echo sequences can be as short as 1 or 2 ms [Figure 7-41].

The echo time, TE, in gradient echo sequences has essentially the same contrast control as spin echo. That is, increasing the TE will increase the T2 – or more precisely, T2* – dependence in the resultant image. The only difference lies in how quickly dephasing occurs. Since gradient reversal techniques do not compensate for all magnetic field inhomogeneity effects, dephasing occurs more rapidly. Therefore, we typically use very short TE values (< 30 ms) for heavily T2* weighted gradient echo images.

By employing gradient reversal, we have enabled the use of shorter echo times within our pulse sequence. The other significant by-product with the elimination of the 180-degree RF pulse is that we significantly reduce the RF power deposition (or SAR) delivered to the patient. Therefore, we can not only acquire data with short echo times, but in general these sequences also involve less risk to the patient.

Shallow Flip Angle

The second principle feature of the gradient echo sequence is the use of a less-than-90-degree RF pulse in order to shorten the required longitudinal relaxation period. The spin echo sequence involves the use of a 90-degree RF pulse for slice selection (or excitation) in order to flip the desired spins into the transverse plane. The 90-degree flip transposes the signal into the transverse plane so that we can measure the signal as it relaxes. A downside of this technique is that we must wait a relatively long time (500 to 3000 ms) to allow for enough signal to undergo longitudinal relaxation before the next excitation of the slice.

The 90-degree RF excitation pulse maximizes the amount of transverse magnetization and therefore the amount of signal available for the echo. However, the full 90-degree flip angle is not required to generate signal [Figure 7-42].

From the figure, we can see that the 90-degree RF pulse flips the entire net magnetization vector

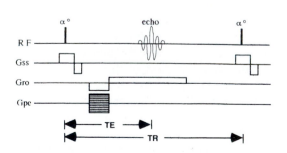

Figure 7-41. Gradient echo sequence.

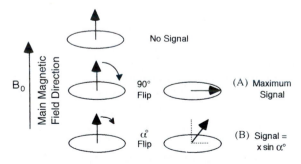

Figure 7-42. Creation of transverse magnetization.

into the transverse plane (A). In example (B) we have flipped the net magnetization at some angle less than 90 degrees. This vector will have a component (or shadow) in the transverse plane though the size of this transverse component will be less than the original vector. This transverse component can be computed from simple geometry as $X \sin \alpha$ where X is the size (or amplitude) of the original vector and α is the angle of our flip.

So, we can now see that a flip of less than 90 degrees will put spins into the transverse plane. Remember, we receive signal from any spins in the transverse plane at the time of the echo, and the flip angle controls how much signal is actually received.

However, this example has also shown us that the amount of signal from this reduced flip is less than we would receive with a standard 90-degree spin echo excitation. Therefore, gradient echo sequences will have less signal-to-noise than spin echo.

The advantage for the gradient echo sequence is that, since we did not flip the spins a full 90 degrees into the transverse plane, the longitudinal recovery (or T1 relaxation) can now occur much more rapidly than would be the case for spin echo. This is particularly important in the case where short TR values are used [Figure 7-43].

With a very short repetition time, the spin echo magnetization does not have sufficient time for relaxation for all spins to return to the longitudinal direction. Therefore, at the next repetition of the sequence, there is significantly less signal available to be flipped into the transverse plane. This continues for each repetition such that the sequence provides poor signal-to-noise performance.

To avoid this problem, we typically try to use TR values on the order of a few times the T1 of the tissues of interest. This relatively long relaxation period provides the required time for longitudinal relaxation. For comparison, the same diagram for gradient echo is shown in Figure 7-44.

In this case, the gradient echo sequence has flipped the spins only partially into the transverse plane. Much of the signal, or net magnetization vector, remains in the longitudinal orientation aligned with the main magnetic field. With only a few spins in the transverse plane, the relaxation process back into alignment with the main magnetic field happens relatively quickly.

Hence, we can now use TR values much shorter than spin echo – on the order of 10 ms. In addition, even if the TR is too short to allow for complete relaxation, more signal is available in the longitudinal orientation for the next repetition than was the case for the spin echo sequence.

Therefore, repetition time (TR) has a similar effect on image contrast as seen in conventional spin echo sequences. Decreasing TR has the net effect of increasing signal dependence on tissues with short T1 values, and therefore directly controls T1 contrast. Decreasing TR increases T1 contrast in the resultant image. However, this will

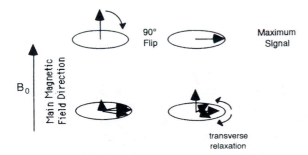

Figure 7-43. 90-degree RF pulse transverse magnetization and longitudinal relaxation.

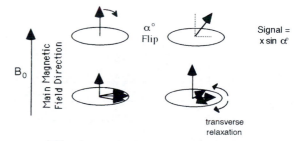

Figure 7-44. α RF pulse transverse magnetization and longitudinal relaxation.

also provide less signal available for the next excitation and therefore decreases signal-to-noise.

Flip angles of less than 90 degrees are another parameter for contrast control in gradient echo sequences. In general, as the flip angle (FA) approaches 90 degrees, the sequence contrast behavior approaches that of standard T1 weighted spin echo sequences. However, the contributing factor of the short repetition time in gradient echo sequences cannot be ignored.

As the flip angle is increased, more signal is converted into transverse magnetization such that fewer spins are available for the next repetition of the sequence. Therefore, the flip angle will play a pivotal role in the resultant signal-to-noise. By increasing flip angle, we are decreasing the amount of signal available for the next repetition; this is the same as decreasing TR, the time allowed for relaxation of the spins in the longitudinal direction.

With larger flip angles, spins with short T1 relaxation rates will have more complete relaxation and contribute more signal to the next sequence repetition. Therefore, increasing flip angle increases T1 dependence in the resultant image.

In summary, very shallow flip angles (less than 10 degrees) flip very little signal into the transverse plane. Hence, such sequences will tend to have poor signal-to-noise performance. The gradient echo pulse sequence is shown in Figure 7-45.

The following trends can be noted for the various contrast control parameters in gradient echo sequences.

Increasing TR
Decreases T1 dependence
Increases signal-to-noise

Increasing TE
Increases T2* dependence
Decreases signal-to-noise

Increasing FA
Increases T1 dependence
Decreases signal-to-noise
Approximately the same as decreasing TR

Gradient echo sequences have increased contrast sensitivity over spin echo due to increased T2* dependence. This can be an advantage or disadvantage depending upon the clinical application, and needs careful consideration.

On the downside, gradient echo sequences are more gradient intensive. That is, the short TE and TR values require rapid gradient switching – an additional burden on the system hardware. In general, gradient echo sequences have the following advantages over spin echo.

Dramatically reduced scan times (due to short TR)
Lower RF power deposition (SAR)
Increased number of slices per unit time (for a given TR)

The Balanced Gradient Echo Sequence

In Figure 7-46 we have redrawn the pulse sequence diagram showing the phase dispersion diagrams in each of the three gradient directions. Looking first at the slice select direction, we see that the phase dispersion increases at the middle of the α RF pulse as we flip the magnetization into the transverse plane. The negative balancing pulse brings the phase dispersion immediately back to zero. No further RF pulses or gradient pulses are employed in the slice select direction so our phase dispersion remains zero through the echo. Therefore, our sequence is balanced in the slice select direction.

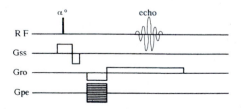

Figure 7-45. Gradient echo pulse sequence.

In the readout direction, the phase dispersion decreases during the first, negative pulse. With the gradient reversal, the dispersion begins a gradual increase and crosses zero precisely at the center of the echo. Note that no 180-degree RF pulse exists so the phase dispersion never becomes inverted about the zero phase line as we saw in spin echo. With zero phase dispersion at the center of the echo, we are balanced in the readout direction.

Finally, in the phase encoding gradient direction, the phase dispersion increases with the application of the gradient pulse. Again, since we have not applied any additional RF or phase encoding gradient pulses, the phase dispersion remains at a constant, nonzero value through the echo. Remember from spin echo that this is actually a desirable condition as it is the means for spatial differentiation of lines within our dataset.

Here is a summary of the advantages and disadvantages of gradient echo imaging.

Advantages

No 90-degree pulse means faster longitudinal relaxation so a shorter TR (faster scan) can be used

No 180-degree pulse means fewer RF pulses and allows the use of a short TR with less RF power deposition to the patient

Short TR provides a quick T2* scan though may be limited in number of slices

Disadvantages

T2* contrast rather than true T2

More work for the gradients and noisier for the patient

Relatively low signal-to-noise but high contrast

Unpredictable contrast was initially a problem but has become something of an advantage now that it's used to give increased sensitivity to hemorrhage

Gradient Spoiling and Rephasing

A technique proposed to gain better contrast control is to manipulate the phase in the transverse plane at the time of the next RF pulse. For example, if we spoil all the transverse magnetization following data collection, we are left with the longitudinal components only for the next RF flip. This is accomplished by adding additional gradient pulses as shown in Figure 7-47.

The figure shows the addition of three gradient pulses – one in each direction – after the echo readout and before the next RF pulse. The goal of these gradients is to spoil the signal in the transverse plane. That is, to make the gradient phase dispersion nonzero [Figure 7-48].

Figure 7-48 shows that the spoiler pulses effectively increase the phase dispersion in all three directions such that there is no coherent signal in the transverse plane at the time of the next RF pulse. This can also be represented by the magnetization diagram [Figure 7-49].

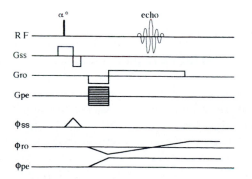

Figure 7-46. Gradient echo sequence phase dispersion.

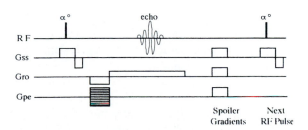

Figure 7-47. Spoiled gradient echo.

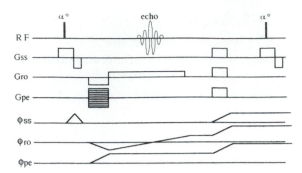

Figure 7-48. Phase dispersion of spoiled gradient echo.

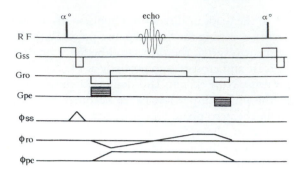

Figure 7-50. Phase dispersion of rephased gradient echo.

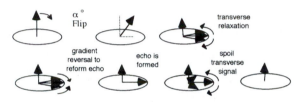

Figure 7-49. Magnetization of spoiled gradient echo.

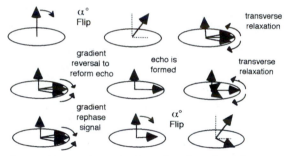

Figure 7-51. Magnetization of rephased gradient echo.

So we see that the only signal left for the next RF pulse is one that has successfully relaxed in the longitudinal direction. Because this is essentially what happens in T1 weighted spin echo imaging, spoiled gradient echo sequences will provide more T1 dependence.

The advantage of gradient echo with spoiling is that for short TR values, one can achieve much higher T1 weighted contrast. Unfortunately, it incorporates additional gradient pulses, which means more work for the gradient hardware and may require lengthening TR or decreasing the number of slices available.

Conversely, we can preserve the transverse magnetization through the use of rephasing gradient pulses [Figure 7-50] and record the changes schematically in a magnetization diagram [Figure 7-51].

In this case, the magnetization in the transverse plane is manipulated such that it is preserved at the next RF pulse and may contribute to the signal in the next repetition of the pulse sequence. The net effect of this scheme is an increase in the T2* contrast in the resultant image even with very short TR values. Again, this technique involves additional gradient pulses so the gradients must work harder, and the TR may need to be increased to preserve the number of slices available.

The rephased technique will basically provide a higher level of T2 contrast with very short TR and TE. Note that for very long TR, the transverse magnetization will eventually relax into the longitudinal direction such that rephased gradient echo becomes equivalent to spoiled gradient echo. At this point, the image contrast becomes dependent upon the flip angle and echo time used. Here is a summary for short TR values.

Spoiled gradient echo

Spoils the transverse signal

Only longitudinal signal contributes to next RF pulse

Increases T1 dependence (weighting)

Rephased gradient echo

Preserves transverse signal

Both signals contribute to the next RF pulse

Increases T2* dependence

FAST SPIN ECHO

There are two ways to speed scan times in MRI: either reduce the amount of data collected, or reduce the time span to acquire the number of data points needed. The first strategy can be achieved using conjugate symmetry or a rectangular field of view in which only a portion of the raw data (or time domain) is sampled while maintaining resolution through zero-filling or a similar scheme.

There are several ways to shorten the time to collect scan data, such as reducing the number of acquisitions or the matrix size. However, these methods tend to negatively affect signal-to-noise and/or resolution. Fast spin echo uses a modifi- cation of existing spin echo concepts – acquiring multiple data lines per sequence repetition – to produce the desired reduction in scan time.

To understand how the fast spin echo tech- nique works, we will first review the physics of conventional spin echo.

Review of Conventional Spin Echo

In traditional spin echo imaging, a 90-degree radio frequency (RF) pulse excites the desired slice. That is, the protons (or spins) within the tissues are flipped 90 degrees from the relaxed state aligned with the main magnetic field, into the transverse plane. Remember that spins aligned with the main magnetic field cannot generate any signal toward the resulting image. The desired spins must be flipped into the trans- verse plane.

Once in the transverse plane, the spins are given a period of time for relaxation to occur – both T1 (longitudinal) and T2 (transverse or dephasing). A 180-degree pulse is then applied to reverse the effects of dephasing and generate an echo. The time between the 90-degree pulse and the echo is called the echo time or TE. Figure 7-52 shows the detail of a conventional multiecho spin echo sequence with the appro- priate timing of the gradients along the slice select (ss), readout (ro), and phase encoding (pe) directions.

Figure 7-52 shows a multiecho sequence whereby two echoes are generated within a single repetition of the sequence by applying a second

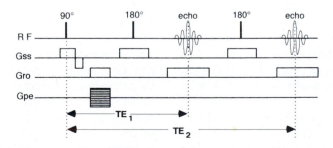

Figure 7-52. Conventional multiecho spin echo pulse sequence.

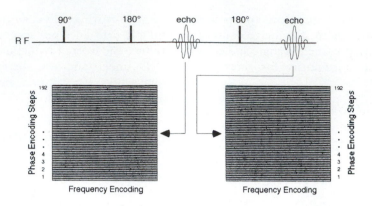

Figure 7-53. Filling of *k*-space.

180-degree pulse following the first echo. Note that the readout gradient is applied during each echo for frequency encoding. However, the phase encoding gradient is applied only once – at the beginning of the sequence – so each echo is acquired at the same phase encode value. The data is filed into two separate raw data files to create two independent images corresponding to the two echoes.

The mathematical name for the raw data file, or time domain, is *k*-space. The collection of the two echoes described above fills one line in each of two *k*-space files [Figure 7-53]. The sequence is then repeated, beginning with another 90-degree pulse and two 180-degree pulses.

The phase encoding gradient is now incremented so the next two echoes are acquired with altered phase, thus filling the next lines in each of the two *k*-space files. The process repeats until *k*-space is entirely filled.

Note that as the data collection continues, the phase encode gradient occurs in incremental steps. The data lines at the top and bottom of the *k*-space file are required with relatively high amplitudes of the phase encoding gradient, while the center lines are acquired with very low or zero amplitudes of the gradient.

Remember that high gradient amplitudes lead to greater phase dispersion during the echo and poor signal-to-noise. Hence, the center lines of *k*-space contribute the most to the resulting

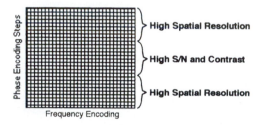

Figure 7-54. *k*-space dependence on SNR and contrast versus resolution.

signal-to-noise and the most toward contrast, while the outer lines contribute high frequency or spatial resolution information, as shown in Figure 7-54. This concept becomes important in understanding the contrast and resolution control of the images in fast spin echo.

Fast Spin Echo

The fast spin echo technique was first developed in 1984 as the RARE (rapid acquisition with relaxation enhancement) method by Dr. J. Hennig and colleagues at the University of Freiberg, Germany, and presented in *Magnetic Resonance in Medicine*, December 1986. While the concept was not new, the implementation gained greater success using improved software and hardware technology (i.e., superior gradient performance and eddy current compensation).

The fast spin echo sequence is similar to conventional spin echo. A 90-degree pulse initiates the sequence, followed by multiple 180-degree pulses to generate echoes. This sequence will typically use many more echoes than conventional schemes, with 4 to 16 echoes acquired. For a simple demonstration, a fast spin echo sequence is shown using five echoes in Figure 7-55 (this is commonly referred to as a five-echo train fast spin echo).

When using fast spin echo, we acquire multiple echoes with successive 180-degree pulses, but a separate phase encoding gradient is applied before each echo. Recall that in conventional spin echo imaging, each echo is acquired with the same phase encoding and sorted into separate k-space files to generate separate images.

Here, each echo represents a different line within the same k-space file to be reconstructed into a single image as shown in Figure 7-56. Hence, for each repetition of the sequence (i.e., each time a 90-degree pulse is applied), five different lines of k-space are filled.

By acquiring several lines of k-space within a single repetition of the sequence, the total time of the scan can be reduced dramatically. This is shown for a 192×256 matrix in Figure 7-57. Remember that each line of data contains 256 points in the frequency encoding direction, while the phase encoding direction is determined by the number of sequence repetitions, in this case 192.

As seen in the example above, conventional spin echo scan time is determined by the product of (1) the repetition time, (2) the number of

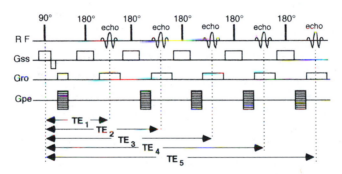

Figure 7-55. A five-echo train fast spin echo sequence diagram.

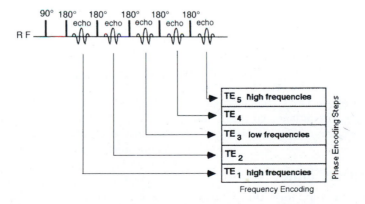

Figure 7-56. Fast spin echo k-space filling.

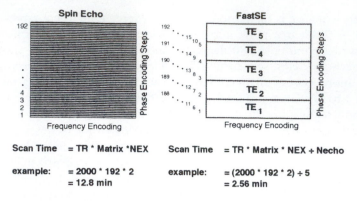

Figure 7-57.   Spin echo versus fast spin echo filling of *k*-space.

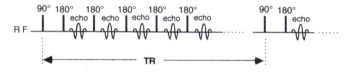

Figure 7-58.   Effect of repetition time (TR).

phase encoding steps (i.e., the number of times the sequence is repeated at a different phase encode amplitude), and (3) the number of acquisitions. In fast spin echo, since each repetition represents the acquisition of five lines of *k*-space, the number of phase encoding steps is divided by the number of echoes acquired for each image.

Overall scan time has been reduced by a factor of 5 in this case without changing the repetition time (TR), resolution (matrix), or the number of acquisitions (NEX).

The time-saving benefits have costs, however, in contrast and resolution of the resulting images. Since one is now using multiple echo times to generate a single image, the contrast results can become mixed. The effects of each of the scan parameters on image contrast and generation will be considered independently.

Effect of Repetition Time

The effect of varying the repetition time in a fast spin echo sequence [Figure 7-58] is similar to that seen with standard spin echo. That is, increasing the repetition time allows more time for longitudinal relaxation, reducing the contrast dependence on T1 values of the tissues. This effect allows more T2-weighting in the image.

The difference between fast spin echo and conventional spin echo lies in the fast spin echo ability to increase the TR values employed as a trade-off against the time savings achieved. Therefore, TR values of 3000 to 5000 ms are quite common with the fast spin echo technique, maximizing the resulting signal.

Effect of Effective Echo Time

In fast spin echo, the term effective echo time (ETE) is used rather than echo time (TE) because multiple echoes comprise the data for a single image. Hence, echo times of 20, 40, 60, 80, and 100 ms may be combined to generate a single image. ETE refers to the echo placed in the center of *k*-space, which contributes the most to the resulting image's contrast.

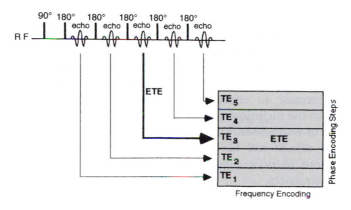

Figure 7-59. Filling of *k*-space.

In Figure 7-59, the center echo is encoded into the center of *k*-space, making this the ETE for this sequence. If the actual echo times are 20, 40, 60, 80, and 100, then 60 ms becomes the ETE. The resulting contrast for the image will be comparable to a standard spin echo sequence with an echo time of 60 ms. Take note, however, that more T1 weighted and heavily T2 weighted information may be mixed in due to the inclusion of the 20 and 100 ms echoes within the image.

The effective echo time is generally not an operator-selectable option, since the sequence must be preprogrammed for optimal signal-to-noise at each echo. That is, specific sequences may include the ability to use flow compensation or low bandwidth techniques. If the user has the option to alter the ETE, this significantly complicates the sequence design and may result in compromises to the sequence effectiveness. A variety of sequences are generally provided with different ETE values giving the operator choice of contrast in the resulting image.

Effect of Echo Train Length

The echo train length (ETL) refers to the number of echoes used to comprise the image. The example of Figure 7-59 has a value of 5, or five echoes within the sequence. This does not always have to be the case, and different

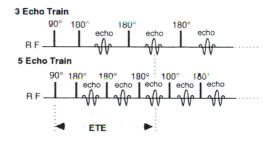

Figure 7-60. Effect of echo train length (ETL).

sequences can be written with different numbers of echoes acquired for each image. Figure 7-60 compares a three-echo train with a five-echo train having the same effective echo.

The obvious benefit of increasing the ETL is a saving in scan time. The scan time is the number of phase encoding steps divided by the number of echoes used, so the five-echo train sequence produces a shorter scan time. But this can have some drawbacks, as well.

Figure 7-60 shows the two sequences with the same effective echo time. Notice that the last echo in the three-echo train is shorter than in the five-echo train. This will result in fewer slices (reduced coverage) available with the five-echo train sequence. This is analogous to the conventional spin echo sequence employing a long TE resulting in fewer slices. We may be able

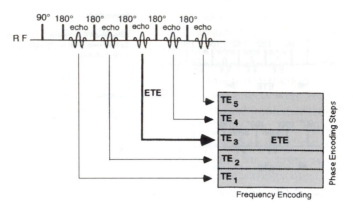

Figure 7-64. Standard order of k-space filling.

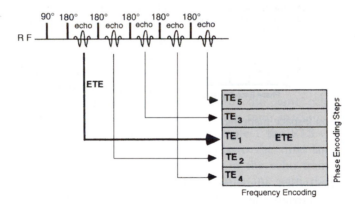

Figure 7-65. Reordered k-space.

the outermost portions of k-space. This creates two desirable effects.

First, we know that the center lines of k-space contribute the most contrast control over the resulting image. Also, due to T2 decay, the first echo within the sequence will have the highest signal available. By reordering k-space (Figure 7-65) the echo with the highest signal is placed in the portion of k-space where it will have the greatest impact on the resulting signal of the image. This echo will also contribute most to the contrast of the image.

Thus, by reordering the filling of k-space, we have direct control over image contrast and the opportunity to have a sequence with a relatively

short effective echo time. This is how T1 or proton density-weighted images are acquired using the fast spin echo technique.

Remember that fast spin echo employs multiple echoes, so that a sequence with an effective echo time of 15 or 20 ms may have more T2 contrast than desired, based on the timing of the later echoes used to make up the image.

Since physical parameters (or timing) within the sequence are free of changes, there are few trade-offs for employing reordered k-space. The only difference is in how the data acquisition system files the data into k-space. This technique is limited only by the capabilities within the system hardware and software to place data anywhere in *k*-space and reconstruct the appropriate image. Reordering is generally preset within the sequence to permit short echo fast spin echo.

In summary, the fast spin echo technique allows for collection of faster images – particularly T2-weighted spin echo contrast. It is also easily implemented on almost any scanner and has become routine for many clinical sites. One drawback is that, due to the successive 180-degree echoes, this technique has reduced sensitivity to hemorrhage. To compensate for this factor, modifications involving the incorporation of gradient echoes in addition to the spin echoes have been proposed to increase the level of magnetic susceptibility effects.

THREE-DIMENSIONAL VOLUME IMAGING

One of the unique characteristics of magnetic resonance imaging is that it is inherently a three dimensional process; there is no fixed relationship between the imaging plane and the apparatus. Images of equal quality and resolution can be formed in axial, sagittal, coronal, or even oblique planes. In the discussion of pulse sequences, we have thus far only discussed the formation of images of a slice or collection of slices. More than one slice was imaged by utilizing the T1 recovery period to interrogate other slices. Now we will introduce the modifications to the pulse sequences that permit truly simultaneous imaging of a contiguous volume.

Pulse Sequence Diagrams

If we start with a basic spin echo pulse sequence [Figure 7-66] we can easily convert it to a volume imaging (3D) sequence [Figure 7-67] by adding another phase encoding function. We have to add it to the slice gradient control because we wish to resolve the selectively excited volume into many slices. For clarity, let us refer to this as slice encoding. The process is identical to that performed in the phase encoded axis. The top two lines are the transmitted RF and the analog-to-digital conversion (where the received signal is captured), respectively.

Figure 7-68 shows the basic pulse sequence diagram for gradient echo imaging. There are two plots for the slice select gradient; one for 2D

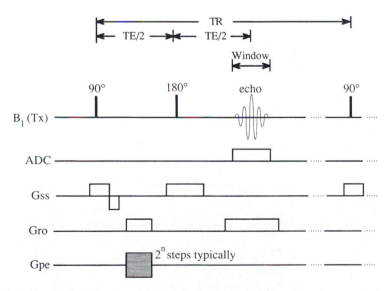

Figure 7-66. Simple 2D spin echo pulse sequence.

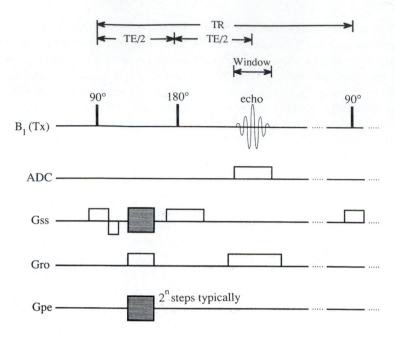

Figure 7-67.   Simple 3D spin echo pulse sequence.

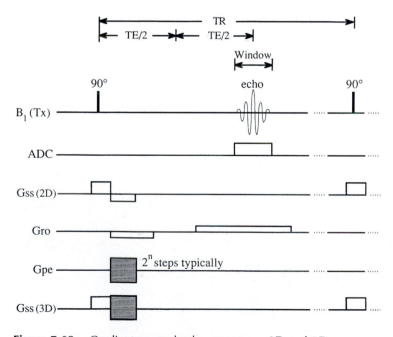

Figure 7-68.   Gradient reversal echo sequences, 2D and 3D.

and one for 3D. Finally, to achieve shorter TE and faster scanning, we generally find that the gradient pulses are maximally overlapped. For example, the slice encoding and balancing (rephasing) portion of the slice select function are most often combined.

In all 3D cases, each of the original phase encoding steps must be applied independently for every slice encoding value. We usually use a number of slice encoding values that is a power of 2, such as 16, 32, or 64, as the fast Fourier transform (FFT) processes them very efficiently, but other values are permissible. The FFT then separates the slices the same way it defines the resolution in the plane along the phase encoded axis.

One drawback of 3D imaging is the minimum scan time for a given TR is longer by a factor of the number of slice encodings. This makes 3D imaging practical in a clinical setting only when very short TR is desired. It is for this reason that the primary use of 3D techniques is in conjunction with gradient refocused echoes and reduced flip angles.

Another (minor) difference in the pulse sequence is that the slice axis gradient pulses during the RF pulses are generally much weaker than for 2D imaging. This is simply because we want to simultaneously excite a thicker volume, sometimes referred to as a slab (as opposed to a slice). A typical 2D slice is 2 to 10 millimeters thick. A typical 3D slab is 16 to 128 millimeters across, sometimes more depending on the number of slices and their individual thicknesses.

This last feature points to an advantage of 3D imaging. The minimum slice thickness is not critically limited by the maximum gradient strength as it is in 2D imaging. Slice thickness in 3D imaging is done by encoding. Thus the gradient pulse length can be increased as well as the strength to achieve higher resolution. Typical sequence conditions provide phase encoding resolution on the order of one millimeter or less. Slice excitation in 2D reaches a practical limit at two or three times that thickness. Further reduction of the 2D thickness requires lengthening the RF pulses and TE significantly.

There are times when we will want to choose a 3D sequence simply because we require very thin slices. There are also reasons that relate to signal strength and to contrast that we need to consider when choosing between 2D and 3D scanning.

Signal-to-Noise Ratio (SNR)

The basic equation for the signal strength in a spin echo sequence (i.e., 90-degree excitation) leads to a maximum signal-to-noise ratio per unit of scan time, $SNR(t)$, at a TR of 1.26 times the T1 for the single tissue being considered[1]. For partial flip gradient refocused echo the maximum $SNR(t)$ can be achieved for virtually any TR by the proper choice of flip angle[1]. Figure 7-69 plots $SNR(t)$ versus TR (expressed as a multiple of T1) for both cases. The spin echo response function is fairly forgiving near the maximum. To maintain efficiency within 90 percent of its maximum the TR for a spin echo sequence only needs to be kept between 0.6 and 2.5 times T1. However, the clinical situation requires that a certain region of the patient be entirely scanned. If the number of slices required is high enough, the minimum TR that can cover the anatomy may be too long from the viewpoint of $SNR(t)$ efficiency.

In typical applications we encounter a strong function of field strength, due in part to a change in the desired signal bandwidth and to the increase in T1 at higher fields. Tissues range in their T1 dependence on field strength from no dependence for CSF (T1 = 4000 ms, T2 = 1600 ms) to approximately the square root of field strength for muscle and brain. For example gray matter has a T1 of 300 ms at 0.064 T, 650 ms at 0.35 T, and 1200 ms at 1.5 T. T2 changes are smaller and less important for what follows.

In the case of an axial series of slices through the brain about 14 cm must be covered. If 7-mm slices are used then 20 slices are required. There is no problem to image 20 slices with a TR = 2000 ms (100 ms/slice) at high or even

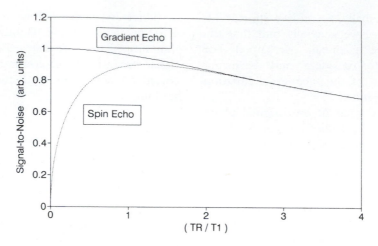

Figure 7-69.   SNR per unit time as a function of the TR interval expressed as multiples of the T1 of interest.

middle field strength. TR = 2000 ms is within its targeted range $(1.67 \times T1)$ at $1.5\,T$ and only slightly long $(3.1 \times T1)$ at $0.35\,T$. In fact, since the lesion relaxation time is longer than that of gray matter often, the sequence will work well. At $0.064\,T$, however the TR is $6.7 \times T1$ – very inefficient. The conditions require a different sequence at low field and at $0.35\,T$ for thinner slices (say 40 slices at 3.5-mm thickness).

These conditions lead to a choice of partial flip gradient reversal 3DFT techniques [Figure 7-68] for most applications at low fields and any applications requiring large numbers of thin slices at all fields. For a more rigorous discussion of these points the reader is directed to Carlson et al[2]. or Kramer et al[3].

Contrast Control

The partial flip gradient reversal echo sequence is becoming one of the most used sequences in routine practice. Because of its inherent speed and flexibility when combined with 3DFT sequencing, this sequence is being adapted to do many new jobs. By choosing the flip angle the contrast due to T1 resembling long or short TR can be achieved in a fixed TR. The higher flip angles are used in angiography applications to suppress stationary tissues and thereby highlight vessels with sufficient inflow of unsaturated spins. By using very short TR and changing the gradient pulse details (such as spoilers) the relative contribution of the standard FID response and the steady-state free precession response (from spins remaining in the transverse plane) can be changed. This allows the contrast from T2 to be had in a very short TR sequence.

Figure 7-70 is a plot of the effective TR versus flip angle for a partial flip gradient reversal sequence. If we consider any two tissues, we can calculate the contrast due to T1 that would be observed for a 90-degree excitation as a function of TR. The definition of contrast for this graph is the ratio of the signal strengths.

For a given actual TR (three are plotted) the contrast equivalent TR is shown for all flip angles below 90 degrees. The graph shows that these sequences can produce the contrast of long TR scans adequately even with a very short TR like 50 ms. An important point is that the slope is very steep at low flip angles, so precision may be crucial if a particular contrast is needed. It need hardly be said that the SNR may not be good enough at very low flip angles.

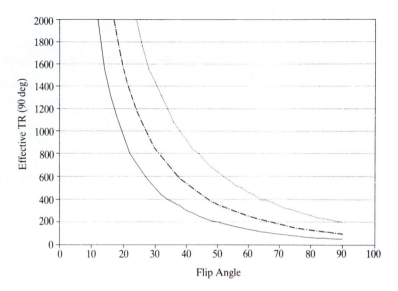

Figure 7-70. T1 contrast and effective TR, T1(a) = 4000 ms, T1(b) = 250 ms: (solid line) TR = 50 ms, (dash-and-dot line) TR = 100 ms, (dotted line) TR = 200 ms.

Slice Profile

The slice definition in 3D imaging arises out of the FFT rather than out of the excitation spectrum of an RF pulse (as is the case in 2D). Therefore the slice response has some sidelobes that are substantially like a sinc function[2]. These can give rise to artifacts in the slice direction. While they may not be easily recognized, they are indeed familiar. The artifacts that are completely analogous and well known are those seen in the plane that look like edge reverberations. They are found near sharp features with high contrast and go by many names. They are the result of insufficient resolution to properly define the sharp edge that was the source of the ringing. The consequence for 3D imaging is that we should always get fewer artifacts with thinner slices. This is a good match since it was for thin slices that we were initially motivated to choose 3D.

There is an advantage to the fact that the raw data has all of its axes Fourier encoded. We can reconstruct images out of the 3D data set at oblique angles and even on curved surfaces without any loss of resolution. This is not to say that all 3D data sets have equal resolution on the three axes. What it does mean is that the information is in a form that permits total preservation of whatever resolution is present onto any desired viewing plane using very standard processing[4].

Summary

Here is a list of advantages and disadvantages for 3DFT techniques.

Technical advantages

Minimum slice thickness not critically dependent on gradient strength

Minimum TE not dependent on slice thickness

Gradient reversal scans much less sensitive to magnet inhomogeneity and bulk susceptibility artifacts

Large numbers of slices can be scanned with short *or* long TR contrast; contrast control by flip angle

Raw data set is inherently well suited for ideal slice reformatting

Technical disadvantages

Efficiency suffers for small number of slices; loss at ends

Contrast variation between slices (especially near ends)

Slice profile/crosstalk

Longer minimum scan time, reconstruction time.

Greater motion sensitivity (same as longer scan?)

RE refocused scanning technically more difficult but can be done

REFERENCES

1. Ernst RR. In: Waugh JS. ed. *Advances in Magnetic Resonance* Vol. 2. New York: Academic Press 1–135, 1966.
2. Carlson JW, Crooks LE, Ortendahl D, et al. Comparing S/N and section thickness in 2-D and 3-DFT MRI. *Radiology* 166:266–270, 1988.
3. Kramer DM, Guzman R, Carlson JW, et al. The physics of thin-section MR imaging at low field strength. *Radiology* 173:541–4, 1989.
4. Kramer DM, Li A, Simovsky I, et al. Applications of voxel shifting in MR imaging. *Invest Radiol* 25: 1305–1310, 1991.

CHAPTER 8

Advanced MR Pulse Sequences

Peggy Woodward

Sequence technology has advanced in leaps and bounds in the past five years. As a result MR imaging sites no longer rely solely on simple T1 and T2 images in multiple planes to make a diagnosis. They tend to produce a wide variety of imaging sequences on the patient and in less time than was realized in the not so distant past.

In this chapter, we describe the more advanced imaging techniques being used clinically today.

FAT SUPPRESSION TECHNIQUES

Historically, clinical MR imaging is based on identifying signal-producing hydrogen, most of which is contained in water and lipid components. Generally, fat is seen as a bright signal on conventional T1 weighted images and less bright on T2 weighted images. It can be very bright on fast spin echo T2 weighted images as well, due to the T1 contributions of early sampled echoes. Fluid filled structures are commonly seen as dark on T1 and bright on T2 weighted images. We know that structures containing significant amounts of free hydrogen, as is found in most simple fluids, are in organized compartments of the body, such as the urinary bladder, ventricular system, and ocular bulb. Fat surrounds many of these structures. In some tissues, fat is a molecular component along with hydrogen in fluids. Increased hydrogen concentration, as it relates to disease processes, is the hallmark of tissue abnormalities. The most common example is found in diseased fatty bone marrow, where an increased amount of hydrogen is found in the fatty marrow and is due in part to the inflammatory response of the body to the pathology. Many times it is difficult to separate the fat from water so that diagnostic ability is hampered[1].

A variety of fat suppression techniques is available, including STIR (short TI inversion recovery), chemical shift sequences that include spectral presaturation (fat sat), out of phase techniques, and water–fat separation. Clinically, chemical shift sequences and STIR have been used for many years. Lack of uniformity of suppression, especially when imaging areas requiring

127

large fields of view (such as the abdomen and pelvis) have resulted in vast improvements in imaging techniques specifically designed to address this issue. In this chapter we will describe both old and new imaging techniques used to suppress fat signal.

STIR

STIR imaging is the simplest form of fat suppression available. The technique is derived from a basic inversion recovery sequence, which uses a short inversion time TI, usually in the range 90–150 ms. If the appropriate TI is chosen where there will be no appreciable signal from fat containing tissues, only fluid containing structures will exhibit high signal. The resultant image will display relatively low signal but high contrast in areas where both fluid and fat resides. For lesion detection and conspicuity, this is necessary, since lesions are commonly associated with high fluid content and may be within or adjacent to fat containing structures. The clinical advantages of STIR are based on its additive T1 and T2 contrast, significant fat suppression capabilities, and the magnetization recovery range that is twice that of a spin echo sequence. This produces images with high lesion contrast and conspicuity[2]. However, since the sequence is T1 dependent, the use of a paramagnetic contrast media is not advised due to additional T1 shortening in the target tissue for which signal may be nulled along with fat. Figure 8-1 shows a typical STIR sequence on an elbow in the coronal plane. Refer to Chapter 7 for a complete description of inversion recovery and STIR imaging.

Chemical Shift Imaging

Chemical shift imaging is so named because the regional chemical differences in closely aligned molecules take on two primary forms: Phase cancellation and spectral presaturation.

Most operators are familiar with the chemical shift phenomena because they see it as an artifact that produces a black line at the fat–water interface that is a result of shifted fat signal in

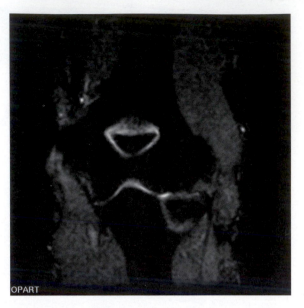

Figure 8-1. Coronal image of the elbow using STIR. (Courtesy Toshiba America MRI, Inc.)

the readout direction. The opposite edge appears as a misregistered bright signal. Both are depicted in Figure 8-2.

This phenomenon is a consequence of a precessional frequency difference of hydrogen in fat and water. When both are contained in the same voxel, Fourier transformation can not separate this chemically based difference from the distribution frequencies produced by the readout gradient. Thus the computer misregisters this as a disparity in spatial location along the frequency encoding direction. An artifactual signal void that is several pixel widths is then visible at the fat–water interface. The artifact becomes worse with increasing field strength and when using narrow bandwidth sequences. And although the artifact exists, it can be used to differentiate fat–water interfaces because of its known anatomic location. Actually, we want to know the chemical shift of certain elements since this is the basis of our ability to determine fat distribution within tissues. It helps us to distinguish a variety of liver and bone marrow diseases such as liver degeneration by fatty

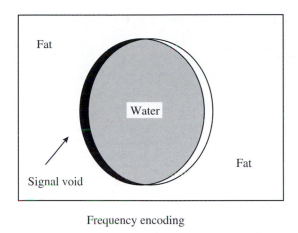

Frequency encoding

Figure 8-2. Illustration of chemical shift artifact depicting spatial misregistration of the fat versus water signal. If a fat molecule were residing in water, the band of signal void versus increased signal would be swapped.

infiltration, cirrhosis, hepatitis, and bone marrow necrosis.

Phase Cancellation

Based on the mechanism of chemical shift origin, chemical shift techniques for fat suppression have been developed that use pulse sequence designs that cancel the signal from fat. The simplest fat suppression technique occurs as a result of fat and water tissues residing in the same voxel when using gradient echo imaging with very specific echo times. These are called "phase cancellation" techniques.

When fat and water are present in the same voxel, a chemical shift between them results in different precessional frequencies. Following RF excitation, at TE = 0, both fat and water are "in phase" with respect to one another. Their signals are additive so that at TE = 0, maximum signal intensity is achieved. As TE increases, the fat and water spins begin to precess at their characteristic frequency. Due to chemical shift, their signals will precess at different rates and eventually move 180 degrees "out of phase" from one another. If

their phase relationship is exactly opposite, their signals will cancel and the signal intensity in the voxel will be minimal. This is called "out of phase." With further increases in TE, the phases of fat and water will cycle in and out with each other. The signal intensities will be brightest when in phase, and darkest when out of phase. This relationship is depicted in Figure 8-3.

By choosing an echo time when the spins' phases are 180 degrees out of phase, signal for fat will be minimal. The degree to which fat suppression occurs is dependent on the amount and proportion of fat and water in a given voxel. If a ratio of 1:1 exists, then complete cancellation will occur when the spins are out of phase. If the voxel contains only fat, then suppression will not occur because there has been no opposing contribution from water signal.

Echo times used to produce in-phase or out-of-phase images are field strength dependent and can be determined by calculating the frequency difference or chemical shift between fat and water at that field strength (water has a chemical shift of 4.7 ppm (parts per million) while most lipids have a chemical shift of 1.2 ppm, hence the 3.5 ppm difference). Multiplying 3.5 by the operating frequency of the field strength in use will yield the chemical shift in Hertz at that field strength. Figure 8-4 shows this frequency difference as calculated for a variety of field strengths.

To determine the appropriate TE for fat signal cancellation, the operating frequency in MHz is multiplied by 3.5 ppm. The inverse of the result is converted to milliseconds, 1/frequency difference = TE ms, and becomes the in-phase TE. One half the in-phase TE and multiples thereof, become the out-of-phase TEs.

For example, with an operating system of 1.5 T, the chemical shift frequency difference is 224 Hz, so that 1/224 = 0.00446 or 4.5 ms. That means that for every 4.5 ms, the phases of fat and water are cycling in and out with one another. For images where fat and water signal is additive and therefore maximum, choosing an echo time of TE = 4.5 ms, in this example, will yield in-phase images. Selecting a TE that is

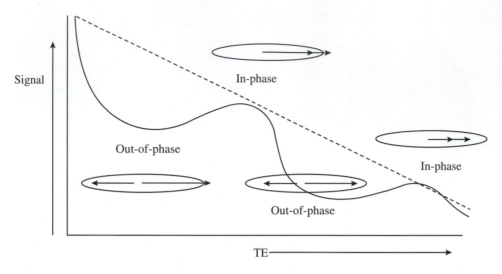

Figure 8-3.   Relationship of TE to spin phases of fat and water.

Field strength in Tesla	Frequency difference in Hertz
0.2	30
0.35	52
0.5	75
1.0	149
1.5	224
2.0	298

Figure 8-4.   Frequency difference between fat and water at various field strengths.

approximately one-half the in-phase TE can generate out-of-phase images, where the signal from fat has been suppressed. Multiples of both the in-phase and out-of-phase TE can be used to generate images. The use of out-of-phase TE would produce the fat suppressed images. Here is a sample in-phase/out-of-phase calculation:

Field strength	1.0 T
Larmor frequency	42.58 MHz/T × 1.0 T = 42.58 MHz ≈ 42.6 MHz
Chemical shift	3.5 ppm × 42.6 MHz = 149.1 Hz ≈ 149 Hz

In-phase TE	$1/149 = 0.0067 =$ 6.7 ms, therefore 6.7, 13.4, 20.1, etc.
Out-of-phase TE	$6.7/2 = 3.35 \approx$ 3.4 ms, then 3.4 + 6.7 = 10.1, 16.8, 23.5, etc.

Figure 8-5 charts these relationships for various field strength.

Out-of-phase chemical shift images appear as if a black line has been drawn about all fat–water interfaces, and the signal from structures containing mostly fat will be suppressed. The advantages of this type of fat suppression include superb edge enhancement of fat–water interfaces, a decrease in the signal from fat containing structures, and a reduction in the chemical shift artifact and therefore confusion arising from the artifact. Furthermore, an increase in the ability to characterize high-signal intensity structures on T1 weighted images such as differences between increased signal normally associated with fat and that from hemorrhage (the fat signal is voided, whereas the signal from hemorrhage remains intense) is advantageous. The disadvantages

In-Phase Versus Out-of-Phase TE

Field Strength (T)	0.15	0.2	0.35	0.5	1.0	1.5	2.0
Frequency (MHz)	6.4	8.5	15	21.3	42.6	63.9	85.2
Chemical Shift (Hz)	22.4	30	52.5	75	149	224	298
In-phase TE (ms)	44.6	33.3	19.0	13.3	6.7	4.5	3.4
Out-of-phase TE (ms)	22.3	16.7	9.5	6.7	3.4	2.3	1.7

Figure 8-5. In-phase and out-of-phase echo times depicted are the calculated times of cycling. Consult the operator's guide for the system to which you are affiliated for exact TE values.

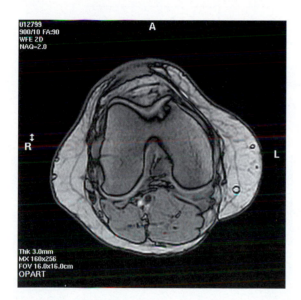

Figure 8-6. Gradient echo out-of-phase image of the knee, using TE = 10 ms at 0.35 T field strength. (Courtesy Toshiba America MRI, Inc.)

include a slight decrease in the apparent size of pathology at the interface due to the size of the pixel shift (which increases with field strength and narrow bandwidth imaging), and a decrease in SNR as a result of gradient echo technology. In addition, magnetic susceptibility increases when gradient echo imaging is performed so that areas where this is more apparent, such as the region of the pituitary, sphenoid and ethmoid sinuses, appear to have significant signal voids. Figure 8-6 shows an out-of-phase image of the knee.

In 1984, Dixon[3] developed a phase cancellation scheme in which a 2DFT hydrogen proton chemical shift technique by which the chemical shift of two spectral lines, water and lipid, could be resolved while maintaining excellent spatial resolution. The original technique, commonly referred to as the *Dixon technique*, was comprised of a pair of spin echo data sets. One set used a conventional 180-degree refocusing pulse to produce in-phase spins, while the other used an offset version of the refocusing pulse and a gradient reversal technique to generate out-of-phase signals. A reference point for the transmitter was set to the precessional frequency of water, then addition and subtraction of the two data sets were performed to yield water only and fat only images, respectively[3]. The amount of offset was determined by a time approximately equal to one-quarter the difference in frequency of the components being evaluated[4]. Figure 8-7 shows a graphical representation of the Dixon pulse sequence.

While the technique produced images based on chemical shift, it also suffered from magnetic field inhomogeneities, motion, and susceptibility effects. Additionally, reconstruction schemes were complicated by factors that affect the phase of the MR signal. Thus, variants of the technique were developed to bypass the usual scheme of double-set acquisition, thereby reducing scan time, and to compensate for factors that have plagued the method. These techniques, based on water–fat phase opposition continue to be used in a limited way, such as to visualized adrenal tumors, as is depicted in Figure 8-8.

Water–Fat Separation Techniques

Water–fat separation techniques are outgrowths of the previous methodology of fat suppression.

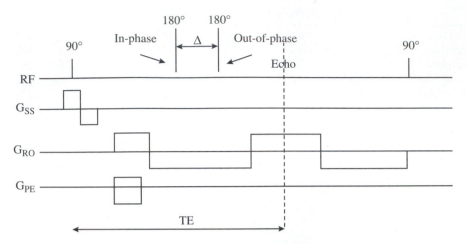

Figure 8-7. Pulse sequence diagram of the Dixon technique.

In this type of technique, all the information necessary for separating water and fat signals can be generated in a single acquisition using a *"sandwich" spin echo sequence* that is also capable of multiple-echo acquisition[5]. The technique was developed not only as an improvement to Dixon's method of fat suppression but as a way to compensate for difficulties in separating fat and water peaks especially laborious at lower field strengths where the frequency difference is small. Because of the longer time period necessary for the phase cycle at lower fields [see Figure 8-5], more *k*-space data can be acquired in a single acquisition.

Water–fat separation techniques are sophisticated versions of fat suppression that have been specifically designed for mid- and low-field MR imaging. They are based on the fundamental relationship between phase and frequency, whereby the bigger the frequency, the faster the phase accumulation. At the mid-low-field range, the precessional differences between fat and water are very slight so that their phase differences build up more slowly. For example, at 0.35 T, dephasing occurs approximately every 10 ms instead of 2 ms generally seen on 1.5 T systems. The close frequency prohibits chemical saturation techniques for this reason.

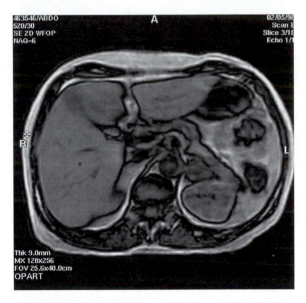

Figure 8-8. Water Fat Opposed Phase (WFOP) spin echo image of the abdomen at the level of the left adrenal gland. (Courtesy Toshiba America Medical Systems, Inc.)

In some water/fat separation techniques, three echoes are acquired at specified intervals that have differing amounts of phase variations between the water and fat components of the

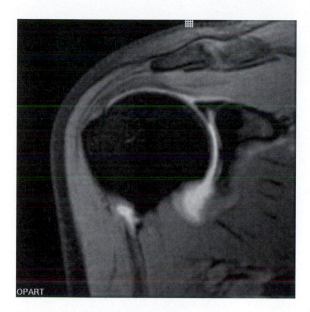

Figure 8-9. Shoulder arthrogram using gadolinium and a 2D FE version of the water/fat separation technique. (Courtesy Toshiba America Medical Systems, Inc.)

MR signal. A single RF echo is sandwiched between two gradient echoes, which are used to produce out-of-phase images and to determine B_O distribution. Correction of static field inhomogeneity is performed using B_O distribution information, prior to any image calculation. By adding and subtracting the echoes representative of water plus fat, and water minus fat, water-only and fat-only images can be generated from the phase images produced. The result is a method of fat suppression based on chemical shift properties instead of T1 relaxation characteristics like STIR. This may be quite beneficial when contrast enhancement is necessary, as is seen in Figure 8-9.

Spectral Presaturation Techniques

Spectral presaturation techniques use variations in the way the RF pulse is applied and when it is applied. Purely speaking, fat is selectively saturated by using a narrow bandwidth frequency-selective prep pulse of long duration. The fat vector is rotated about the direction of the

applied RF field while T1 and T2 relaxation is occurring so that the signal from fat is driven to zero. A conventional pulse sequence is then acquired which results in signal from water only. This method not only is time consuming but it requires high RF power, thus increasing SAR levels. Variations of this method use a short duration frequency selective 90-degree pulse and spoiler gradients in the transverse plane to force continued dephasing of the fat spins. But, fat saturation methods have their own set of difficulties. Even though theoretically, only water's magnetization in the z-axis is available for signal, it is impossible completely to saturate the signal from fat without affecting that of water. This may be a result of non-pure RF sidebands that cause incomplete fat saturation and/or partial saturation of water components. Other problems, related to T1 contrast of brain, seen differently on fat sat images when compared to conventional images, make fat sat techniques somewhat unreliable.

Solutions to these problems have been developed in more sophisticated fat saturation sequence designs. In one method a narrow bandwidth 90-degree pulse is used in conjunction with a reduced strength in the slice select gradient. This induces an exaggerated chemical shift misregistration in the slice direction. It is followed by a gradient reversal of the slice select gradient during the 180-degree refocusing pulse. Fat protons are shifted out of the slice plane and therefore do not receive both 90-degree and 180-degree pulses. That leaves only the water component, which has been stimulated by both RF pulses, to produce signal.

Other techniques have been developed to suppress the signal from fat while preserving the tissue T1 contrast. An example of this type of technique, PASTA, is based on polarity altered spectral and spatial selective acquisitions. This sequence uses a narrow band spectral selective 90-degree pulse to eliminate fat signals and an altered polarity for 90 degree and 180 degree gradients to avoid contamination of fat signals[6]. When compared to conventional fat sat techniques, PASTA can suppress the signal from fat without affecting the signal from water. An example is seen in Figure 8-10.

Uniform fat suppression in anatomic regions where large fields of view are necessary, such as the chest and abdomen, is difficult to obtain due to widely varying frequencies that are encountered in these tissues. High order shims may resolve some of this problem but are not clinically practical. First-order shimming is effective, but when the slices move from the isocenter, the frequency is shifted in the readout direction. A fat suppression method that addresses this issue was developed for multislice imaging, which uses an off-resonance pre-pulse for each slice. The sequence is called *MSOFT* (multislice off-resonance fat suppression technique)[7].

MSOFT uses slice selective off-resonance fat saturation with multidirectional first order shimming in the *x*, *y*, and *z* direction, prior to acquisition. During this time, frequency domain information is quickly sampled and recorded for each slice. A fat suppression pulse that is specific to each frequency offset is preset and applied for each slice. When multislice imaging is performed over large areas such as the chest and abdomen, where large frequency shifts are common as a result of susceptibility effects, this scheme provides uniform fat suppression throughout the entire imaged volume. Figure 8-11 shows an MSOFT image of the abdomen. MSOFT also is beneficial when imaging smaller FOVs due to its precision in fat suppression[1].

With the advent of fast spin echo imaging came the need to develop a method by which the bright signal from fat could be minimized. Modified versions of fast spin echo, such as *DIET*, (dual interval echo train) effectively minimize the high signal from fat without adversely affecting scan time or contrast[8]. This scheme uses an echo train spacing at the beginning of the pulse sequence that is much longer than the ensuing echoes, as is seen graphically in Figure 8-12. This allows for sufficient T2 decay of fat before subsequent data acquisition. Successive echoes are then acquired using equal and short echo train spacing. The generated images minimize

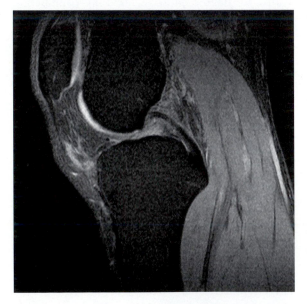

Figure 8-10. PASTA fat suppression used in extremity imaging. (Courtesy Toshiba America Medical Systems, Inc.)

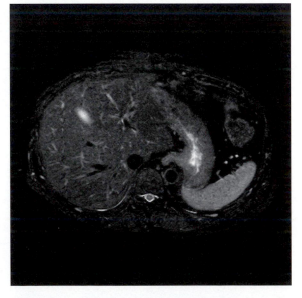

Figure 8-11. Abdomen image using MSOFT. (Courtesy Toshiba America Medical Systems, Inc.)

the bright signal seen from fat. While the fat signal is not totally eliminated, it is reduced in comparison to conventional fast spin echo images. An additional benefit of its use is the potential for increased sensitivity to hemorrhage due to the increased spacing between refocusing pulses[9]. Using a longer echo train spacing for the first echo only, followed by shorter spacing also allows for an increase in the echo train length without adversely affecting scan time.

Dual echo variants, which allow for the collection of proton density and T2 information, are obtained by incorporating the odd, large echo spacing in the middle of the sequence instead of at the beginning. Equal and small echo train spacing is used at the beginning of the echo train for data collection to allow for generation of a proton density image[9]. The remaining echoes that will contribute to the T2 weighted image are acquired using a large, initial echo spacing followed by smaller and equal spacing. Figure 8-13 shows this relationship.

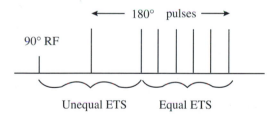

Figure 8-12. Graphic representation of the DIET scheme.

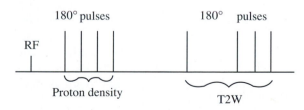

Figure 8-13. Simple graphic illustrating a variant of the DIET technique in which a proton density image can be collected while minimizing the bright signal from fat.

ADVANCED FAST IMAGING TECHNIQUES

Echo Planar Imaging

In the 1980s, an ultrafast gradient echo imaging technique called echo planar imaging (EPI) was developed by Dr. Mansfield, who elaborated on the fast field echo (see Chapter 7) technique by generating sub-second imaging using multiple gradient reversals that followed one set of RF pulses. The original sequence used a single RF excitation followed by long echo trains with rapidly switching readout gradients. Each echo was phase encoded separately using a very fast and brief gradient application or a weak but constant phase encode gradient. Figure 8-14 shows a typical EPI pulse sequence diagram. A complete image could be acquired in less than 30 ms. These gradient echo variants made imaging such as cine heart scanning viable, since a cine study could be acquired in a single heartbeat.

The technique, although the fastest of the MRI sequences, had significant limitations. Included were the extra cost of additional hardware and software, artifacts related to chemical shift and eddy currents, and physiological effects that may be provoked when much larger electric currents are induced by high-speed time-varying magnetic fields[1]. As a result, development of sequences such as RF refocused EPI, multi-shot EPI, and hybrid EPI technology ensued.

One example of this resulting technology can be defined as half-Fourier fast spin echo imaging. A technique called FASE (fast advanced spin echo technique) uses an extremely long echo train followed by a single 90-degree RF pulse. Half of *k*-space is filled up after this pulse, the rest is filled by HFI (half Fourier imaging) extrapolation, as seen in Figure 8-15.

By applying HFI, both the effective TE and the acquisition time can be reduced. Scan time for these sequences is often less than 1 s per image, resulting in a dramatic decrease in motion artifacts. Clinical functionality is enabled using EPI-type sequences primarily due to these scan

T2 signal and decay

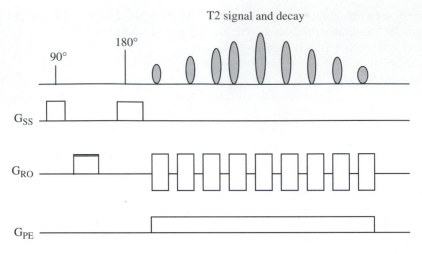

Figure 8-14. EPI pulse sequence diagram.

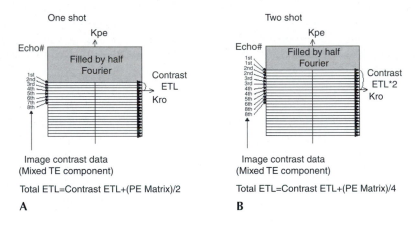

One shot

Two shot

Total ETL=Contrast ETL+(PE Matrix)/2

A

Total ETL=Contrast ETL+(PE Matrix)/4

B

Figure 8-15. Acquisition order and *k*-space tracking of FASE. (Courtesy Toshiba America Medical Systems, Inc.)

time reductions which allow breath-hold imaging while obtaining highly T2 weighted contrast. Exams such as MR cholangiopancreatography (MRCP) [see Figure 8-16] and MR urography become less specialized and more routine. An additional effect of this reduction in data acquisition time is not only an increase in the number of multislices but also a reduction in image blur[10].

Inherent problems associated with RF refocused EPI type sequences include a decrease in signal with progression of echo train length, edge blurring at lower TE values and edge enhance-

ment at higher TEs, and subtle blurring in the phase encode direction. However, the sequence is not limited by gradient power, does not produce artifacts associated with eddy currents and chemical shift and does not produce the acoustic noise, all which are present with gradient echo EPI sequences.

Functional Imaging Techniques

Diffusion and Perfusion MRI is basically a spatial distribution map of signal intensities

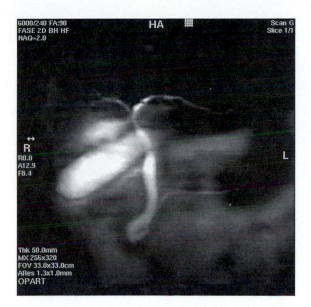

Figure 8-16. 2D MRCP using RF refocused EPI type sequence. (Courtesy Toshiba America Medical Systems, Inc.)

found in a heterogeneous tissue sample. The five main tissue factors that affect the MR appearance are spin density (PD), T1, T2, flow and chemical shift. Spin density, T1 and T2, do not always sufficiently characterize the pathological condition. There can be large differences in signal intensities in patients with the same pathology as well as overlap of values seen in different pathologies. Flow and chemical shift may only provide interesting information in a small set of tissues.

There are two additional tissue parameters that change with physiological condition or pathological state: diffusion and perfusion. Although similar at the macroscopic level (voxel) they are very different at the microscopic (capillary) level. Diffusion is the movement of molecules due to random thermal motion and may give us more static, anatomic/pathologic information. Perfusion is the passage of fluid through vessels of the target organ where change in blood oxygenation will occur, thus gives us more dynamic physiologic/pathologic information. Historically, both have been difficult to evaluate.

Diffusion Brownian motion, or random translational motion of molecules in fluid, is responsible for molecular diffusion. In the presence of magnetic field gradients, loss of phase coherence produces a spin echo attenuation in addition to that produced by spin–spin relaxation. Contrast from molecular diffusion is achieved because phase coherence of in vivo water protons undergoing random motion is reduced resulting in MR signal attenuation. However, in standard MR imaging, the gradients used are not significant enough to produce a noticeable attenuation of the signal. By deliberately applying a strong encoding gradient in a particular direction, signal attenuation, can be exploited to produce useful diffusion variations. For example, when cells swell due to loss of ionic pump mechanism, such as occurs in strokes, diffusion is restricted so that signal gets brighter. Restricted diffusion results in less spin dephasing and brighter signals; when diffusion is not restricted, spin dephasing with concomitant loss of signal results. In this way, diffusion weighted MRI (DWI) can be used for the early detection of acute strokes, ischemic lesions, and other brain and body abnormalities.

In order to accomplish diffusion weighted imaging, an attenuation factor, B is calculated and used to produce diffusion based MR signals. It can be expressed as $B = \exp(-bD)$ where b is a factor depending only on the gradient pulse sequence (gradient intensity and duration) and D is the diffusion coefficient (a function of the diffusing molecule and the liquid's viscosity and temperature). Clinically useful b-factor (diffusion weighted gradient factor) selections appear to be in the $500-1000 \, \text{s/mm}^2$ range.

Diffusion imaging suffers from extreme sensitivity to motion, particularly that related to involuntary patient macroscopic motion and pulsatile motion. The reason for this is that conventional imaging sequence gradients are usually only strong enough to compensate for small orders of flow sensitivity, not those that are associated with cardiac activity. Consequently, the shortest possible DWI sequences must be performed. Single-shot EPI sequences, although very fast (typically about 10 ms), suffer from limited in-plane resolution, low SNR, and a variety of artifacts other than motion. Multishot EPI, by acquiring several sets of data, provides much improved spatial resolution and reduced static magnetic field inhomogeneities. However, it suffers from reduced temporal resolution. Because acquisition time is increased over single-shot EPI methods, ECG gating often times is a necessity[11]. Both EPI versions require high maximum strength gradients with fast switching speed and rise time. Other diffusion sensitive pulse sequences, that do not particularly require extensive hardware upgrades, can be used to create DWI images. Sequences such as steady state free precession (SSFP) have less stringent hardware requirements but suffer from significant loss in SNR. Spin echo technology, with the ability to apply a strong gradient in one or more directions and with the use of ECG gating techniques, can provide diffusion weighted images with acceptable diagnostic value, at the cost of increased acquisition time.

Current applications for DWI include the early detection of stroke (where aggressive treatment options may be implemented for reversible tissue damage); edema; ischemia; cancer; cyst differentiation in the cases where high paramagnetic protein content may have T1 and T2 behavior like that of a solid tumor; and real-time temperature image creation for cancer treatment by hyperthermia[12]. Figure 8-17 shows an example.

Perfusion In the early 1990s, researchers, although acknowledging great hopes for dynamic contrast studies in the assessment of ischemic disease, pinpointed serious problems that had to be overcome. It had long been known that conventional MRI could not detect cerebral infarct until several hours after onset, when secondary signs such as edema were present. Perfusion imaging was based on the rapid bolus injection of contrast media that could be followed to identify potential areas of ischemia literally

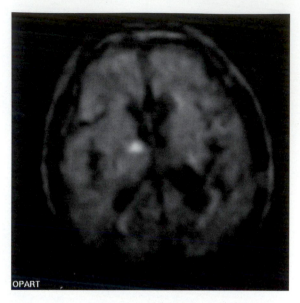

Figure 8-17. Diffusion weighted image using SE sequence. (Courtesy Toshiba America MRI, Inc.)

while the patient was present in the scanner. Early limitations included the need for rapid scan techniques to resolve bolus passage of contrast media; dispersion of the bolus unrelated to local anatomy (e.g., heart); variation in speed of bolus injection; and small signal variations. Additionally, contrast media enhancement from blood brain barrier (BBB) abnormalities could be mistaken for perfusion. Techniques that needed to be developed were those that would measure perfusion instead of blood volume; would enhance small perfusing signals; and would account for BBB variables.

Although similar to diffusion at the macroscopic or voxel level, perfusion can be thought of more as microcirculation of blood in the capillary network. If a typical voxel size is about 5 mm^3 ($1 \times 1 \times 5$ mm) it may contain several thousand capillary segments, so that the microcirculation can be described as intravoxel motion[13]. This poses a very different challenge since the diffusion phenomenon is much smaller.

In an attempt to assess cerebral perfusion without the use of contrast, several methods have been proposed. In general, they fall into two categories; continuous arterial spin labeling (CASL) and pulsed arterial spin labeling (PASL)[14]. In both, the approach is to tag the arterial spins outside of the imaging volume by either inversion or saturation. The tagged spins are then allowed to flow into the slice and the image is acquired. Using a control image without tagging, signal differences are calculated and an estimate of cerebral blood flow is made. CASL has higher SNR than PASL but is limited by arrival time delays and magnetization transfer effects. Because tagging is performed closer to the imaging slice in PASL, it appears to be better suited to the task.

An example of a PASL technique is known as FAIR or flow-sensitive alternating inversion recovery. In this technique, the imaging slice is inverted before each acquisition using a slice-selective inversion pulse. The inflowing spins are uninverted. The control image is acquired with a nonselective inversion pulse so that both the imaging slice and the inflowing spins are uninverted. Uninverted methods (UNFAIR) acquire a flow sensitive image following inversion of all spins outside the imaging volume and a control image without spin labeling. In this method the control image is independent of flow and need only be acquired once. Figure 8-18 is acquired without contrast media.

Magnetization Transfer Contrast

Magnetization transfer (MT) is a method by which tissue contrast can be manipulated such that the measurements are not solely dependent on T1, T2, and proton density. It is based on the premise that because protons in tissues exist in essentially two pools, the free pool and the bound pool, their magnetization can be transferred. By transferring magnetization from one pool to another, it is possible to design pulse sequences to produce substantial changes in tissue contrast. The most common use of this phenomenon is in the brain to visualize better

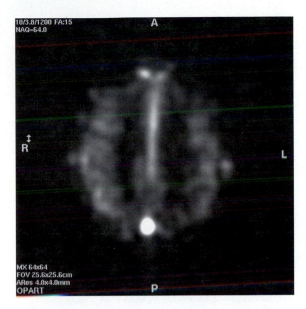

Figure 8-18. PWI using 2D FFE with TE 3.8 and adiabatic RF pulse for 180 inversion spin labeling on a normal volunteer, without the use of contrast. (Courtesy Toshiba America MRI, Inc.)

peripheral vasculature by improving the saturation of background tissue. However, its use in increasing conspicuity of lesions such as recurrent meningiomas and basic ganglia calcifications, has become more evident. The free proton pool is composed of mobile protons such as those found in water. The pool has a narrow spectral line and a long T2 and provides the bulk of MR detected signal. The bound pool contains protons bound in proteins and other large macromolecules and membranes. This pool has a wide spectral band and a short T2, thus its signal is not directly detected by conventional MR techniques.

Magnetization from the two pools can be transferred by dipole–dipole interactions between the spins or by transfer of nuclei by direct chemical means. Because of the difference between spectral lines of the two pools, it is possible to apply an off-resonance frequency to the bound pool to saturate its spins without affecting those in the free pool. The process can destroy bound pool longitudinal magnetization so that transfer to the free pool cannot occur. As a result, there is a reduction in signal intensity that is different for different tissues. This phenomenon can be used to create pulse sequences in which tissue contrast can be maximized.

Magnetization transfer saturation pulses can be applied to most conventional MR sequences. The specific sequence type will have an ultimate affect on how well tissue contrast can be manipulated. In conventional T1 weighted SE sequences with MT, lesion contrast can be either increased or decreased depending on lesion T1. For example, in the brain, T1 contrast changes markedly with fat appearing brighter, and gray matter of the central sulcus, putamen, caudate, periaquaductal area, and substantial nigra increasing in brightness. In IR sequences, such as STIR, the use of magnetization transfer may induce further reductions in tissue signal intensity or greater contrast. This may allow the use of a shorter TE that will decrease motion artifacts, a major barrier to IR sequence technology. In gradient echo sequences, MT can be used to increase endogenous contrast of the cervical spine, especially useful for evaluating degenerative diseases, where gradient echo sequences alone can be insensitive to intrinsic cord disease or may overestimate foraminal stenosis[15]. When using vascular imaging techniques such as time-of-flight (TOF), MT is useful for decreasing background tissue sufficiently to enhance peripheral blood vessel signal. This beneficial effect is the result of unsaturated blood moving into the imaging volume and the fact that the MT effect of blood is lower than that of brain parenchyma.

Other areas that show increased applications in the use of MT sequences are those in which short T1 lesions are seen in T1 weighted sequences, such as basal ganglia calcification, chronic hepatic encephalopathy, subacute hematoma, fatty lesions, and hemartomas. This is because the signal intensity of the lesion is usually equal to or greater than surrounding tissue, which can be effectively reduced by MT application.

MT can also be used synergistically with gadolinium chelates to improve lesion conspicuity. With T1 weighted spin echo sequences, T1 of the lesion is further decreased (if the blood–brain barrier has been crossed, there is already a decrease in lesion T1 from paramagnetic use so its signal intensity increases). Due to saturation effects of the bound pool, background tissue intensity is reduced. The effect may also be useful, with an additional benefit, when performing TOF MRA. Since gadolinium shortens intravascular T1 relaxation times, the sensitivity of blood to the saturation effects of normal RF pulse application is diminished. This results in an increase of the vessel-to-background contrast[16].

MT pulses when applied concomitant to contrast enhanced studies must be done so with caution, or in addition to a noncontrast comparison. In some cases, normally enhancing structures may appear much brighter than usual, confusing interpretation. Examples of such cases include the normally enhancing choroid plexus, pituitary, pineal, and dural sinuses as well as demyelinating lesions, which may appear to be enhancing when in fact it is only the MT effect[15].

This chapter has been devoted to giving the reader a more profound understanding of the sequence technology available for clinical use today. By knowing the general mechanism of sequence design and its intended use, the operator can employ knowledge gained to provide the radiologist and clinician with the most useful diagnostic tools available.

REFERENCES

1. Woodward PJ, Orrison WW Jr. *MRI Optimization: A Hands-On Approach.* New York: McGraw-Hill, 1997.
2. Porter BA. Short TI inversion recovery (STIR) imaging: a technical review and current uses. 1st Annual Magnetic Resonance Imaging for Technologists, 19–21 Feb. 1993, San Francisco, CA, pp. 41–45.
3. Williams SCR, Horsfield MA, Hall LD. True water and fat MR imaging with use of multiple-echo acquisition. *Radiology* 173:249–253, 1989.
4. Young IA. In: Stark DD, Bradley Jr WG, eds. *Magnetic Resonance Imaging.* St Louis: CV Mosby, 1988.

5. Zhang W, Goldhaber DM, Kramer DM, Kaufman L. Separation of water and fat images at 0.35 Tesla using the three-point Dixon method with "sandwich" echoes. *SMR Abstracts*, 656, 1995.
6. Miyazaki M, Takai H, Tokunaga Y, Hoshino T, Hanawa M. A polarity altered spectral and spatial selective acquisition technique. *SMR Abstracts*, 657, 1995.
7. Miyazaki M, Kojima F, Igarashi H. Uniform fat suppression in multislice imaging: a multislice off-resonance fat suppression technique (MSOFT). *SMR Abstracts*, 796, 1994.
8. Kanazawa H, Takai H, Machida Y, Hanawa M. Contrast naturalization of fast spin echo imaging: a fat reduction technique free from field inhomogeneity. *SMR Abstracts*, 494, 1994.
9. Butts K, Pauly JM, Glover GH, Pelc NH. Dual echo "DIET" fast spin echo imaging. *SMR Abstracts*, 651, 1995.
10. Kassai Y. FastASE and its clinical applications. *Toshiba Medical Review*, No. 64, May 1998.
11. Mitsuoka H, Makita J. Diffusion-weighted imaging using multi-shot EPI. *Toshiba Medical Review*, No. 64, May 1998.
12. Bihan DL, Delannoy J, Levin RL. Temperature mapping with MR imaging of molecular diffusion: application to hyperthermia. *Therap. Radiol.* 171:853–857, 1989.
13. Bihan DL. Magnetic resonance imaging of perfusion. *Magn. Reson. Med.* 14:283–292, 1990.
14. Tanabe JL, Yongbi M, Branch C, Hrabe J, Johnson G, Helpern JA. MR perfusion imaging in human brain using the unfair technique. *J. Magn. Reson. Imag.* 9:761–767, 1999.
15. Van Buche M. Magnetization transfer: clinical applications in neuroradiology. In *Multiple Perspectives in MRI Contrast*. Bracco Education Forums, 1997.
16. Elster AD, King JC, Mathews VP, Hamilton CA. Cranial tissues: appearance at gadolinium-enhanced and nonenhanced MR imaging with magnetization transfer contrast. *Radiology* 190:541–546, 1994.

CHAPTER 9

MR Angiographic Imaging

Ralph E. Lee

INTRODUCTION

The use of magnetic resonance angiography (MRA) has become a routine part of diagnostic magnetic resonance imaging (MRI). The widespread clinical acceptance of MRA has brought with it, however, an ever expanding array of specialized MRA sequences, techniques, and protocols. MR angiographers today are faced with a wide variety of "new-and-improved" MRA acquisition protocols; and the number and variety of these "must-have" imaging options seems to grow alarmingly with each new software release. Fortunately, however, most of these "new" techniques can be easily recognized as simple variations (and/or improvements) of a manageably small number of basic MRA imaging approaches[1–7]. And most of these basic MRA imaging concepts can themselves be recognized as simple modifications of routine MRI concepts with which most technologists are already familiar.

The term "MRA" can be applied to almost any MRI scan that is specifically designed to differentiate between flowing spins and stationary spins[8]. Almost any image that yields a minimum level of tissue contrast between blood (moving spins) and non-moving background tissue (stationary spins) can be considered an MRA image. Five of these specialized imaging approaches will be discussed here.

How Do We Image Blood Vessels?

In routine MRI imaging (such as the routine imaging of the gray/white matter of the brain) there are two major mechanisms of tissue differentiation, T1 and T2[5,6,9–11]. In MR angiography too there are two major approaches that have achieved widespread clinical acceptance: the time-of-flight (TOF) approach; and the phase-contrast (PC) approach[12]. One of these approaches, TOF, is dependent on T1 contrast mechanisms, and the second approach, PC, emphasizes T2 tissue differences. In addition to these two main techniques (and their 2D and 3D variations) we will be discussing two techniques (dark-blood and magnitude-contrast) that are used as adjuncts to TOF and PC; and a fifth technique, gadolinium contrast-enhanced (CE) MRA, which has the potential to propel body MRA into the clinical mainstream once and for all[13–16].

A familiarity with the benefits and limitations of each of these MRA sequence types can prove extremely helpful to the clinical MRI practitioner. This is especially true when it is necessary to decide on a specific clinical protocol (series of MRA acquisitions) that will best address an individual patient's needs. MRA is an interactive technology. It begins with a review of the patient's history (as related to the blood flow velocity and flow characteristics of anticipated pathology), continues with the selection of the appropriate imaging sequence, and finishes with appropriate image processing and filming[17,18,19].

It is not unusual for a vessel to appear differently on an MRA image from how it does on a conventional angiogram[20]. In X-ray angiography (XRA) a catheter is introduced into a specific vessel and a contrast agent is injected into that vessel under pressure. As it flows downstream the contrast agent displaces the blood within the vessel [Figure 9-1]. This "blood displacement" makes imaging of the vessel lumen possible no matter what the natural flow dynamics of the vessel may be. This is not the case with MRA[21–24].

MRA is a physiologic record of blood flow. If there is no blood flow, no blood vessels will be seen. And if there is a disturbance in the pattern of blood flow, as is common at a stenotic site, the resulting "turbulence" may be recorded as an area where the vascular signal is reduced or even lost. XRA produces images that are an anatomical map of the vessel lumen. MRA does not. In MRA we do not depict the vessel lumen at all. We

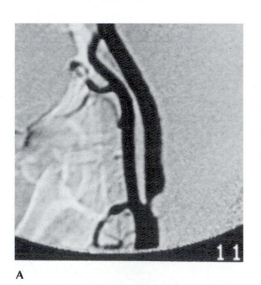

A

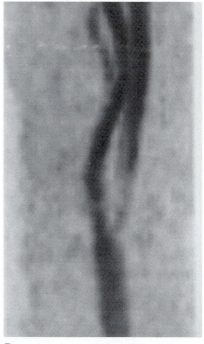

B

Figure 9-1.   A An X-ray angiogram (DSA) of a patient's carotid bifurcation shows a substantial narrowing at the origin of the internal carotid artery. **B** An MRA MIP image shows a similar narrowing in a much more exaggerated way. It could be argued that this apparent hypersensitivity to pathology makes MRA an ideal screening tool.

record the movement of the blood that flows within that vessel.

Dark-Blood "Flow-Void" MRA

Dark-blood (DB) MRA is a perfect example of the paradox that exists between conventional X-ray angiography (XRA) and MRA. In the dark-blood technique, also known as the flow-void technique, blood is not actually imaged at all. In DB MRA the presence of flowing blood is inferred when the images do not show any MR signal at all in the area of blood vessels. DB MRA, in its most often used form, is a spin-echo (SE) based technique. Therefore, one of its strengths is that DB images can be acquired on a wide array of MR magnet types and field strengths. DB MRA takes advantage of the fact that a spin-echo is only produced when the tissue being imaged experiences *both* a 90-degree excitation pulse, *and* a subsequent 180-degree refocusing pulse. If tissue experiences a 90-degree pulse, but never has the phase coherence of its spins brought back into focus by a subsequent 180-degree pulse, no echo is produced. The result is an area of the MRI image that is completely absent of signal. This signal loss is called a "flow void" [Figure 9-2].

Tissue must experience both the 90- and 180-degree pulses within the same slice location in order to elicit signal. This is because the radio-frequency (RF) pulses used to set up the echo phenomena are slice-selective. Consequently, tissue must remain within the same slice location long enough to experience both the 90- and 180-degree pulses; so, if a moving bolus of blood is physically located within slice number one when it experiences the 90- but has flowed into slice position three when the 180-pulse is given, then the blood will give off no signal. The vessel appears black in contrast to the surrounding tissue that (because it is not moving) retains its normal, brighter, signal intensity. Since non-moving (static) tissue retains its normal signal characteristics, DB MRA images are often

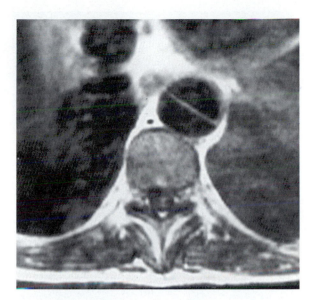

Figure 9-2. Dark flow voids are seen on this axial spin-echo (gated TE 27 ms) on either side of a dissection flap (thin white line crossing the vessel) in this patient's descending thoracic aorta.

capable of visualizing both the vessel lumen *and* the muscular walls of the blood vessel. This means that a DB imaging approach can often be used to directly visualize clot or plaque within the walls of a blood vessel.

BACKGROUND SUPPRESSION TECHNIQUES

As previously mentioned, there are two major approaches to "bright-blood" MR angiographic image acquisition. The first of these techniques, time-of-flight (TOF) MRA, falls into the general category of a background suppression technique. Background suppression techniques (for the purposes of this chapter) are those techniques that seek to minimize the signal intensity of static background structures (minimize the background intensity as opposed to mathematically subtracting it out of the image completely). Blood, a "bright" flow-enhanced signal, is seen

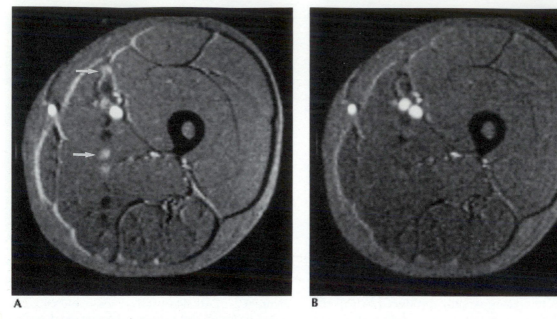

A   B

Figure 9-3. Axial image of arteries and veins of a subject's leg. **A** Note the phase mismapping of arterial signal (arrows) in this image without flow compensation. **B** The arterial signal is more accurately mapped within the vessel walls on this flow-compensated image of the same subject.

against the darker background of stationary material. Background suppression techniques do not attempt to remove all of the signal from non-moving tissues, they simply seek to minimize it to the point where the background does not obscure the greater brightness of the blood vessels [Figure 9-3].

Time-of-Flight MRA

Time-of-flight (TOF) techniques currently form the backbone of diagnostic MRA. In TOF MRA, the imaging volume is pulsed so rapidly that only a small portion of the tissue's longitudinal magnetization can be regained between excitations. Since only that portion of a tissue's T1 signal that has been recovered between pulses is capable of giving off signal with subsequent pulses, the result of this rapid pulsing is an overall loss of signal intensity within the imaging volume [Figure 9-4]. The phenomenon responsible for this loss of signal is known as saturation[12,25–27].

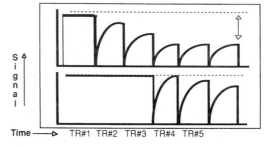

Figure 9-4. Graphic depiction of time-of-flight; the upper line depicts stationary background signal and the lower line represents blood flowing into the volume with a large proportion of its longitudinal signal still intact.

Muscles, cartilage, and other tissues that remain within the imaging volume (long enough to experience multiple RF pulses) quickly become saturated and thereby lose most of their signal intensity. Rapidly moving blood flowing into the volume, by virtue of having spent a portion of the total imaging time outside the excitation volume, experiences fewer "signal dampening" RF pulses. Therefore, the MR signal intensity of blood remains high as it enters and moves rapidly through the imaging volume. Stationary tissue (background tissue remaining within the volume for an extended time) gives up most of its signal. Blood retains most of its longitudinal T1 signal. Therefore blood appears bright against a background of lower signal stationary background structures[19,28–39]. It is the reliance of this approach on magnetic spins, flowing "over time" into an otherwise stationary volume, that gives rise to the term time-of-flight MRA.

3D Time-of-Flight MRA

3D time-of-flight (3D TOF) MRA sequences offer the angiographer a practical approach to the rapid acquisition of high resolution images. The approach is particularly useful for imaging anatomic structures that exhibit a rapid blood flow velocity; and they are especially useful when that blood flow is complex and multi-directional. A perfect example of this type of vascular anatomy is the circle of Willis of the intracranial arterial circulation [Figure 9-5]. Intracranial MRA is, at the time of this writing, far and away the most often requested type of MRA examination in routine clinical practice. Therefore, 3D TOF is arguably the most often used type of MRA imaging sequence[12,40,41].

3D TOF MRA is a volume acquisition approach. The imaging sequences are designed to excite a thick 3D volume (3–6 cm) and then subdivide that large volume into a number of individual partitions of approximately 1 mm each. The 3D approach offers the angiographer a substantial increase in image resolution, compared with 2D MRA techniques. This increase in resolution results from the fact that

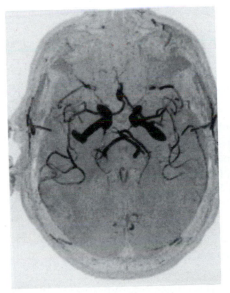

A

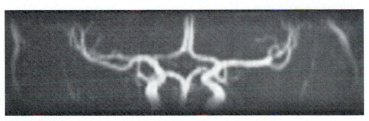

B

Figure 9-5. **A** 3D TOF axial of the cranial arteries in the area of the circle of Willis. **B** Coronal projection from an axial 3D TOF (a single 5 cm thick slab) acquisition. Notice how the slab has been positioned so that blood enters just proximal to the circle of Willis. This positioning is critical to prevent loss of vascular signal (and loss of sensitivity for small basilar-tip and berry aneurisms) due to saturation effects. If a greater area of coverage is required (i.e., the entire basilar artery), a 3D multi-slab acquisition might be a better choice than the single-slab "COW screening" scan shown here.

all 3D sequences offer a substantial increase in signal-to-noise ratio, when compared with 2D imaging techniques. The use of a 3D approach causes signal-to-noise ratio (SNR) to increase proportional to the square root of the number of partitions into which the 3D volume is divided. For example, a 1 mm partition acquired as 1/64th part of a 64 mm 3D volume, will have 8 times the SNR of an otherwise identical 1 mm slice acquired with a 2D imaging approach. This substantial increase in SNR can be utilized, in the case of 3D MRA, to support high resolution imaging (i.e., small voxel sizes on the order of $0.75 \, mm^3$ or less). 3D TOF is, however, not a perfect technique.

3D TOF is a good technique selection, for instance, for the imaging of rapidly moving blood, such as that in the carotid arteries or the intracranial vessels. But 3D TOF would not be a good selection for imaging of the slow moving veins in the same anatomic areas[12]. It is a good selection in the case of rapid flow because the large size (thickness) of the 3D imaging volume requires that blood be moving fairly rapidly in order for it to pass through the volume quickly. Rapid flow is a must because if blood stays in the volume too long it will loose its bright signal[19,28]. Loss of vascular enhancement (in the case of slow moving blood) is the result of the same saturation effects that reduce the signal of non-moving background tissues. 3D TOF is, therefore, not a good choice for imaging slow moving blood flow in structures such as veins or low-velocity arteries such as those in the legs. Furthermore, 3D TOF is not likely to succeed in a situation where rapidly flowing arterial blood is destined to remain within the imaging volume "too long" (e.g., a long axis sagittal acquisition of a carotid artery) [Figure 9-6]. If blood stays within the imaging volume as long as one might expect stationary tissue to stay in the imaging volume (a period of several times TR), blood too will take on the signal characteristics of stationary tissue and it too will become saturated [Figures 9-7 and 9-8].

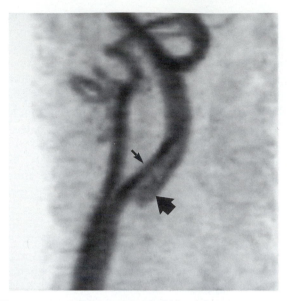

Figure 9-6. MRA is a record of blood flow, so any disturbance in flow will be recorded in the image. Note the area of faster blood flow (small arrow) and slower flow (large arrow) in this 3D TOF image of a patient's carotid artery.

2D Sequential Time-of-Flight MRA

Premature loss of vascular enhancement, due to saturation effects, can be a concern when using 3D TOF techniques. Another variation on the TOF technique is the 2D sequential time-of-flight (2D TOF) approach. This approach is far less susceptible to vascular saturation effects. This technique acquires a set of thin 2D slices (often 50–80) one after the other in a "sequential" series (i.e., acquiring lines 1 through 256 of one slice before moving on to line 1 of the next slice)[40]. Most routine 2D imaging approaches (e.g., those techniques one might select for 2D imaging of an abdomen or a knee, etc.) acquire raw data line one of slice one first. Then they acquire line one of slice two followed by line one slice three and so on. This means that each slice in the imaging volume is exposed to RF excitation many times throughout the image

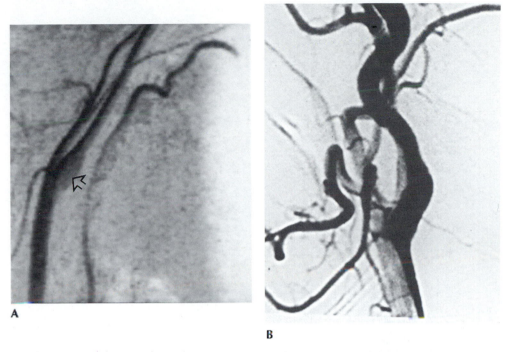

Figure 9-7. **A** An area of decreased signal (arrow) is commonly seen in the carotid bulb of normal volunteers. **B** Similar area of slow wash-out of X-ray angiographic contrast material is also seen in this post-injection DSA image of a different patient's normal carotid bulb.

acquisition. Repeated RF excitation of each slice is counter productive in the case of 2D MRA.

The use of a sequential acquisition approach is critical to successful 2D TOF MRA [Figure 9-9]. This approach ensures that the vascular signal within any one slice has not been saturated (or partially saturated) by having first experienced multiple RF excitations as the blood flows through any proximal slice[19]. Since blood passing through a 2D slice, assuming the MRA slices are positioned perpendicular to the flow of blood, only needs to traverse a single thin 2 or 3 mm slice, there is little chance that blood will remain in the slice long enough to become saturated[29,33,42]. Therefore, 2D sequential TOF (unlike 3D TOF) can visualize slowly flowing venous blood as well as fast-flowing arterial blood [Figure 9-10].

Although 2D TOF has the ability to image both rapidly moving and slowly moving blood, the technique suffers from low resolution in the slice direction. Consequently, when a 2D acquisition is projected from the side (i.e., when viewing an axial acquisition reformatted into a sagittal MIP) the resulting images can appear a bit coarse. Additionally, there are other technical factors to be considered when choosing between a 2D TOF and a 3D TOF acquisition. 2D TOF MRA has a tendency to exhibit a larger area of signal loss following a stenosis (exaggerated signal loss in the presence of turbulence) [Figure 9-11]. This increase in apparent severity of pathology is the combined result of 2D TOF's requirements for comparatively longer minimum TE times, stronger slice encoding gradients, and larger voxel sizes that result from relatively thick 2 or 3 mm slices.

Again, however, there is a trade-off to be considered when deciding between 2D and 3D TOF. 2D TOF has the ability to rapidly image

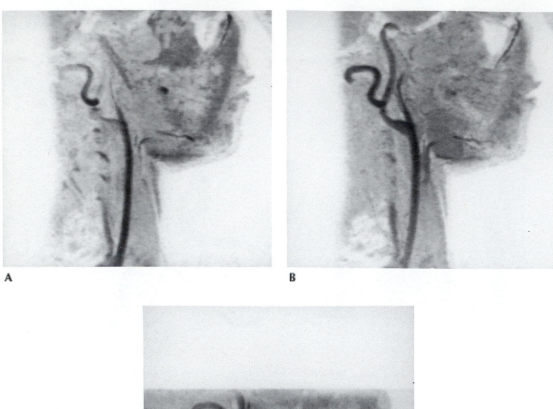

A

B

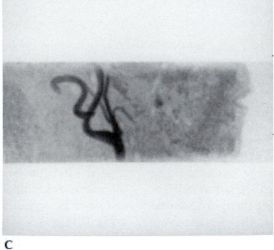

C

Figure 9-8. **A** Saturation of vascular signal is seen to occur quite rapidly on this short TR sagittal 3D TOF image. **B** Less saturation of vascular signal is seen on this long TR sagittal 3D TOF image of the same subject. **C** Maximum vascular signal is seen on this intermediate TR axial 3D TOF image of the same subject.

large areas of vascular anatomy. 2D can successfully image much larger areas of anatomy than 3D TOF can (i.e., a single 3D TOF axial slab at the level of the carotid bifurcation might cover 6 cm of anatomy, however, a series of 80 axial 2D TOF slices might provide a gross screening of 12 cm of the neck vessels in about the same acquisition time). This is the result of 2D TOF's use of the sequential acquisition approach. Since each 2D TOF slice is basically a complete scan in itself, vascular saturation effects are rarely a problem[12,41] [Figures 9-12 and 9-13].

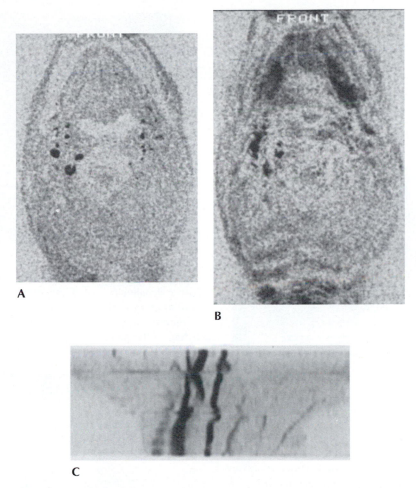

Figure 9-9. **A** This single 2D TOF image shows good vascular signal in the patient's right external, internal, and vertebral arteries. No vessels are seen on the patient's left side due to total occlusion. **B** An adjacent slice is degraded by gross patient movement. **C** A sag. MIP image shows horizontal misregistration artifacts resulting from the patient's intermittent movement during the acquisition.

The larger the number of slices one acquires, the larger the anatomic area of interest that can be covered (albeit with a doubling of imaging time with each doubling of the number of slices to be acquired). This ability of the 2D approach to image large areas is one of the principal strengths of the technique; and it is this ability that makes 2D TOF the second most often used type of MRA acquisition approach. To recap, 2D TOF can screen large areas of anatomy but

suffers from low resolution; 3D TOF provides high resolution imaging of vessels but tends to suffer from a rapid loss of vascular signal.

3D Sequential Multislab Time-of-Flight MRA

Two major advantages of the 3D TOF approach are its ability to acquire high resolution images, and its tendency not to exaggerate the apparent

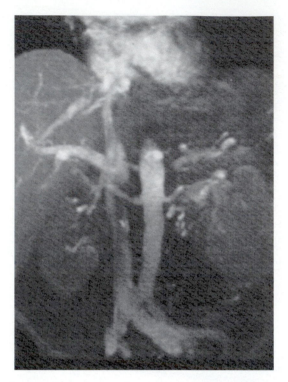

Figure 9-10. A coronal MIP image produced from a series of abdominal breath-hold 2D TOF coronal images shows both arteries and veins.

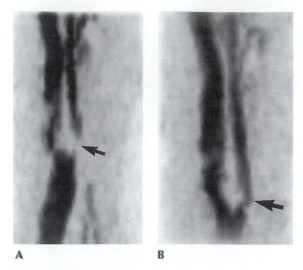

A   B

Figure 9-11. **A** This 2D TOF image shows a complete loss of signal following an area of plaque in the external carotid artery of the patient. **B** A 3D TOF acquisition of the same patient more accurately depicts the true extent of the patient's disease.

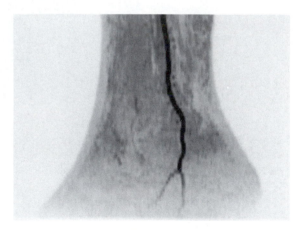

Figure 9-12 This 2D TOF axial acquisition has been projected into the sagittal plane and shows good vessel contrast even in the slowly flowing arteries of this subject's foot.

severity of stenoses[43]. Two of the major advantages of the 2D TOF approach are its ability to successfully image (without suffering from saturation of vascular flow) large areas of anatomy, and its ability to image blood moving more slowly than thick 3D TOF slabs are capable of imaging[19,43,44]. The 3D multislab approach (3D MS) incorporates the good features of both 2D and 3D TOF MRA. In its original form multiple "thick" slabs were acquired [Figure 9-14]. This approach failed to reach widespread clinical acceptance [Figure 9-15]. It was not until the multislab concept was modified to feature a series of "thin" 3D slabs acquired in a sequential fashion (like 2D TOF) that the technique became a truly practical one. Another name for 3D MS is multiple-overlapping-thin-slab-acquisition or "MOTSA."

In the 3D MS approach several "thin" overlapping 3D slabs (often 16 to 32 partitions of 1 mm each) are acquired in a sequential fashion; and then the best (center) slices from all of the slabs are combined into one composite

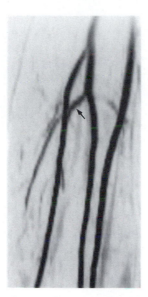

Figure 9-13. This 2D TOF axial acquisition has been projected into the coronal plane and shows areas of decreased image resolution (arrows) as vessels traverse the volume in a diagonal direction.

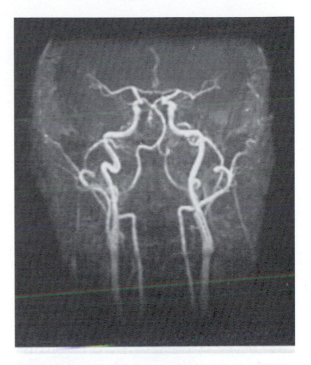

Figure 9-14. An early (January 1990) coronal MIP image derived from three thick (approximately 6 cm each) coronal 3D TOF images. (Courtesy Charles Anderson, David Saloner, and Ralph E. Lee, UCSF School of Medicine, VA Medical Center Campus)

data set for MIP processing. As with the 2D sequential approach, the operator can selectively acquire as many or as few slabs as may be needed in order to cover the area of anatomy required (and scan time requirements will vary directly with the number of slabs to be acquired). Many of the exquisite MRA images seen in publications and product brochures have been acquired using this technique. It is, however, important to remember that many patients will find it difficult to keep still for the extended periods required to acquire excessively large areas of anatomy [Figure 9-16].

3D sequential multislab is similar to 2D sequential in that it combines multiple thin sections, in this case thin 3D slabs, in order to take advantage of the fact that thin excitation volumes are less likely to suffer from saturation of vascular signal. 3D multislab combines the high spatial resolution (and short TEs) of 3D TOF with larger areas of anatomic coverage. 3D MS, by successfully combining the best attributes of

the TOF approach, has achieved a good degree of clinical acceptance[12,40,41].

Gadolinium Contrast Enhanced 3D MR Aortography

Contrast enhanced 3D MRA (CE) is a recent addition to the body MRA arsenal[45]. 2D TOF techniques can image abdominal vessels. However, attempts to adequately image large areas of vascular anatomy (i.e., all of the major vessels of the abdomen) can prove problematic at best. CE MRA protocols are beginning to be used clinically with increasing frequency in the assessment of a wide range of aortic (large vessel) disorders. And now that breath-hold 3D CE MRA capabilities are commercially available, this technique has the potential to assure abdominal MRA

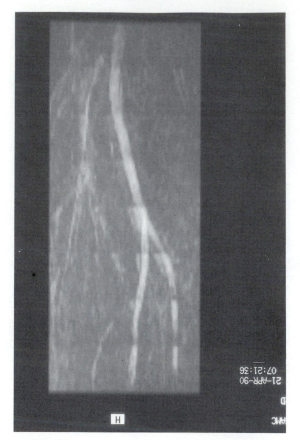

Figure 9-15.   An early example (April 1990) of a thin slab 3D sequential acquisition of the arteries of a subject's leg. Note the areas of signal loss that have resulted from inadequate overlap of 3D slabs (arrow). (Courtesy Charles Anderson, David Saloner, and Ralph E. Lee, UCSF School of Medicine, VA Medical Center Campus)

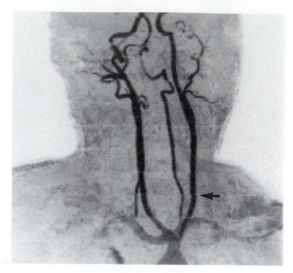

Figure 9-16.   This 3D sequential "show image" (excessively long acquisition time) covers so large an area of anatomy that the patient is seen to have moved slightly (arrow) between consecutive slab acquisitions.

a key position within the clinical mainstream[46]. This technique has been used successfully for rapid assessment (25 s 3D breath-holds) of aortic dissection, aortic arch, and subclavian artery stenosis, stenosis of the proximal renal arteries, and to evaluate AAA (abdominal aortic aneurysms).

The contrast mechanism of gadolinium-enhanced 3D MRA is based on bright (T1 shortened) blood, in contrast to dark (normal T1) stationary tissue. The "darkness" of stationary background tissues is the result of T1 saturation effects (as discussed in the TOF section of this chapter). Bright vascular signal is the result of the T1 shortening of blood signal in the presence of a high dose of (rapidly administered) gadolinium contrast agent [Figure 9-17].

When gadolinium-enhanced blood is timed to pass through a standard 3D volume acquisition during acquisition of the center 20% of raw data (k-space), the brightness of the blood will dominate the image. This contrast domination results from the fact that the center 20% of k-space is responsible for over 90% (in a 256 matrix acquisition) of an image's contrast. That is to say, that when only the center 20% of raw data is used (under experimental conditions) to form an image, that image can be readily identified as a T1 or a T2 image. The remaining data provides most of the edge-definition capabilities of the image.

the scan) must be completed during the "arterial bolus" phase of contrast enhancement.

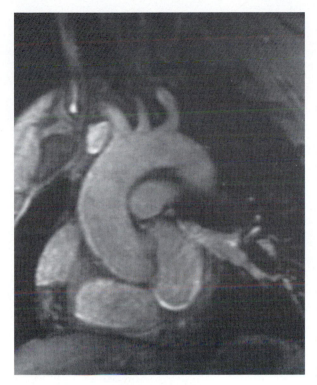

Figure 9-17. A single image (not an MIP image) acquired in a paracoronal "candy cane" projection, showing excellent detail in the area of the origins of the major aortic vessels. Note that much of the interpretation of body MRA is done from individual slices, with MIP images providing only an overview of gross vascular anatomy.

Injection/acquisition timing is a critical factor in CE MRA technique. Images must be acquired with appropriate timing in order to ensure maximum vessel/background contrast; and because of the fact that images that are acquired too long after contrast injection have a tendency to suffer from a confusing overlap of arteries and veins. This is true because blood (e.g., contrast enhanced blood) cycles out of the "bolus" arterial phase and into an equilibrium phase, within both the arteries and the veins, within about 2 min. Therefore, in order for a 3D CE aortogram to be successful, the entire scan (or at least the center 20% of *k*-space portion of

BACKGROUND SUBTRACTION TECHNIQUES

Background Subtraction Techniques: A Historical Perspective

Once upon a time (more than 25 years ago when this author began his angiographic career) unwanted structures were removed from conventional contrast X-ray angiographic images (XRA) through optical/film subtraction techniques. In order to do an optical (film–film) subtraction two films were required. A precontrast "mask" X-ray was made with everything identical to that which will be used in the angiographic run. Immediately following acquisition of this mask image the iodine contrast was injected and the contrast enhanced angiographic XRA images were acquired.

The result of this two-step procedure was two nearly identical images. One image, the "mask," showed the patient's non-vascular anatomy (e.g., the pelvic bones). The second image showed all of the patient's non-vascular anatomy as well as a superimposition of contrast-enhanced blood vessels.

The mask image was then taken into the darkroom and optically reversed (copied onto a reversal film that changed the original X-ray "negative" film into an identical "positive" film). This reversal mask image was then sandwiched together with the unaltered contrast enhanced XRA image and a copy film was then made of this "film sandwich." For each "white" area of bone on the contrast enhanced XRA image there now exists (in the "film sandwich") an identical "black" area on the reversal mask. Consequently, when a light was projected through the "film sandwich" (a copy film) all of the light that would have come through the white (bone) areas was now blocked by an identical black area on the reversal mask. The bones were, in effect, subtracted out of the resulting image leaving only the vessels to be printed on the final copy film.

Background Subtraction Techniques

The "subtraction" concept is critical to an understanding of the two topics that follow, magnitude-contrast and phase-contrast MRA. Optical (film based) subtraction techniques are largely a thing of the past. The concept is presented here (above) in order to emphasize the point that many basic elements of MRA are simply modifications of processes with which many technologists have already become familiar. Contemporary image subtraction is, for the most part, accomplished through computer-based techniques. Optical subtraction's more contemporary "computer based" counterpart is digital subtraction angiography (DSA) [Figure 9-18]. In DSA a digital mask image is mathematically subtracted from an otherwise identical contrast enhanced XRA image and the result is a digital subtraction image. Like its optical counterpart, this DSA image does not suffer from a confusing overlap of anatomic structures (like bones) because all unwanted anatomy has been subtracted.

In DSA the digital pixel values of a pair of images are subtracted. That is to say, the signal intensity of a pixel on image one (e.g., an intensity of 100 on the mask image) is subtracted from the signal intensity of the same pixel location on image two (e.g., 100 on the angiographic image). If there is no blood vessel located at that pixel location the signal intensities should mathematically cancel each other out completely. If there is a blood vessel in that location the pixel should be brighter (e.g., 300) on the angiographic image than it was on the mask. There should, therefore, be a residual signal in the area of the blood vessel when the two numbers are subtracted.

Background subtraction MRA techniques also seek to minimize background signal through mathematical (digital) means. Background subtraction techniques attempt to mathematically "subtract" unwanted structures from the image in much the same way as DSA. This means that background subtraction techniques are less likely to suffer from the same level of premature saturation of vascular signal. This lack of signal loss is not so much the result of "less" loss of vascular signal, as it is the result of a "more" efficient approach to the removal of competing background signal. In order to be seen (e.g., on a MIP image) the signal intensity of the vessel must be greater than the signal intensity of the background. If the background signal has been effectively reduced to zero, a vessel need only exhibit a tiny bit of flow enhancement in order to appear as "bright" on a MIP image.

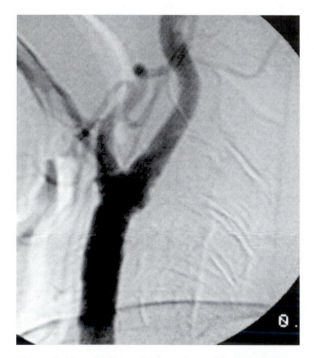

Figure 9-18. An X-ray DSA angiographic image of a patient's carotid bifurcation shows the vessels (full of X/R contrast media) and subtle impressions of the vertebral bodies (as a result of slight movement between the acquisition of the digital mask image and the acquisition of the matching contrasted image).

Magnitude-contrast MRA

The magnitude-contrast (MC) approach to MR angiographic imaging is an older less sophisticated technique than the other background subtraction techniques (phase-contrast) that we will be discussing in this chapter[34,47-51]. Its clinical usefulness is, therefore, somewhat limited. Magnitude-contrast is however, because of its relatively straightforward conceptual basis, an ideal teaching tool for the introduction of the background subtraction approach[41].

Magnitude-contrast (MC) sequences approach removal of background signal in a fundamentally different way from time-of-flight (TOF) techniques. In TOF the background signal is still there, it is simply suppressed to a point at which the signal from flowing blood appears bright in comparison. In MC, also known as rephase-minus-dephase (RD), a "mask" image (flow dephased: a dark-blood type "flow-void" in the area of blood vessels) is matched with a second "flow" image (flow rephased: image with bright GMR "flow compensated" blood signal in the area of blood vessels). The two images are mathematically subtracted in a process not unlike digital subtraction angiography [Figure 9-19].

If we assume that the stationary background signal remains constant during the acquisition of both images, then a subtraction of the two images should result in total removal of background signal. Blood vessels, however, should experience the subtraction of zero signal intensity (dephased: flow-void) from a bright signal intensity (rephased: bright blood signal) resulting in a high signal remainder within the vessels. The resulting subtraction images can then be combined through the use of a standard maximum-intensity-projection (MIP) algorithm.

In TOF MRA background objects are suppressed, not actually subtracted. This means that, in a few limited circumstances, objects that exhibit unusually short T1 values may fail to become effectively saturated (i.e., methemoglobin and gadolinium contrast). If these objects remain bright they could be mistaken for areas of flow enhancement (blood vessels) [Figure 9-20]. Background subtraction sequences do not suffer from this potential artifact because they remove all "non-moving" structures.

Background subtraction MRA approaches (MC and PC) have two characteristics that the technologist must keep in mind when selecting between them and a TOF acquisition: first, background subtraction techniques have the benefit of being able to image blood moving at a slower velocity than 3D TOF [Figure 9-21]; and second, background subtraction techniques have the limitation of minimum TE times that are substantially longer than 3D TOF acquisitions[8]. Background subtraction techniques, therefore, exhibit an increased area of turbulent

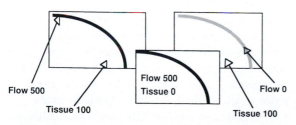

Figure 9-19. This is a graphic depiction of the RD background subtraction technique. Note that the background signal from nonmoving objects should remain constant and therefore be completely subtracted out of subsequent MIP images.

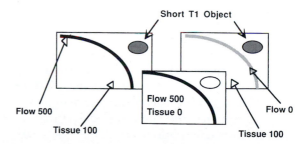

Figure 9-20. Even materials with extremely short T1 characteristics (background objects that often remain bright on TOF images) are efficiently subtracted out of subsequent MIP images by MC sequences. Other background subtraction techniques, such as PC, also provide the MR angiographer with this capability.

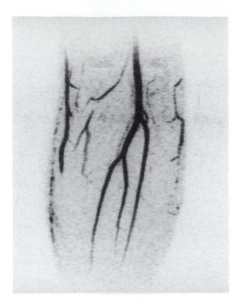

Figure 9-21   As seen in this coronal MC acquisition of a patient's leg, this type of sequence is often capable of imaging blood flow that is too slow for a 3D TOF acquisition.

signal dropout (loss of vascular signal) following a stenosis. MC's (and PC's) longer TE times result in a noticeable increase (as compared to 3D TOF) in the apparent severity of vascular stenoses.

Phase Contrast MRA

Phase contrast (PC) MRA does not attempt to achieve vascular/background contrast through manipulation of longitudinal signal characteristics like time-of-flight (TOF) MRA[52]. PC MRA approaches the problem of image contrast in a fundamentally different way from either TOF or MC MRA[52]. PC MRA sequences are designed to be sensitive to the inherent differences in transverse magnetization (rates of T2 phase dispersion) that occur between stationary and moving tissues[53–59]. PC MRA sequences seek to quantify those spins experiencing a velocity induced phase shift, and to present those "flowing" spins in contrast to stationary background tissues.

The amount of phase shift, in the presence of a flow encoding gradient, is directly dependent on the local strength of the gradient and the velocity at which the spin is moving[60]. Spins situated at different locations along a gradient experience different levels of gradient strength. In the case of phase contrast MRA, a pair of flow encoding gradients are utilized (producing a pair of images for subtraction). These flow encoding gradients render the acquisition sensitive to flow occurring along the plane of the gradient. Each pair of flow encoding gradients is sensitive to flow only in one plane of sensitivity. For example, a flow encoding gradient set might be sensitive to right/left or left/right flow but not flow occurring in the up/down direction. Consequently, sequences must utilize multiple pairs of flow encoding gradients in order to visualize multidirectional (complex) areas of vascular anatomy. Therefore, because scan time is increased each time an additional flow encoding gradient is applied, 3D PC acquisitions will always take longer to acquire than similar 3D TOF acquisitions.

In the original 3D PC approach, multiple pairs of flow encoded images were acquired during one image acquisition (three sets of gradients, one for each of the three orthogonal directions of blood flow). For each of the three directions a pair of two "raw-data" images were acquired. One of the images in the pair would have a flow encoding gradient in a positive direction, and the second "mirror image" would have this gradient reversed into the negative direction. The image data from one of these paired images would be subtracted from its mirrored mate and a subtraction image would result. In order to achieve sensitivity to flow in all three directions (as is mandatory for MRA of the intracranial vessels) each scan would need to employ three flow sensitive gradient pairs (six raw-data image sets), which would take substantially longer than a 3D TOF volume to acquire. It should be noted, however, that current 3D PC imaging schemes are much more efficient than the original six-image system (now requiring only the acquisition of three flow images and one magnitude image). Consequently, current applications of 3D PC only require two to three times as long to acquire a volume with multi-directional flow sensitivity.

Imaging time requirements aside, the 3D PC MRA approach can (under certain circumstances) succeed in situations where 3D TOF is less likely to provide adequate images[12,41]. For instance, flow encoding gradients have no effect on stationary objects. Moving spins, however, will show a residual signal when the pair of flow encoded raw-data images is subtracted. Therefore *only* blood vessels will show on the subtraction images [Figure 9-22]. This is not always the case with 3D TOF MRA images.

There are a couple of instances where a non-flowing object can artificially exhibit a bright, seemingly flow enhanced, signal intensity on a 3D TOF image. Most common among these artifactual situations is the case where a "non-moving" gadolinium-enhanced mass (i.e., a tumor) can appear as a "bright" object on a 3D TOF MIP image [Figure 9-23]. This phenomenon can occur as the result of the extreme T1 shortening of tumor tissue. Contrast-induced T1 shortening can cause non-moving tissue to regain more of its longitudinal signal (in a given TR) than non-enhanced background tissue; and this tissue will, therefore, appear brighter than adjacent tissue despite the fact that it is in no way "flow-enhanced."

Because phase contrast techniques "subtract" unwanted background structures as opposed to simply "suppressing" their signal intensity (as is the case with TOF MRA techniques) they do not suffer from artifactual enhancement of MRI contrast-enhanced structures[60]. Consequently, even non-moving objects with artifactually short T1 relaxation times (like contrast-enhanced tumors and methemoglobin-containing blood clots) are effectively removed before the final MIP images are created.

Phase contrast sequences (both 2D PC and 3D PC) offer the ability to acquire MRA images both before *and* after the injection of gadolinium MRI contrast. This is not the case with either 2D or 3D TOF sequences, which suffer from a confusing overlapping of arteries and veins after contrast injection (gadolinium renders most vascular saturation bands ineffective). However, it should be noted that the need for PC sequences to acquire pairs of flow sensitive images, causes them to have minimum TE times that are substantially greater than those needed for 3D TOF sequences. And, as a general rule, the longer the minimum TE, the greater the likelihood that vascular signal will be lost completely for a short distance following a stenosis (much like when 2D TOF images are compared to the shorter TE images from a 3D TOF scan)[10,11]. This exaggerated signal loss can make a stenosis artifactually appear more severe on a 3D PC MIP (or a 2D PC MIP) than on a similar 3D TOF MIP of the same stenosis. It is critical to note, however, that the 3D PC MRA approach has, as perhaps its most clinically important features, the ability to acquire high-resolution images of blood flow moving far too slowly for 3D TOF techniques to image; and image large areas of blood flow with a relative insensitivity to the length of time that blood remains within the excitation volume.

2D Phase Contrast MRA

The 2D phase contrast (2D PC) technique is based on the acquisition of thick 2D slices (a single 2D PC slice is often as thick as an entire 3D slab might be in most other applications, i.e. single 2D PC slices of 3–8 cm each are not uncommon in routinely recommended MRA protocols). Once acquired, 2D PC slices are projected from one direction only. For instance, the projection of a 2D PC image is limited to the same dimensional plane as the one it was acquired in (i.e., if acquired axially, the resulting image is an axial image that can not be reformatted into a sagittal or coronal image). The strength of this "thick slice" approach is speed of acquisition. When the thickness of the excitation volume is not subdivided into smaller partitions (as it is in a 3D volume acquisition), the time

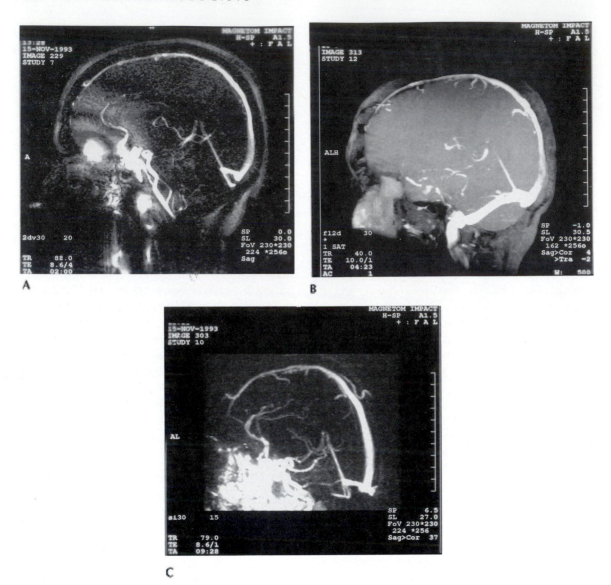

Figure 9-22 **A** Example of a 2D PC angiogram of a patient's sagittal sinus. The acquisition time for this image was 2 min and the image can be viewed in straight sagittal projection only. **B** Example of a 2D TOF sagittal acquisition on the same patient. Acquisition time for this image was 4 min 23 s and the image scan can be viewed as a series of single slices or any variety of angled MIP projections. **C** Example of a 3D PC of the same patient. Acquisition time for this image was 9 min 28 s and the image scan can be viewed as a series of single slices or any variety of angled MIP projection.

required for spatial encoding (in the slice direction) is *substantially* minimized[52].

Additional strengths and weakness of the 2D PC approach are similar to those of the 3D PC approach (albeit at a *much* lower resolution): the benefit of the ability to be used successfully both before and after the injection of gadolinium contrast; and the limitation that the apparent

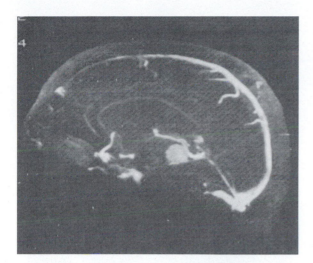

Figure 9-23. A gadolinium-enhanced tumor artifactually appears as a bright, presumably flowing, object in this patient's head (2D TOF MRA).

severity of vascular narrowings will tend to be exaggerated due to the relatively long TE times characteristic of the technique; also the ability to image large areas of blood flow with a relative insensitivity to the length of time that blood remains within the excitation volume[10,11,60]. And it is this last feature, the ability to *rapidly* image large areas of anatomy, that makes 2D PC the imaging sequence of choice for most MRA "scout" or "localizer" imaging applications.

Under most implementations of the 2D PC technique the angiographer can elect to view the final image with all flowing objects shown as "bright" (a "magnitude" or "speed" image) or in a form where movement in one direction (e.g., from right to left) is "bright" and flow in the opposite direction is "dark." This second, or "phase," imaging approach offers the additional benefit of being able to document the direction-ality of blood flow. Phase contrast sequences also require that the user preset (i.e., pre-select before the scan is run) the range of blood flow velocities for optimal visualization of the vessel of interest. That is to say, the operator must decide in advance if the resulting images will be used to

visualize fast moving arterial structures, or slowly moving venous structures. This pre-selection operation is called selecting a velocity-encoding-factor (VENC) by some equipment manu-facturers; and it is called selecting an "optimum-velocity" (V-Opt.) by others.

Velocity Encoding

There is an additional technical consideration of which we must be aware with phase contrast (2D PC and 3D PC). The operator must, in advance, select the range of blood flow velocities that the acquisition will most effectively image. With PC it is possible to image only slowly flowing structures, such as veins, or only rapidly flowing structures such as arteries. The range of possible velocities that can be accurately imaged in one acquisition is fixed, however, at 360 possible degrees of phase shift. Therefore, it is not often possible to encode the full physiologic range of velocities contained within both arteries and veins all within a single image[52,60].

The imaging factor that determines the optimum range of blood flow velocities that a PC sequence can image is the velocity-encoding-factor, or VENC (also known as optimum-velocity V-Opt.). The selection of a V-Opt. of 20 cm/s will, for example, cause blood flowing at exactly 20 cm/s to be assigned the maximum (brightest) possible pixel intensity. Care must be taken, however, to select an optimum velocity factor slightly greater than the anticipated peak velocity of blood within the volume. For example, if the operator anticipates that the renal arteries will be flowing no faster than 35 cm/s, then selection of a V-Opt. 40 sequence might be appropriate.

Great care must be taken in the selection of an appropriate VENC because the signal from blood moving at a higher rate than the chosen VENC can not be seen as the greater than the "brightest possible" pixel. For example, if 40 cm/s is the VENC value chosen but the flow velocity is really 42 cm/s the signal will alias (wrap around). The "42" signal will be recorded

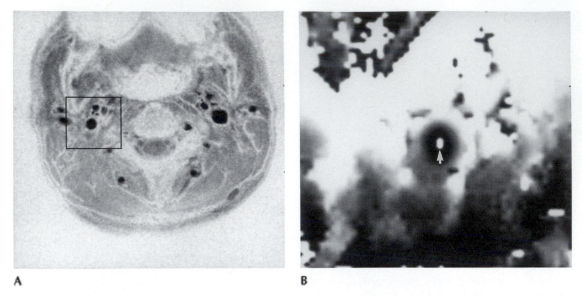

A   **B**

Figure 9-24. **A** A magnitude image showing the area (box) containing the vessel seen in image B. **B** A white dot (small arrow) is seen as evidence of phase wrap on this axial 2D PC angiogram of a patient's jugular vein (large arrow).

as a velocity two units greater than the darkest end of the available range. Phase wrap on PC images can be thought of as conceptionally similar to the phase wrap sometimes seen in the phase encode direction of routine MRI images. In a velocity encoding situation in which there are only 360 degrees of phase encoding possible, a shift of two greater than the maximum possible will be recorded as 362 degrees shift. The scanner will interpret 362 degrees as the same as 2 degrees of phase shift. The scanner will "see it" in much the same way as we see a clock (with no hour hand) as appearing identical at one minute after noon, and 61 minutes after noon. The signal from the vessel will "phase-wrap" from very bright to very dark [Figure 9-24].

IMAGE PROCESSING

Maximum Intensity Projection

A maximum-intensity-projection (MIP) is a record of a "maximum intensity ray" (as generated through a mathematical algorithm) as it passes through an angiographic volume (a series of 2D or 3D MRA source images)[8,61]. Each pixel on a MIP image represents the highest intensity voxel experienced in that location on any partition within the imaging volume. A MIP is not unlike a subtraction image in conventional X-ray angiography (XRA). In XRA (either digital subtraction angiography, DSA, or conventional cut-film XRA) a pre-injection mask image (containing everything except blood vessels) is used in conjunction with the post-injection images to remove unwanted structures (see background subtraction). This has the effect of removing complicating structures, such as large bones, thus leaving an unobstructed image of only the blood vessels. Similarly, the MIP algorithm is often used in MRA to create a new set of images in which the vessels can be viewed as if from a different direction than the original plane of acquisition.

The MIP algorithm could be thought of as working in this way. Imagine a 3D volume five partitions deep with a matrix of 10×10. Now visualize a ray passing through a point three steps in and three steps down from one corner of this cube. This ray would pass through each of the five partitions (at this same location) and end with the creation of a separate 6th, MIP, partition. Let's further imagine that at position 3–3 of this 6th, or MIP, partition the ray records a signal intensity. The intensity of the signal is equal to the highest intensity the ray encountered at point 3-3 in all five partitions it passed through. A ray passing through vascular anatomy should retain a high "maximum intensity" as it encounters a bright blood vessel; and a ray passing through non-moving tissue only should record a low background intensity[41]. The result would be a high-contrast "angiographic" projection image emphasizing only high signal intensity blood vessels [Figure 9-25].

An individual 3D MRA acquisition can contain 60 or more images. Use of a MIP algorithm is one approach to reducing the quantity of MRA information to a manageable dozen or so processed images. MIPs are also a means of excluding unwanted structures from the image. As MRA techniques become more efficient at imaging a wide range of blood velocities (e.g., both arteries and veins) within the same image, the selection of small a subset of

the MRA volume (through the use of selective regions-of-interest) is a practical approach to limiting the confusing overlap of vessels [Figure 9-26].

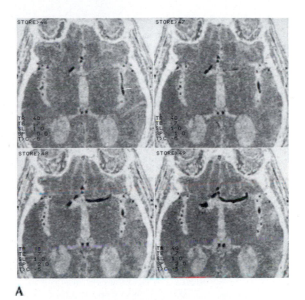

A

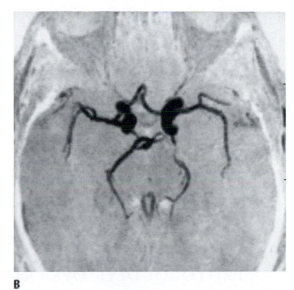

B

Figure 9-26. **A** The cranial arteries pass through multiple partitions from this 3D TOF axial acquisition. **B** An MIP image allows the viewer to more easily appreciate the anatomy of this patient's circle of Willis.

Figure 9-25. Graphic depiction of an MIP "ray" passing through several partitions from a 3D acquisition, then ending in the creation of a projection image.

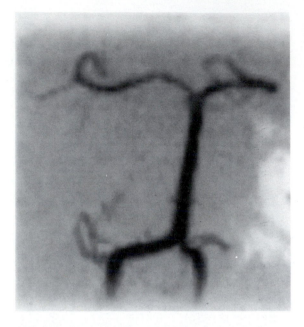

Figure 9-27.   High-resolution axial 3D TOF MIP images of the distal vertebral arteries and basilar artery of a patient show excellent small vessel detail and good vessel to background contrast. However, it should be noted that a review of the unprocessed "source" images continues to provide critical additional information.

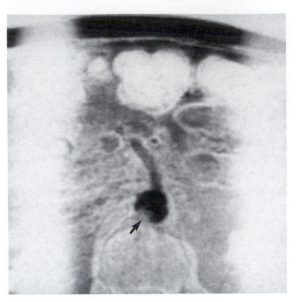

Figure 9-28.   This axial 2D TOF image of a patient's aorta in the area of the SMA shows a minor blockage (arrow). There is a large area of intestinal gas overlying the area that would make the use of ultrasound difficult in this case. Note again that much of the interpretation of body MRA is done from individual slices, with MIP images providing only an overview of gross vascular anatomy.

It must be remembered, however, that the information contained in a MIP image [Figure 9-27] is never as detailed as that in the unprocessed "source" images [Figure 9-28]. A MIP can be thought of as a highway map. It provides a quick and easy view of the relative location and shape of the vessels. But a detailed "street map" is still the best way to find a specific address. And, likewise, a review of the unprocessed source images is often the best way to find (and quantify) specific areas of pathology.

MRA PROTOCOL DEVELOPMENT

Far and away the best advice I can give about exactly how best to develop MRA protocols is to "begin with *your* equipment manufacturer's recommended protocols[8]." In the beginning pages of this chapter we have laid the foundation for the optimization of your equipment manufacturer's protocols to fit better into a variety of clinical situations. So far we have become familiar with the fundamentals of time-of-flight MRA (TOF), phase-contrast MRA (PC), magnitude-contrast MRA (MC), gadolinium contrast-enhanced 3D MRA (CE), dark-blood "flow-void" MRA (DB), and maximum-intensity-projection (MIP) image processing[19,28,52,54,62,63]. These six items will now begin to function as our basic "tool set" for MRA protocol development. In this final section of the chapter we will discuss what attributes to look for in a quality MRA image. We will also learn how to quickly diagnose potential causes of suboptimal images. Finally, and perhaps most importantly, we will discuss practical approaches to improving the diagnostic accuracy of our MR angiographic examinations.

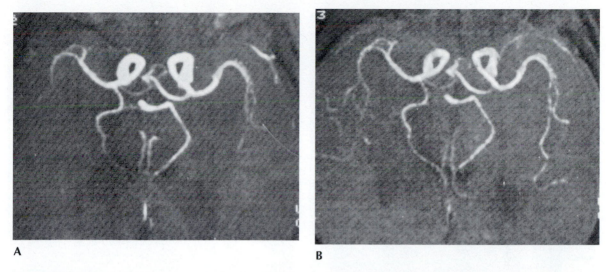

Figure 9-29. **A** 3D TOF image acquired with a "higher" flip angle. **B** 3D TOF image of the same patient acquired with a "lower" flip angle. Note: Small vessel detail is better on the "lower" flip angle image.

It is difficult, because of the wide array of MRI equipment configurations, magnet field strengths, and available computer software packages, to make specific imaging suggestions. The problem with making specific TR and TE recommendations [see Figure 9-8] becomes apparent when one considers the fact that a protocol that is ideal for use on one magnet, is almost sure to fail on another equipment manufacturer's magnet. This chapter will, therefore, make suggestions like "decrease the flip angle slightly" [Figure 9-29] or use a "MOTSA" type technique [Figure 9-30] "if possible." Equipment manufacturers are usually quite good at suggesting appropriate "routine" imaging protocols. So start with one of your manufacturer's suggested protocols, and make *minor* adjustments to the imaging parameters as needed.

Intracranial arteries

A 3D MRA approach in this area is required because of the overriding need for high-resolution images. The intracranial vessels (ICV) of the circle of Willis are small vessels. Failure to successfully identify small areas of pathology, like a

5 mm aneurysm, can have a devastating effect on patient morbidity. 3D TOF is the approach most often used in clinical practice. A single 5 or 6 cm 3D axial slab [see Figure 9-5A] is usually sufficient for screening purposes. Ideally, this size volume will be divided into 60 to 70 partitions and will utilize a ramped flip angle "TONE"-type RF profile[62,63]. Position the axial slab so that the lower edge of the imaging volume is placed slightly below the level of the infraclinoid siphon [see Figure 9-5B] of the internal carotid artery.

A *3D* sequential *multi-slab* (MOTSA) protocol is a better approach if visualization of small distal vessels is of key clinical importance[43]. The MOTSA approach may also be the best selection when the angiographer wishes to screen a large area of anatomy [see Figure 9-16] like the distal vertebral arteries *and* the entire length of the basilar artery *and* the circle of Willis all in one acquisition[12,28,44]. A 256 matrix is the most common selection for nonspecific screening examinations and the use of a head coil is mandatory for all ICV imaging. A matrix increase to 512 may be prudent for aneurysm screening cases that present with a positive family history of

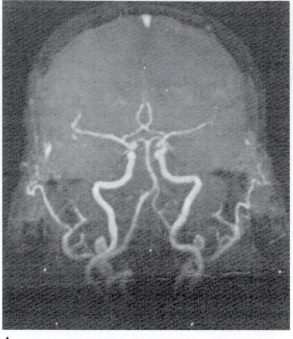

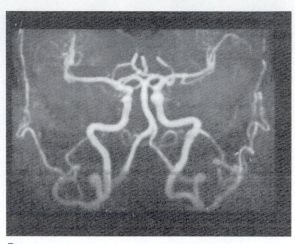

B

A

Figure 9-30. **A** Since 3D TOF coronal slab acquisition with an inappropriately large area of coverage. **B** Coronal projection from an axial 3D MS acquisition of the same patient. Note how the basilar artery appears narrow and pathologic on the single-slab acquisition when it is in fact shown to be widely patent on the 3D MS image. Note also that the distal portions of the middle cerebral arteries are poorly seen on the single-slab image (both artifacts are due to saturation effects resulting from the use of an inappropriately large imaging volume).

intracranial aneurysms or in the case of individuals with known polycystic disease of the kidneys. Low resolution MRA imaging approaches (i.e., 3D matrixes as low as 128, and most forms of 2D imaging) are generally considered below the minimum standards of clinical reliability.

The use of an axial 3D phase-contrast (PC) slab acquisition is also an appropriate selection[60]. Use of this approach for screening purposes has largely fallen out of favor in recent years because of its tendency to exaggerate the apparent severity of stenotic pathology. 3D PC meets the requirement for high resolution imaging of the ICV. *Additionally*, the ability of 3D PC to image blood that is flowing at too low a velocity for 3D TOF to image, makes it an ideal selection for

imaging areas of redundant flow (like giant aneurysms) or extremely slow flow (like AV fistulas). The 3D PC approach is a bit more time consuming to acquire than 3D TOF, despite the fact that PC sequences can be acquired with the minimum TR possible without an adverse effect on vascular contrast (unlike TOF).

It is common in clinical practice to reduce the number of 3D PC phase encode steps (along with a simultaneous reduction in FOV sufficient to maintain image resolution) or to reduce the number of image partitions (3D slices). Imaging time can be reduced still further, either for 3D TOF or 3D PC, by placing the phase encoding direction from side to side and acquiring a rectangular (asymmetric) FOV matrix. This approach works well in ICV acquisitions because of the elliptical shape of the head. This approach has the additional benefit of displaying any motion artifacts from patient eye movement across the face, instead of backwards into the area of the ICV.

Intracranial veins

The intracranial veins are low velocity structures. Therefore, only an imaging approach that is sensitive to the presence of slow flow is likely to succeed. The two "slow flow" sequences that we have in our MRA tool-box are 2D TOF and phase contrast (either 2D PC or 3D PC).

The use of series of 2D TOF slices [see Figures 9-22B and 9-23] is one common approach to imaging the intracranial veins. The most important decision the MR angiographer must make, in the case of 2D TOF, is from what orientation to acquire the images[19,28]. If thrombosis or invasion of the sagittal sinus is the question, a coronal series of slices (perpendicular to the sagittal sinus) will be most effective for identifying a clot or other pathology. However, if the cortical veins are the area of interest, acquisition of slices in a transverse plane may be best. One practical approach to this type of examination is simply to acquire a set of axial and coronal slices. This "double set" approach is practical because each series of 3 or 4 mm 2D slices (256 matrix, head coil) should take no longer than four or five minutes to acquire. And the combination of both axial and coronal acquisitions greatly increases the likelihood that all of the slow moving veins will be successfully imaged without fear of artifact[64].

A second, and perhaps more efficient, approach to the imaging of the draining intracranial veins is to acquire several quick 2D PC slices[52,60]. One of these slices might be a 5 or 6 cm axial slab positioned to contain the transverse sinuses; and another of these slices could be a sagittal 3 or 4 cm slab [see Figure 9-22A] positioned to contain the sagittal sinus. One of the strengths of the PC approach is its rapidity. Acquisition of each of these slices (even when

several excitations, or NEX, are used) should take only 2 or 3 minutes. This speed of acquisition can be used to facilitate the acquisition of two axial slices and two sagittal slices. This two-slice approach allows one acquisition in each direction to be acquired with a low VENC (like 10 or 20 cm/s) and another slice at a higher VENC (such as 40 or 60).

All manufacturers include in their PC applications guide (or should include) a chart of a listing of normal blood flow velocities. In the case of the sagittal sinus, a normal range of 15 or 20 cm/s might be listed. Therefore a VENC selection of 20 would be an appropriate selection. However, in the presence of pathology (i.e., a tumor partially occluding the sinus and thereby causing an increase in blood flow velocity through the narrowed vascular opening) it is often wise to image with a range of velocity-encoding factors.

Arteriovenous Malformations

MRA evaluation of arteriovenous malformations (AVM) is another area in which the imaging of slowly moving intracranial blood becomes necessary. In this case, however, only a portion of the blood that the angiographer must visualize will be moving slowly. As its name implies, AVMs contain both an arterial component and a venous component. Consequently, a minimum of two MRA acquisitions are required in order to fully evaluate this kind of pathology[19,28,60].

The arterial component is most often imaged in much the same way as any other fast flowing intracranial vessel. The most common approach is through the use of an axial 3D TOF acquisition (preferable a 3D slab without a ramped flip angle or TONE configuration, 256 matrix, head coil). An alternate, although lower resolution approach, would be to utilize an axial 2D PC slice with a high VENC. However, due to the unpredictability of the blood flow velocity ranges common within AVMs it would be wise to acquire several 2D PC slices, each with a different VENC (perhaps 60, 80, and even 100 cm/s).

The use of a series of 2D TOF slices, or a series of several 2D PC slices (at different VENCs), is the most widely used approach to visualizing the draining veins of an AVM. The appropriate plane of acquisition for 2D slices will depend entirely on the anatomy involved. But it should be noted that the use of an incrementing (traveling or walking) saturation region in conjunction with 2D TOF slices is NOT recommended. The use of saturation regions in the case of an AVM can be problematic because of the unpredictability of the direction that arteries and veins will be flowing. In fact, it is virtually guaranteed that at some point within the AVM both arteries and veins will be flowing in the same direction at the same time.

Carotid Artery

A screening examination of the carotid arteries is, in almost all cases, a series of axial 2D TOF slices acquired in a neck coil. This "quick screening" approach is often, as a matter of clinical efficiency [see Figure 9-9], scheduled as an "add on" series in addition to another MRI examination (i.e., a routine brain scan plus a series of 2D carotid images). The diagnostic aim of this type of examination is to classify patient pathology into gross categories such as normal, mild to moderate, or severe to critical[64]. Despite the obvious time savings temptation, it is not technically advisable to attempt this type of examination in a standard head coil (no matter how firmly the patient is thrust into the coil). The extreme outer edge of a head coil is an extremely inefficient location to place the area of interest of any diagnostic examination; and the quality of the resulting MRA images will suffer.

Most carotid acquisitions are, therefore, performed with a neck coil (preferably one with a "wrap-around" Helmholtz or phase-array type design)[8]. Acquisition of a single series of 50–60 axial 3 mm slices with an overlap of 30%, or 60–80 axial 3 mm slices with an overlap of 50%, is the approach that has achieved the widest clinical

acceptance[13–16,19,28]. The stack of slices should be positioned to cover the anatomy from the mid-common carotid artery through the mid-internal carotid artery. An image matrix of approximately 256 is usually considered sufficient for carotid imaging. The use of voxel sizes larger that those commonly used for ICV MRA is usually considered adequate because of the relatively large caliber of the carotid vessels.

Use of a parallel vascular saturation region (sat band) positioned distal to each of the 2D TOF slices is standard. This configuration allows for the effective removal of blood signal flowing in the head to feet direction (i.e., veins), and thereby prevents the resulting images from appearing as a confusing mass of overlapping arteries and veins. The use of a saturation band option that moves the band incrementally (i.e., keeps the band at a fixed distance from each slice in a "walking" or a "traveling" configuration), is ideal. Some manufacturers also suggest that the order of slice acquisition be arranged in such a way that slices are gathered first in the most distal locations (nearest the patient's head) and then sequentially incremented in a more proximal direction. This distal-to-proximal approach insures that blood cannot become partially saturated by having experienced RF excitation while passing through a more proximal slice.

Studies have shown that the diagnostic accuracy, and specificity, of carotid MRA examinations increases significantly when a combined 2D TOF and 3D TOF approach is employed[13]. A multi-scan approach usually begins with a standard axial 2D TOF screening acquisition as described above, except that the number of 2D slices and/or the percentage of slice overlap may be reduced slightly to reduce scan time. 2D TOF images have a characteristic tendency to exaggerate the apparent severity of carotid stenoses [see Figures 9-11 and 9-20]. Consequently, the use of 2D TOF to locate the presence of pathologies is highly dependable on other factors. However, 2D's ability accurately to quantify the degree to which a stenosis may reduce a vessel's diameter is somewhat limited. The solution to this problem is to use 2D TOF to locate areas in need of further evaluation using a 3D TOF acquisition. A single axial 3D TOF slab, positioned with the area of pathology within the lower third of the volume, is the most usual approach (at high field). 3D TOF images, owing to their shorter TEs, are less likely to artifactually exaggerate the appearance of pathology and are therefore better able accurately to depict the true severity of a stenosis.

Basivertebral Arteries

The use of a high resolution 3D acquisition is a must in cases in which the patient is being evaluated to rule out basilar stenosis or basilar tip aneurysm, occlusion of the small arteries that supply the posterior fossa (like the inferior cerebellars), or dissection of the distal vertebral arteries[14,28]. Axial 3D multislab TOF acquisition of the intracranial, basilar, and distal vertebral arteries [see Figures 9-14 and 9-30B] works well in the head coil, and is the most widely accepted approach for screening of the basivertebral system. Because the anatomic distance to be screened in these cases (from the distal third of the vertebral arteries to the basilar tip) is quite large, most practitioners choose to acquire these images with only a 256 matrix, thus limiting the use of high resolution 512 matrix imaging to a single slab 3D TOF acquisition only after an aneurysm or specific area of dissection has been located.

An exception to this high resolution 3D TOF recommendation is in cases where the patient is known to have a large basilar aneurysm with slow blood flow. In this case a 2D PC, or even 3D PC approach might be best. A second exception would be in instances where the examination is intended to establish the patency of the vessels, with no expectation of quantification of stenoses or identification of possible vertebral artery dissection. In the case of this type of gross screening examination, a series of three or four coronal 2D PC slices (6, 7, or even 8 cm thick) acquired with a range of

velocity-encoding-factors (i.e., VENC 20, 40, and 60) is the most commonly selected approach.

A series of axial 2D TOF slices can also be used to answer questions of gross patency. However, 2D TOF of the distal vertebrals is never a good selection with which to evaluate traumatic vertebral dissection. The distal vertebral arteries turn, for a short distance, from a vertical to transverse course and then turn back to vertical again. Blood flow signal is routinely lost completely in this transverse area. This is the same area in which one would expect to find a traumatic dissection. 2D TOF is also not a good choice (in any anatomic location) for the evaluation of fibromuscular dysplasia (FMD, a condition where blood vessels are distorted into a tortuous course by pathologic growth of surrounding musculature). Also, patient movement on 2D TOF causes the apparent path of blood vessels to artifactually take on a serpentine appearance. This characteristic 2D TOF motion artifact has been seen to mimic the appearance of FMD.

Aortic Arch

The use of an axial 3D multislab acquisition [see Figures 9-2 and 9-16] is the tried-and-true approach to imaging this area of anatomy[28,64]. The selection of a 3D approach provides a boost in signal-to-noise ratio that is much needed in body coil imaging. Body imaging requires the use of a relatively large field-of-view. Consequently, a minimum of a 256 matrix (or a asymmetric "rectangular" field of view with a similar voxel resolution) is the clinical standard; and many imaging centers, especially those with access to a phased-array or similar wrap-around body coil, use a 512 matrix.

The newest and most efficient way to image any large abdominothoracic vessel is with gadolinium contrast-enhanced 3D (CE)[46]. This approach, however, requires an entire 3D volume to be acquired within a single 25–30 s patient breath-hold. In this approach a large field-of-view coronal 3D slab is positioned to include the aortic arch in its lower third and entire aortic outflow tract and subclavian arteries; or a para-sagittal slab is positioned to include the ascending aorta [see Figure 9-17] in its upper third and as much descending aorta as possible. A slab thickness of 3.5 to 4.5 cm is then acquired. The principal image contrast mechanism in CE MRA is the timing of a large bolus of gadolinium contrast material to pass through the imaging volume at just the right moment. The target time for the gadolinium-enhanced blood to pass through the volume is during the acquisition of the center 20% of raw data (*k*-space).

Timing is critical in 3D CE MRA. It is often wise first to acquire a "timing run" using a test dose of about 1 cc of gadolinium. In this process an axial 2D GRE slice is positioned so that it crosses the aorta at the area of principal clinical interest (i.e., the aortic arch). A test dose of contrast is given and a single image is repeatedly collected (i.e., one image each second) until an increase in aortic signal intensity is seen (until the test bolus arrives). With the time delay between injection and the arrival of the contrast in the area of interest now known, it then becomes possible to calculate any delay time that may be necessary in order to ensure that the next gadolinium bolus passes through the area of interest at the optimum time.

Abdominal Veins

These studies are most commonly performed utilizing a 2D TOF breath-hold approach[8]. This is because of the requirement the patient hold their breath; and because of the need to select an imaging sequence that is capable of successfully visualizing slowly moving venous blood (a task for which 2D TOF is ideally suited)[65–68]. The angiographer may choose either a coronal acquisition [see Figure 9-10] which provides a high resolution antero–posterior projection (but suffers from in-plane saturation); or an axial acquisition, which yields stronger in-flow contrast for most abdominal veins but yields a poor quality MIP projection. The axial acquisition nearly always yields a better diagnostic result[69]. A careful review of the un-MIPed axial source images often proves to be the key to accurate clinical interpretation; and MIP images of the abdominal vasculature, although often striking to look at, are frequently not as diagnostically valuable as the unmanipulated source images.

For a gross screening (to rule out deep vein thrombosis) the axial 2D TOF breath-hold approach is definitely the best. A series of 5–7 mm thick slices can be acquired at intervals of 1 cm (allowing for a gap between slices) from the heart to the upper thighs in a relatively short time. Breath-holding during slices acquired in the abdomen is mandatory. However, breath-holding in the area of the pelvis is often not necessary (especially if a tight binder is placed across the lower abdomen to minimize abdominal wall motion). The thickness of the slices and the presence of an intra-slice gap precludes the creation of useful MIP images.

It should be noted that the use of axial (parallel) vascular saturation regions in combination with acquisition of axial 2D TOF breath-hold images of the abdominal veins is often not advisable. This is because portions of the abdominal vessels wind across the abdomen in such a way that portions of the veins normally flow in the same direction as arteries might be expected to flow[8]. These portions would, even in normal individuals, appear artifactually absent of blood flow if they were to encounter an "arterial" saturation band. Since abdominal MRA images are often (usually) interpreted in a slice-by-slice rather than MIP format, visualization of both arteries and veins on the same axial image (i.e., imaging without saturation bands) usually does not create confusion.

Renal Arteries

No clear consensus has been reached as to whether the TOF or PC approach is better for imaging the renal arteries[69,70]. 2D TOF breath-hold imaging (either with or without the addition of cardiac gating/triggering) was the first approach to be seriously investigated; and this approach continues to be an effective [see Figure 9-28], albeit technically challenging, imaging strategy. A series of 5–7 mm 2D TOF slices can be acquired coronally (in a body coil) with the patient suspending their breathing in end-exhalation. These images can be acquired one at a time with a between slice shift of 2–3 mm less than the slice thickness (to allow for an overlap in slice coverage). When using a conventional body coil it is often advisable to acquire thicker (7 mm, 256 matrix) slices to ensure a sufficient level of MRI signal. The relative thickness of these slices (as compared to the anatomy in interest) can be somewhat offset through the use of a substantial overlap in slice positioning. Imaging centers that have access to a phased-array of other type of "wrap-around" body coil may wish to use thinner (5 mm, 256 matrix) slices (or a series of 6 or 7 mm slices with a 512 matrix).

The coronal 2D TOF breath-hold approach [see Figure 9-10] frequently yields images of surprisingly high clinical effectiveness (considering the simplicity of the approach). However, image registration problems (due to patient difficulties in repeatedly suspending their respiration in exactly the same phase of end-expiration) are common. This type of image registration problem can significantly degrade MIP image quality. This is more of an aesthetic limitation than a diagnostic accuracy problem because many (most) abdominal MRA diagnoses are made for a review of individual source images, not MIPs.

The use of 3D TOF for imaging the renal arteries has been met with somewhat less enthusiasm than the other angiographic approaches discussed here. This approach is most often attempted using a single axial 3D TOF (or 3D TOF with a ramped flip angle TONE configuration) slab. A slab of 4 or 5 cm (40 to 60 partitions) is positioned such that the renal origins are located about a third of the way from the inflow side of the slab. If sufficient MRI signal is available (i.e., with a wrap-around body coil) use of a 512 matrix is often advisable. The use of a 3D multislab MOTSA approach is an alternative to the single slab approach; however, the axial saturation regions commonly employed in this method can prove problematic at times. Both 3D TOF approaches do not require breath-holding, and as such, can suffer from a loss of vascular edge definition in distal areas of the renal arteries; and visualization is often limited to the proximal 1–2 cm of the renal arteries.

The use of 3D PC for imaging the renal arteries is the method of choice at a large number of MRI imaging centers. Like 3D TOF, an axial 3D slab is positioned to include the renal origins. The number of partitions and related matrix sizes are usually similar to those described for the 3D TOF technique; and it is not uncommon for images to be acquired using VENCs of 25, 35, or even 45 cm/s. Owing to the time constraints that are common within the clinical environment, it is often a good idea first to acquire a series of two or three low resolution (fast) axial 2D PC images from which to select the optimum VENC for high resolution 3D imaging of the renal arteries.

Gadolinium contrast-enhanced 3D MRA techniques (CE) are rapidly becoming the clinical standard in abdominal MRA. This technique (as described in the MRA theory chapter of this text, and briefly recapped in the aortic arch section of this chapter) combines the high resolution characteristics of 3D MRA with the superior vascular edge definition capabilities of 2D breath-hold techniques. In this approach a coronal 3D slab (again as described above) is positioned to include the anterior wall of the aorta and an area of anatomy extending several centimeters beyond (more posterior than) the posterior wall of the aorta. The preliminary use of a timing run (with the axial test slice positioned at the level of the renal origins) is strongly advised. Contrast transit times can vary, in this author's experience, by as much as 200–300 percent depending on patient body habitus and cardiac efficiency.

Lower Extremities

The slow rate of blood flow that is characteristic of the arteries of the legs (thighs to ankles) makes this a difficult area to image[19,28,70]. And these difficulties are further compounded by the huge anatomical distance that a successful examination must cover. The low rates of blood flow in the extremities preclude the use of 3D TOF techniques. The anatomic distance to be covered (in a reasonable amount of time) precludes the use of 3D PC techniques.

The use of thin transverse 2D TOF slices (multiple stacks stepping up the legs) is the approach that has been most thoroughly investigated[65–68]. In this approach the use of a high signal-to-noise ratio coil such as the knee or head coil is of critical importance in the lower legs [see Figures 9-13 and 9-14] and ankles. The need for thin slices (perhaps 3 mm or less in the feet and 3–4 mm in the lower legs, with thickness largely dependent on imaging time constraints) is mandated by the small diameter of the vessel[12,26].

Choice of flip angles for 2D TOF acquisition will vary with the degree of vascular signal pulsatility. For instance, if your manufacturer's suggested protocol uses a 35- or 40-degree flip angle for body coil imaging of the pelvis/aortic bifurcation, a 45- or 50-degree flip angle might be appropriate for body coil imaging of the calf and for head/extremity coil imaging of the lower leg, and 55- or 60-degree for extremity coil imaging of the ankle and proximal vessels of the foot.

As is true with most areas of body MRA imaging, the 3D CE approach appears to be gaining in clinical utility in this application. However, issues of run-off timing (e.g., table movement delay increments) continue to be technically challenging.

REFERENCES

1. Hawkes R, Holland G, Moore W, et al. Nuclear magnetic resonance (NMR) tomography of the brain: a preliminary clinical assessment with demonstration of pathology. *J Comput Assist Tomogr* 4:577–586, 1980.
2. Young I, Burl M, Clarke G. Magnetic resonance properties of hydrogen: imaging in the posterior fossa. *AJR* 137:895–901, 1981.
3. Crooks L, Mills C, Davis P, et al. Visualization of cerebral and vascular abnormalities by NMR imaging: the effects of imaging parameters on contrast. *Radiology* 144:843–852, 1982.
4. Felmlee JP, Ehman RL. Spatial presaturation: a method for suppressing flow artifacts and improving depiction of vascular anatomy in MR imaging. *Radiology* 164:559–564, 1987.
5. Haacke E, Lenz G. Improving MR image quality in the presence of motion by using rephasing gradients. *Am J Roentgenol* 148:1251–1258, 1987.
6. Pattany PM, Phillips J, Chiu L, et al. Motion artifact suppression technique (MAST) for MR imaging. *J Comput Assist Tomogr* 11:369–377, 1987.
7. Edelman R, Atkinson D, Silver M, et al. FRODO pulse sequences: a new means of eliminating motion, flow and wraparound artifacts. *Radiology* 166:231–236, 1988.
8. Saloner D, Anderson CM, Lee RE. Magnetic Resonance Angiography. In: Higgins CV, Hricak H, Helms C, eds. *Magnetic Resonance of the Body*. New York: Raven Press, 679–718, 1991.
9. Xiang QA, Nalcioglu O. Differential flow imaging by NMR. *Magn Reson Med* 12:14–24, 1989.
10. Nishimura DG, Macovski A, Jackson JI, et al. Magnetic resonance angiography by selective inversion recovery using a compact gradient echo sequence. *Magn Reson Med* 8:96–103, 1988.
11. Schmalbrock P, Yuan C, Chakeres DW, et al. Volume MR angiography: methods to achieve very short echo times. *Radiology* 175:861–865, 1990.
12. Chien C, Anderson CM, Lee RE. Principles of Blood Flow and MRA. In Edelman R, Hesselink J, and Zlatkin. *Clinical MRI* 2nd edn. Philadelphia: Saunders, 1995.
13. Saloner D, Anderson CM, Rapp JH, et al. MR imaging of carotid endarterectomy specimens: implications for MRA. In: Proceedings of a meeting of the Society of Magnetic Resonance in Medicine, Berlin, Germany, 1992.
14. Anderson CM. Carotid and vertebral arteries. In Anderson, Edelman, Turski, eds. *Clinical Magnetic Resonance Angiography*. New York: Raven Press, 309–340, 1993.
15. Anderson CM, Saloner D, Lee RE, et al. Magnetic resonance angiography and conventional angiography of the carotid bifurcation: comparison of stenosis assessment in

40 bifurcations. In: Proceeding of a meeting of the Society for Magnetic Resonance Medicine, San Francisco, 1991.

16. Xian MP, Anderson CM, Reilly LM, et al. MRA of the carotid artery combining 2D and 3D acquisitions. In Proceedings of a meeting of the Western Vascular Society, Maui Hl, 1992.

17. Lee RE, Anderson CM, Saloner D, et al. Evaluation of carotid MRA examinations: novice vs. experienced readers. In: Proceedings of a meeting of the Society for Magnetic Resonance in Medicine, San Francisco, 1991.

18. Lee RE, Anderson CM, Saloner D. Novice vs. experienced readers in 58 carotid arteries. In: Proceedings of the Tenth Annual Meeting of the Society for Magnetic Resonance Imaging, New York, 1992.

19. Anderson CM, Lee RE. Time-of-flight angiography. In: Anderson, Edelman, Turski, eds. *Clinical Magnetic Resonance Angiography*. New York: Raven Press, 11–41, 1993.

20. Anderson CM, Saloner D, Tsuruda JS, et al. Artifacts in maximum-intensity-projection display of MR angiograms. *Am J Roentgenol* 154:623–629, 1990.

21. von Schulthess G, Higgins C. Blood flow imaging with MR: spin-phase phenomena. *Radiology* 157:687–695, 1985.

22. Podolak MJ, Hedlund LW, Evans AJ, et al. Evaluation of flow through simulated vascular stenoses with gradient echo magnetic resonance imaging. *Invest Radiol* 24:184–189, 1989.

23. Evans AJ, Hedlund LW, Herfkens RJ, et al. Evaluation of steady and pulsatile flow with dynamic MRI using limited flip angles and gradient refocused echoes. *Magn Reson Med* 5:475–482, 1987.

24. Motomiya M, Karino T. Flow patterns in human carotid artery bifurcation. *Stroke* 15:50–56, 1984.

25. Haacke EM, Masaryk TJ, Wielopolski PA, et al. Optimizing blood vessel contrast in fast three-dimensional MRI. *Magn Reson Med* 14:202–221, 1990.

26. Saloner D. Intensity dependence of flow signal in slice selective velocity measurements. *Magn Res Imaging* 7:61–67, 1989.

27. Gao JH, Holland SK, Gore JC. Nuclear magnetic resonance signal from flowing nuclei in rapid imaging using gradient echoes. *Med Phys* 15:809–814, 1988.

28. Anderson CM, Lee RE. Time-of-flight MRA. In: Finn JP, ed. *Radiologic Clinics of North America*. Philadelphia: Saunders, 1993.

29. Gullberg GT, Wehrli FW, Shimakawa A, et al. MR vascular imaging with a fast gradient refocusing pulse sequence and reformatted images from transaxial sections. *Radiology* 165:241–246, 1987.

30. Laub GA, Kaiser WA. MR angiography with gradient motion refocusing. *J Comput Assist Tomogr* 12:377–382, 1988.

31. Frahm J, Merbolt KD, Hanicke W, et al. Rapid line scan NMR angiography. *Magn Reson Med* 7:79–87, 1988.

32. Lenz G, Haacke E, Masaryk T, et al. In-plane vascular imaging: pulse sequence design and strategy. *Radiology* 166:875–882, 1988.

33. Keller PJ, Drayer BP, Fram EK, et al. MR angiography with two-dimensional acquisition and three-dimensional display. Work in progress. *Radiology* 173:527–532, 1989.

34. Kim JH, Cho ZH. 3-D MR angiography with scanning 2-D images: simultaneous data acquisition of arteries and veins (SAAV). *Magn Reson Med* 14:554–561, 1990.

35. Nishimura DG. Time-of-flight MR angiography. *Magn Reson Med* 14:194–201, 1990.

36. Brown DG, Riederer SJ, Wright RC, et al. High-speed line scan MR angiography. *Magn Reson Med* 25:475–482, 1990.

37. Dumoulin CL, Cline HE, Souza SP, et al. Three-dimensional time-of-flight magnetic resonance angiography using spin saturation. *Magn Reson Med* 11:35–46, 1989.

38. Ruggieri PM, Laub GA, Masaryk TJ, et al. Intracranial circulation: pulse-sequence considerations in three-dimensional (volume) MR angiography. *Radiology* 171:785–791, 1989.

39. Lee JN, Riederer SJ, Pelc NJ. Flow-compensated limited lip angle MR angiography. *Magn Reson Med* 12:1–13, 1989.

40. Anderson CM, Lee RE. MRA: Time-of-Flight Techniques, Ch. 17. In *Categorical Course on Cardiovascular Imaging*. American College of Radiology, 1995.

41. Lee RE. MR Angiographic Imaging Theory for the Technologist. In Woodward P, Freimarck R Eds. *MRI for Technologists*. New York: McGraw-Hill Publishing, 1995.

42. Hennig J, Mueri M, Friedburg H, et al. MR imaging of flow using the steady state selective saturation method. *J Comput Assist Tomogr* 11:872–877, 1987.

43. Marchal G, Bosmans H, Van Fraeyenhoven L, et al. Intracranial vascular lesions: optimization and clinical evaluation of 3D TOF MRA. *Radiology* 175:443–448, 1990.

44. Parker DL, Yuan C, Blatter DD. MRA by multiple thin slab 3D acquisition. *Magn Reson Med* 17:434–451, 1991.

45. Prince MR. Gadolinium-enhanced MR Aortography. *Radiology* 191:155–164, 1994.

46. Prince MR. Body Angiography with Gadolinium Contrast Agent. *In MRI Clin N Am* 4:11–24, 1996.

47. Wedden V, Meuli R, Edelman R, et al. Projective imaging of pulsative flow with magnetic resonance. *Science* 230:946–948, 1985.

48. Meuli RA, Wedeen VJ, Geller SC, et al. MR gated subtraction angiography: evaluation of lower extremities. *Radiology* 159:411–418, 1986.

49. Axel L, Morgan D. MR flow imaging by velocity compensated/uncompensated difference images. *J Comput Assist Tomogr* 11:31–34, 1987.

50. Tasciyan TA, Lee JN, Riederer SJ, et al. Fast limited flip angle MR subtraction angiography. *Magn Reson Med* 8:261–274, 1988.

51. Laub G. Magnetization recovery angiography. In: Proceedings of the Eighth Annual Meeting of the Society for Magnetic Resonance in Medicine, Amsterdam, 153.

52. Turski PA, Korosec FR. Phase contrast angiography. In: Anderson, Edelman, Turski, eds. *Clinical Magnetic Resonance Angiography*. New York: Raven Press, 11–41, 1993.

53. Moran P. A flow velocity zeugmatographic interlace for NMR imaging in humans. *Magn Reson Imaging* 1:197–203, 1982.

54. Dumoulin CL, Hart HJ. Magnetic resonance angiography. *Radiology* 161:717–720, 1986.

55. Dumoulin CL, Sonza SP, Hart HR. Rapid scan magnetic resonance angiography. *Magn Reson Med* 5:238–245, 1987.

56. Dumoulin C, Souza S, Walker M, et al. Three dimensional phase contrast angiography. *Magn Reson Med* 9:139–149, 1989.

57. Dumoulin CL, Yucel EK, Vock P, et al. Two- and three-dimensional phase contrast MR angiography of the abdomen. *J Comput Assist Tomogr* 14:779–784, 1990.

58. Merboldt K, Hanicke W, Frahm J. Rapid Fourier flow imaging using flash sequences. *Magn Res Med Biol* 1:137–148, 1988.

59. Nayler GL, Firmin DN, Longmore DB. Blood flow imaging by cine magnetic resonance. *J Comput Assist Tomogr* 10:715–722, 1986.

60. Turski PA. Intracranial MRA: stroke, aneurysms, AVMs, and venous thrombosis. In Anderson, Edelman, Turski, eds. *Clinical Magnetic Resonance Angiography*. New York: Raven Press, 181–308, 1993.

61. Rossnick S, Laub G, Braeckle R. Three dimensional display of blood vessels in MRI. In: Proceedings of the IEEE Computers in Cardiology. New York: Institute of Electrical and Electronic Engineers, 193–195, 1986.

62. Wolff S, Balaban R. Magnetization transfer contrast (MTC) and tissue water proton contrast in vivo. *Magn Reson Med* 10:135–144, 1989.

63. Purdy D, Cadena G, Laub G. The design of a variable tip angle slab selection (TONE) pulses for improved 3D MR angiography. In Proceedings of the 11th annual meeting of the SMRM. Berlin: SMRM, 882, 1992.

64. Anderson CM, Lee RE. MRA of the Aortic Arch and Carotid Arteries. In *Categorical Course on Cardiovascular Imaging*, American College of Radiology, 1995.

65. Gehl HB, Bohndorf K, Klose KC, et al. Two-dimensional MR angiography in the evaluation of abdominal veins with gradient refocused sequence. *J Comput Assist Tomogr* 14:619–624, 1990.

66. Kim D, Edelman RR, Kent KC, et al. Abdominal aorta and renal artery stenosis: evaluation with MR angiography. *Radiology* 727–731, 1990.

67. Steinberg FL, Yucel EK, Dumoulin CL, et al. Peripheral vascular and abdominal applications of MR flow imaging techniques. *Magn Reson Med* 14:315–320, 1990.

68. Edelman RR, Zhao B, Liu C, et al. MR angiography and dynamic flow evaluation of the portal venous system. *Am J Roentgenol* 153:755–760, 1989.

69. Lee RE, Anderson CM, Saloner D. Optimization of MR angiography in the abdomen and extremities. In: Proceedings of the Eighth Annual Meeting of the Society for Magnetic Resonance Imaging, Washington 1990.

70. Edelman RR, Hochman MG. Body MRA. In: Anderson, Edelman, Turski, eds. *Clinical Magnetic Resonance Angiography*. New York: Raven Press, 399–462, 1993.

CHAPTER 10

MR Contrast Media

Eric Hohenschuh and Alan D. Watson

INTRODUCTION AND BACKGROUND

Contrast agents are pharmaceuticals used to increase the information content of diagnostic images. Image contrast is the difference in signal intensity between two tissues, and contrast enhancement is the process by which this difference is increased. The term enhancement is also generally applied to any pharmaceutically based manipulation of tissue as manifested on a diagnostic image. Image contrast may be enhanced by increasing or decreasing the signal intensity of one tissue relative to another. Image contrast may be altered by manipulation of the physical parameters inherent to the imaging method, or through the administration of a pharmaceutical to alter the physical characteristics of tissue itself. For example, the low keV X-rays utilized in mammography are selected to maximize contrast between calcium and breast tissue.

This chapter is intended to provide an explanation of the physical principles of contrast enhanced magnetic resonance imaging (MRI), to describe the current generation of MR contrast enhancing agents and to touch upon new directions in MR contrast media development[1-5].

Pharmaceutical contrast agents have been used with every clinical diagnostic imaging method developed to date. The purest form of pharmaceutically based image enhancement is nuclear medicine (scintigraphy) where the imaging method is inseparable from the administered drug. The scintigraphic image is a direct representation of drug distribution alone with no contribution to the image from the tissue itself.

All other diagnostic modalities rely upon inherent tissue properties which are generally sufficient to produce an acceptable medical image. Diagnostic pharmaceuticals are used to modify the appearance of tissues in that their effects are superimposed upon the intrinsic tissue effects.

The contrast enhancement agents used in MRI and X-ray computed tomography (CT) operate by entirely different mechanisms. X-ray CT agents function *directly* through their ability to scatter or absorb X-ray photons. The observed

X-ray attenuation is simply the weighted average of native tissue attenuation plus attenuation caused by the contrast agent. Conversely, MR contrast agents function *indirectly* through their alteration of the local magnetic environment of tissue. These agents influence the magnetic resonance phenomenon primarily by altering tissue relaxation rates.

The physics which distinguish the various clinical diagnostic modalities (nuclear medicine, X-ray, MR and ultrasound) dictate that fundamentally different materials must be used as contrast media. Representative agents, currently used in each of these imaging modalities, along with selected properties, are presented in Table 10-1.

The recognition of the importance of magnetic materials and their effect on the relaxation times of resonating protons occurred almost simultaneously with the discovery of the magnetic resonance in 1946[6]. Paramagnetic ferric ions in solution were shown to reduce the T1 nuclear relaxation rate of water protons.

Paul Lauterbur was not only responsible for the seminal development of the magnetic resonance imaging technique[7], but also the conception and subsequent development of contrast enhancing media. In 1978, he published the first use of paramagnetic ions and chelate complexes to alter relaxation times in canine heart tissues[8].

During the early years of magnetic resonance imaging, the need for a contrast enhancing medium was strongly debated. Initially, one of the primary reasons for adopting MRI over alternate imaging modalities was its noninvasive nature, combined with the exceptional quality of unenhanced T1 and T2 weighted images (with respect to anatomical resolution and inherent contrast). These advantages seemed sufficiently compelling to obviate the need for additional (invasively provided) contrast enhancement.

The development of the first commercial contrast enhancing agent, gadolinium diethylenetriaminepentaacetic acid dimeglumine, abbreviated as GdDTPA [Figure 10-1] or gadopentetate dimeglumine (Magnevist®), commenced around 1981 and its first reported use in humans occurred in 1984[9-11]. It was soon recognized that additional enhancement of image contrast between normal and diseased tissue could significantly increase the sensitivity and specificity of MRI diagnosis. Unenhanced magnetic resonance studies often poorly delineated, or missed completely, a variety of pathological tissue conditions including some meningiomas[12]

Table 10-1

Comparison of Basic Chemical and Biological Properties of Pharmaceuticals for Diagnostic Imaging

	Magneto-pharmaceuticals	X-ray/CT Pharmaceuticals	Radio-pharmaceuticals	Ultrasound Pharmaceuticals
Representative agent	Gd-DTPA-BMA Omniscan®	Iohexol Omnipaque®	Tc99m Tetrofoxmin Myoview™	Human albumin microspheres Optison®
"Active" components	Paramagnetic gadolinium ion	X-ray absorbing iodine	Gamma-ray emitting technetium isotope	Echogenic octafluoropropane gas
Water solubility	High	High	High	Low
In vivo stability	High	High	High	Low (minutes)
In vivo metabolism	No	No	Yes	No
Dosage (in grams "active" component)	1.5–5.0	20–45	10^{-9}–10^{-11}	10^{-4}
Biodistribution	Extracellular	Extracellular	Intracellular	Blood pool

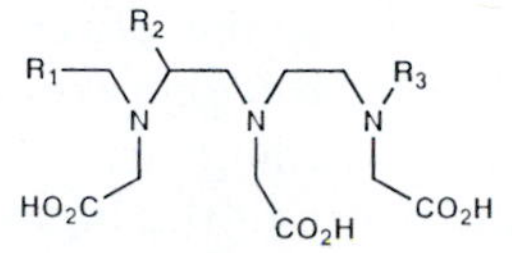

R₁	R₂	R₃	Acronym
$-CO_2H$	$-H$	$-CH_2CO_2H$	DTPA
$-CONHCH_3$	$-H$	$-CH_2CONHCH_3$	DTPA-BMA
$-CO_2H$	$-H$	$-CHCO_2H$ $\quad\mid$ $CH_2OCH_2C_6H_5$	BOPTA
$-CO_2H$	$-CH_2C_6H_4OC_2H_5$	$-CH_2CO_2H$	EOB-DTPA

Figure 10-1. Schematic diagram of DTPA-based acyclic ligands DTPA, DTPA-BMA, BOPTA, and DTPA-EOB.

and small metastatic lesions with little associated edema[13,14]. MR contrast enhancement offered the hope of identifying smaller lesions earlier in the progression of disease, discriminating tumor mass from edema and recurrent tumor from fibrous tissue.

Finally, the intrinsic sensitivity and resolution inherent in body organ imaging, although improved through the use of surface coils, is lower than that seen in brain imaging due to the large field of view and the effects of body motion. Therefore, clinical applications of body MRI have been relatively slow to develop despite the apparent deficiencies of CT and ultrasound techniques. These factors, along with the enormous market potential of magnetic resonance contrast media, have provided the necessary impetus for further research and development to produce a range of extracellular and tissue- or organ-specific contrast media.

MECHANISMS OF CONTRAST ENHANCEMENT

Differences in the magnetic resonance signal intensities of tissues being imaged define *MR image contrast*. The difference needs to be of sufficient magnitude to visualize and clearly define anatomic and pathologic features of interest.

The contrast observed in unenhanced magnetic resonance images arises as a consequence of differences in the intrinsic tissue properties of spin density, $N(H)$, relaxation times, T1 and T2, resonant frequency, chemical shift, magnetic susceptibility, flow/perfusion, and other molecular motions. An effective contrast enhancing medium alters the proton spin density $N(H)$ or the relaxation times T1 and/or T2 such that a measurable change in signal intensity is observed.

In many circumstances, the biophysical properties of native (unenhanced) tissues are not sufficiently dissimilar to produce an appreciable difference in the signal intensities of different tissues. To resolve the isointensity demonstrated by such tissues, a material may be administered which alters, in one tissue more than another, one or more of the intrinsic MR properties; this provides contrast enhancement. Positive contrast enhancement occurs when the tissue of interest appears brighter in an image after the administration of a contrast enhancing agent. Negative contrast enhancement occurs when the target tissue darkens in an image following administration of a contrast enhancing agent.

Signal intensity will increase when $N(H)$ increases, T1 decreases, or T2 increases. Signal intensity will decrease when $N(H)$ decreases, T1 increases, or T2 decreases. For example, some gases (CO_2), perfluorocarbons, and deuterated water serve as contrast agents for proton MR imaging because they possess no hydrogen nuclei and thereby reduce the total spin density within volume elements (image voxels). Paramagnetic materials, such as the metal ions Gd^{3+}, Fe^{3+} and Mn^2, molecular oxygen, and free radicals, all decrease both T1 and T2, potentially increasing or decreasing the signal dependency on local drug concentration and the pulse sequences employed in imaging. Magnetic particles and ^{17}O cause a reduction in T2 that is many times greater than the reduction in T1, resulting in a dramatic drop in signal intensity. Recently small superparamagnetic particles, based on single nanocrystal cores, have been shown to behave more like paramagnetic species, decreasing both

T1 and T2 in similar proportions[15]. The alteration of the relaxation times (T1 and T2) has been the most important avenue of development for magnetopharmaceuticals to date.

The effect of a paramagnetic species on the observed T1 and T2 relaxation times arises as a consequence of interactions between the unpaired electrons of the paramagnetic ion and the hydrogen nuclei of water molecules[16], for which a theoretical explanation is available[17,18].

In the absence of a paramagnetic compound, the intrinsic proton relaxation rates of tissue, $1/T_{1(intrinsic)}$ and $1/T_{2(intrinsic)}$, govern the overall tissue signal intensity. Following the administration of a paramagnetic compound, the observed relaxation rates are a linear combination of the intrinsic and paramagnetic relaxation rates due to the tissue and to the agent[19].

$$1/T_{1(observed)} = 1/T_{1(intrinsic)} + 1/T_{1(paramagnetic)}$$

$$1/T_{2(observed)} = 1/T_{2(intrinsic)} + 1/T_{2(paramagnetic)}$$

The concentration of paramagnetic species is critical to the degree of observed relaxation enhancement. The relationship between the concentration of a paramagnetic species and the observed $1/T_1$ or $1/T_2$ is represented by the equation

$$1/T_{1,2(observed)} = 1/T_{1,2(observed)} + r_{12}[c]$$

in which c is the concentration and r_{12} is the T1 or T2 relaxivity of the paramagnetic species. Relaxivity (r) is a measure of the ability of a paramagnetic species to influence relaxation rates and is expressed in units of $mM^{-1}s^{-1}$ where the concentration of a species is expressed in units of millimoles per liter (millimolar, mmol/L, or mM) and the relaxation rate enhancement produced by such a quantity of a magnetopharmaceutical is expressed in reciprocal seconds (s^{-1}). Relaxivity is measured experimentally at a given magnetic field strength and temperature in a single (specified) medium such as water, a physiological fluid such as plasma, or in tissue.

Paramagnetic species reduce both T1, which results in a signal intensity increase, and T2, which results in the loss of signal intensity. At lower concentrations, the effects of T1 shortening predominate; at higher concentrations, the effects of T2 shortening are more significant. This is a consequence of the biexponential signal intensity equation, the choice of TR and TE and the ratio $r_2 : r_1$. Figure 10-2 shows the effect of varying the concentration of the nonionic paramagnetic gadolinium chelate complex GdDTPA-BMA [Figure 10-1] or gadodiamide (Omniscan®) on the signal intensity for a defined spin echo pulse sequence.

The impact of magnetopharmaceuticals on the choice of pulse sequence needs to be considered[20,21]. The optimal pulse sequence will provide the best signal-to-noise ratio (SNR) and the best contrast-to-noise ratio (CNR), and will vary depending on the chosen contrast enhancing agent. Paramagnetic materials have a strong effect on T1, thus T1 weighted imaging protocols,

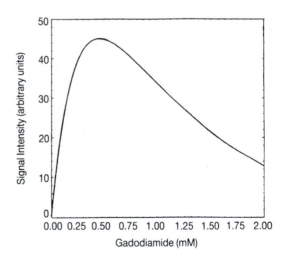

Figure 10-2. Change in signal intensity versus concentration (mM or mmol/L) of a gadodiamide injection calculated using the equation, $SI = 100(1 - e^{-TR/T_1})e^{-TE/T_2}$. T1 and T2 values were measured in vitro at 10 MHz. Within clinical dosage ranges (0.01 to 0.3 mmol/kg) currently used for paramagnetic agents, the reduction in T (which results in a loss of signal intensity) is dominated by T1 reduction, leading to an overall increase in signal intensity.

which minimize competing T2 effects, are desirable. Conversely ferromagnetic, superparamagnetic (T2), and susceptibility (T2*) enhancing agents rely on T2 weighted imaging sequences[22] to maximize contrast enhancement.

Several principles guide the development of MR contrast agents.

- The drug must have the ability to alter the signal intensity of protons in its vicinity, as outlined above. Relaxivity is the measure of a compound's potency at altering T1 and T2 relaxation rates.
- The drug must demonstrate differential distribution to either normal or abnormal tissues. Tissue-specific distribution is a sought-after characteristic of effective contrast media.
- The amount of material injected per unit of body weight (the dosage expressed as mmol/kg) must not induce excessive adverse reactions (i.e., toxicological responses in recipients experienced at a rate presenting unacceptable risk in the target patient population).

BIOLOGICAL FACTORS

Distribution

Achieving selective distribution of the signal modifying entity, be it a paramagnetic ion or superparamagnetic particle, has been an extremely active area in contrast media research. The first class of contrast agents to be developed for MRI included a series of small metal chelates containing paramagnetic gadolinium ion, Gd^{3+}. The ligands incorporated into these agents include the linear DTPA and DTPA-BMA [Figure 10.1] and the cyclic DOTA and HP-DO3A [Figure 10.3]. The compartmentalization of contrast enhancing agents and the equilibration over time between intravascular and extravascular fluid spaces in the body determine the efficacy of these agents in enhancing their specific target tissues. The kinetics of redistribution of the

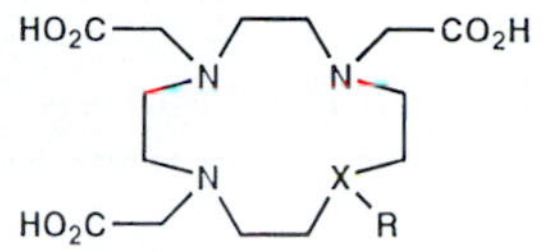

X	R	Acronym
N	-CH$_2$CO$_2$H	DOTA
N	-H	DO3A
N	-CH$_2$CH(OH)CH$_3$	HP-DO3A
N	-CH(CH$_2$OH)CH(OH)CH$_2$OH	DO3A-THB
O		DOXA

Figure 10-3. Schematic diagram of the tetraaza-based macrocycles DOTA, DO3A, HP-DO3A, DO3A-THB, and DOXA.

agents play a major role in predicting the degree of enhancement and its development over time. The pharmacokinetics of these four commercially available small metal chelates are essentially the same with apparent volumes of distribution in the range 0.2–0.3 L/kg (20–30 percent of body weight) similar to the volume of the extracellular fluid (ECF)[23].

Distribution into the ECF is a result of the hydrophilic nature of these agents. The agents do not cross an intact blood–brain barrier (BBB), but will accumulate in brain and CNS regions with a pathologically compromised barrier, providing enhancement of a wide range of conditions including primary and metastatic brain tumors, infections and other inflammatory processes, and cerebrovascular insults[24–26].

Clearance and excretion

The route of elimination and excretion of the ECF agents in man is well understood, and the resultant impact on their efficacy, due to rapid washout and renal excretion, is similar to that of well-known iodinated contrast media. The transient impact of these extracellular contrast agents on soft tissue (in vivo) contrast provides the basis for clinical applications based on the dynamic or

Table 10-2

Kinetics and Distribution of Various Contrast Media in Man

Compound	CNS Dosage	Volume of Distribution, V_d (L/kg)	$t_{1/2}$ Distribution, α (min)	$t_{1/2}$ Elimination, β (min)	Renal Clearance Rate, Cl_r (mL/min/kg)	Plasma Clearance Rate, Cl_p (mL/min/kg)
Diatrizoate	306 mg/kg	0.19	6.8	155.6	1.76	ND*
Iohexol	375 mg/kg	0.27	21.5	123	128**	127**
GdDTPA	0.1 mmol/kg	0.27	7.2	94.8	1.76	1.94
GdDOTA	0.1 mmol/kg	0.17	7.2	91.2	ND	1.31
GdDTPA-BMA	0.1 mmol/kg	0.19	3.7	77.8	1.70	1.78
GdHP-DO3A	0.1 mmol/kg	0.20	12.0	94.2	1.41	1.50

*ND = not determined.
**Determined as mL/min.

temporal nature of contrast uptake and wash-out following administration. Table 10-2 provides elimination and excretion data using the concepts defined below.

- CNS dosage is the dosage of contrast media required for CNS applications.
- V_d is the volume of distribution of the drug; a hypothetical volume of body fluid that would be required to dissolve the total amount of drug at the same concentration as that found in the blood.
- $t_{1/2}\alpha$ is the distribution phase half-life; the time necessary for drug concentration to reduce by one-half in the central compartment of a two compartment model.
- $t_{1/2}\beta$ is the elimination phase half-life; the time necessary for the drug concentration to reduce by one-half in blood, plasma, or serum, after equilibrium has been reached.
- Cl_r is the renal clearance rate; the hypothetical plasma volume of the unmetabolized drug which is cleared in 1 min through the kidneys.
- Cl_p is the plasma clearance rate; the volume of plasma from which a drug is extracted,

per minute, as a result of all elimination pathways.

Nonspecific contrast media are characterized by lack of tissue selectivity, short plasma half-lives, and simple distribution throughout the extracellular (ECF) fluid space. Clearance of contrast media from the body can occur by glomerular filtration, active secretion, or a combination thereof. The extent of clearance from the ECF and the rate of systemic clearance and elimination through the kidneys is controlled primarily by the molecular weight of the agent; the glomerular filtration molecular weight cutoff is approximately 40 kD. All low molecular weight complexes currently in use for MR contrast enhancement are rapidly cleared from the intravascular space (elimination half-lives on the order of 100 min)[27–29] and excreted by the kidneys. The charge and lipophilicity of an agent play a significant role in controlling its rate of clearance from the plasma, since binding to indigenous proteins (e.g., serum albumin) may alter biodistribution and delay clearance.

GdDTPA-BMA, demonstrates clearance and elimination characteristics typical for agents in this class. In the preclinical evaluation of GdDTPA-BMA, rats were injected with

[153]GdDTPA-BMA. In 2 h, 71.6 percent of the label was excreted in urine, and by 24 h, 88.1 percent of the label had been recovered in urine, while 3.7 percent was recovered in feces. A small fraction of the residual gadolinium label is found in the liver. In mice, at seven days post injection, the amount of gadolinium in the liver was 0.043 percent of the administered dose, which decreased six-fold over the next two weeks[30].

Toxicity

Assessment of the safety of a magnetopharmaceutical is carried out through detailed toxicological studies. The four main purposes of toxicity testing are as follows.

1. To assess the toxic potential of a material.
2. To determine the type of hazard a material might represent.
3. To elucidate mechanisms of toxicity.
4. To generate reliable data for use in risk–benefit assessment.

The sources of toxicity following the introduction of foreign drug substance into the body are manifold and are dependent on both the route and rate of administration. The terms acute and chronic are often used in connection with toxicity and refer to the time span after which toxic effects are manifested.

Acute toxicity is a measure of exposure to a material, and is generally determined on the basis of one or more short, high intensity dosages to an animal within a defined time span (up to 24 h). It is a common misconception that acute toxicology is only concerned with death as an outcome of exposure. Acute toxicology is concerned with all effects resulting from acute exposure to materials; generally it is the adverse effects that are of most concern in toxicology, but beneficial effects may also be important. One example of a beneficial toxicologic effect currently under investigation is the mitochondrial superoxide dismutase (SOD) mimetic activity of MnDPDP, a manganese based liver directed MRI contrast agent. It has shown SOD-mimetic activity in animal models and may be useful as a cardioprotective agent[31].

Chronic toxicity is a longer-term phenomenon, generally including multiple dosages at a predetermined level to assess the effects of long-term buildup of a test substance over a period of weeks (out to years) on an appropriate animal model. The dosage and time periods tested are usually scaled as some multiple of the intended clinical use. For example, therapeutic agents require more intensive chronic toxicity testing than diagnostic agents that are primarily used only once.

Subacute or subchronic exposures are referred to as both multiple exposures and continuous exposure over a short time span, but in excess of 24 h. It is generally accepted that these exposures extend over a period not exceeding 10 percent of the target species life span. Diagnostic MR contrast agents are generally subjected to subchronic toxicity testing over a period of 21 to 28 days.

Metabolism of drugs may be beneficial if the metabolites are nontoxic and rapidly eliminated. However, in some situations, a metabolite may be more toxic than the parent compound. While some drugs are rapidly metabolized either by enzymes in the plasma (in the case of intravenously administered drugs) or by various target organs, others pass through the mammalian system essentially unaltered (notably such compounds as GdDTPA and GdDTPA-BMA).

Toxicity can arise from six primary sources, the first two of which are of critical importance in the design of magnetopharmaceuticals.

Chemical Interactions Chemotoxicity is broadly defined as the inherent toxicity of a particular chemical structure, having the ability to alter the structure or function of biological matter. Contrast media, on a dose-dependent basis, manifest toxicity in a variety of ways which include the inhibition of platelet aggregation, mechanisms of coagulation, erythrocyte fragility and morphology, and the inhibition of enzymes such as lysozyme and acetylcholinesterase[32–34]. Physical effects of mass, such as osmolality or cardiovascular effects of intravascular volume overload, are considered separately (see below), independent of potential chemical interactions. Immunoreactivity, carcinogenicity, mutagenicity, and teratogenicity are often classified separately, in order to organize analysis of a complex series of biological phenomena initiated by some (often unknown) chemical event.

Paramagnetic MR contrast enhancing agents generally consist of a metal ion bonded with an organic moiety (ligand) to provide a metal chelate complex. The metal ion and ligand have their own inherent toxicities, determined by the abilities of each to bind to endogenous metals and ligands (often proteins or cofactors) in the body. Both the ligand and its metal chelate complex are susceptible to a variety of enzymatic processes in the body, notably hydrolysis, amide and ester degradation, and reduction or oxidation. These processes generate metabolized products which can have a radically altered biodistribution compared with that of the parent compound.

In addition the dissociation of a metal chelate complex releases free, often highly toxic, metal ions into the body[35]. The different charge, lipophilicity or hydrophilicity, and binding avidity to other donor atoms in the body determine the extent of the toxicity of an individual metal ion. Similarly, the innate toxicity of ligands freed by dissociation from the metal ion to which they are initially bound is determined by the same factors, as well as by the extent of their ability to bind to the variety of metal ions which in vivo are already fulfilling vital tasks (primarily Zn^{2+}, Cu^{2+}, $Fe^{2+/3+}$ and Ca^{2+}).

Osmolality and Viscosity A separate contribution to the toxic effect of intravenously injected drugs results from the alteration of the osmotic balance of plasma, which is normally around 290 mOsm/kg. A material that is injected without perturbing this osmotic balance will have little osmotoxic effect. However, chemically inert or benign matter such as glucose or mannitol, when injected in sufficient concentration to shift

serum osmolality can cause hyperosmotic shock. Charged contrast media, which by definition include two or more charged particles, such as gadopentetate dimeglumine (a three particle system) can have osmolalities (depending on their concentration) as high as 2000 mOsm/kg in a solution provided for injection. Intravenous injection of sufficient quantities of hypertonic material will transiently increase serum osmolality. The natural response to osmotic load is dilution by diffusion of extracellular and intracellular water into the vascular space, accompanied by urinary excretion of the osmotically active material. Hyperosmotic shocks include hyponatremia, hyperkalemia, and kidney failure, while passage through the brain of a bolus of a hyperosmolar solution can disrupt the blood–brain barrier, causing severe nausea and even death[36]. Conversely, a bolus injection or slow infusion of large volumes of a hyperosmolar solution (under 290 mOsm/kg) can cause hemolysis.

These issues, and associated adverse events, have been well documented for a variety of iodinated X-ray contrast media[36,37] and newer generations of radiographic and MRI contrast media are lower osmolality (primarily nonionic) agents. Table 10-3 indicates the extent to which ionic and nonionic hypertonic contrast media can impact the osmotic balance in plasma (calculations assume 2.5 L of plasma in circulation).

The viscosity of an agent is often an important consideration, relating to patient comfort and efficacy. Viscosity limits the rate of injection in a manner inversely proportional to the syringe needle or catheter diameter.

Anaphylactic Reactions Anaphylactic reactions that can result from the administration of contrast media are generally not associated with antibody-related responses, so the term anaphylactoid is used to describe anaphylactic-like reactions with contrast media. Minor anaphylactoid reactions, for example mild flushing, erythema, and scattered urticaria are relatively common events with ionic X-ray contrast agents; 5–6 percent of patients experience a mild

Table 10-3

Contrast Agent Osmolality

Agent	Stock Solution (mOsm/kg)	Dose (mL)	Percent Change in Osmolality of Plasma
Diatrizoate	1500	150	+24%
Iohexol 300	616	150	+9%
GdDTPA	1940	10	+2%
GdDTPA-BMA	790	10	+1%

reaction[34]. Moderate anaphylactoid reactions occur in less than 2 percent of examinations and severe life-threatening reactions occur at the rate of 1–2 per 1000 examinations[38]. Mortality rates range from 1 per 10,000 to 1 per 75,000 examinations[39].

There is no agreement concerning the etiology of the anaphylactoid reaction. Several inciting factors may exist, any of which can potentially trigger a reaction, however, the final determinant is the individual patient's reactivity. Stress and fear, histamine release, complement activation and coagulopathy have all been implicated. It has been suggested that the CNS may be a common initiator (or a mediator) of these adverse reactions. Some segments of the population exhibit a higher rate of anaphylactoid reactions; these include patients with a history of atopy, patients between the ages of 20 and 29, and patients who have previously experienced anaphylactoid reactions[38].

Anaphylactoid reactions including cutaneous, respiratory, and cardiovascular elements have been observed in response to gadolinium contrast agent administration[40,41]. Some of these adverse events have been severe. Researchers have shown that gadopentetate dimeglumine (under experimental conditions which have been optimized for antibody production) is capable of inducing an IgG response in rats[42]. Current recommendations for the use of these agents advocate caution, particularly in the case of patients with a known clinical hypersensitivity, a

history of asthma, or other allergic respiratory disorders. In general, diagnostic pro-cedures involving the use of contrast agents should be conducted under the supervision of a physician trained in the management of adverse reactions.

Carcinogenicity and Mutagenicity The potential hazard of materials which, due to their interaction with genetic mechanisms, result in an inheritable change (mutation) is a further source of toxicity which is assessed in preclinical evaluation. Tests usually performed on MRI contrast agents include the Ames test, mammalian cell forward gene mutation assay, rat hepatocyte primary culture/DNA repair study, and cytogenetic assay.

Teratogenicity Developmental toxicity studies, referred to as teratology or segment I, II, and III studies, assess the impact of contrast media on the development of a new organism from conception through birth and beyond. The first guidelines for these studies were promulgated by the U.S. Food and Drug Administration in 1966. A segment I, or fertility and reproduction, study is designed to assess effects on male and female fertility, general reproductive function, and the development of offspring. A segment II study assesses test animals for potential adverse effects from chemical exposure during major organogenesis in embryo and fetal development, including the production of structural alterations (teratogenic effects). The segment III, or perinatal and postnatal, studies involve the treatment of pregnant animals from a certain day of gestation through lactation: parturition, litter size and weight, and growth and viability of offspring are monitored.

Formulation The composition in which the MR-active component of a contrast enhancing agent is introduced into an organism has a major bearing on its distribution and toxicity. In order to function safely and effectively as an MR contrast enhancing agent, materials need to be soluble (at least to provide 100 mM to 1 M solutions), or dispersed homogeneously in a predominantly aqueous medium. Contrast agents need to have acceptable viscosity (in the range 0–3 cP) and osmolality (in the range 300–2000 mOsm/kg). All materials included in the injected formulation must be stable in vivo, or their metabolized products need to be nontoxic. It is necessary for these agents to have a shelf life of at least one year while maintaining a sterile, pyrogen-free, concentration-constant composition. Various components which are not MR-active are used to adjust the above properties to provide physiologically tolerable and safe media and are known as excipients.

In the case of metal chelate complexes, additional quantities of free ligand (often as a calcium or sodium salt) or the calcium complex of the ligand are added to bind any excess free metal[35]. This excess ligand has been observed to have a surprisingly large effect on the acute toxicity characteristics of these formulations. Sodium chloride (to elevate osmolality) and various other excipients are commonly included to control the pH of contrast media formulations to prolong shelf life, to ensure stability, and to alter viscosity.

Very often paramagnetic chelate complexes are formulated as quaternary amine salts, i.e., an amine or amino sugar is protonated to provide a counterion with a single positive charge. N-methylglucamine (meglumine, abbreviated NMG) and lysine counterions are typical examples. These cations appear to have a beneficial effect on

the toxicity of metal chelate complex anions such as $Gd(DOTA)^{1-}$ and $Gd(DTPA)^{2-}$.

MAGNETOPHARMACEUTICALS

The development of contrast media for enhancement of MR images has progressed significantly beyond the early focus on low molecular weight ionic paramagnetic metal chelates[43] such as $MnEDTA^{2-}$ and $GdDTPA^{2-}$. In recent years, polymeric materials, metalloporphyrins, stable organic free radicals, hyperpolarized gases, liposomal formulations, metal particulates, molecular oxygen, and chelates connected to monoclonal antibodies or target-specific proteins, fragments, and small peptides have been studied.

These developments, in many respects, parallel the development of radiopharmaceuticals from the late 1960s where nonspecific agents (with an emphasis on the demonstration of pathologic anatomy) gave way to second-generation scintigraphic agents targeted at specific organ function or disease. Early animal and human imaging studies of simple metal ion salts[8,44] and chelates[45,46] rapidly led to the recognition that the exquisite resolution afforded by MRI could be further enhanced, potentially even coupled with true functional or metabolic imaging, through the use of contrast agents designed to target a specific organ or disease state.

Metal Salts

The first true MRI contrast enhancing agent examined in vivo was $MnCl_2$. It was used to demonstrate contrast enhancement of canine myocardial tissues[47] due to the uptake by myocytes of the paramagnetic manganous ion, which contains five unpaired electrons coupled with the longest electron spin relaxation time of the transition elements[48]. Ferric ion, which also contains five unpaired electrons, is less effective than manganese as a proton relaxation enhancing (PRE) agent, but has been utilized as a gastrointestinal contrast enhancing agent[44]. However, ferric ion produced gastrointestinal irritation and further studies were discontinued. Gadolinium chloride showed efficacy early as a PRE agent[49], but unresolved questions regarding its in vivo distribution and toxicity precluded its further development.

Biodistribution The distribution of the transition metal elements in the body has long been studied due to the essential nature of these elements as trace elements (outside iron) in mammalian nutrition. The biological roles of iron and manganese have been long studied[50–53], and the impact of small added quantities (as MRI contrast enhancing agents) of these chelated metal ions (or even simple salts such as $MnCl_2$ or $FeCl_3$) to the metabolic pool of these elements has so far been shown to be minor. The transport and storage of ferric iron (utilizing hemoglobin, transferrin and other proteins, and ferritin) as well as its biological distribution and function is well understood. Manganese concentration in whole blood ranges from 8 to 9 µg/L, and its comprehensive biodistribution (from 3 min to 24 h) as $^{54}MnCl_2$ has been determined. Manganese localizes primarily in mitochondria hence its presence in pancreas, liver, kidney, and heart[54,55].

Simple metal salts such as ferric ammonium citrate[59] (Geritol) have been used as contrast enhancing agents for gastrointestinal imaging. Technetium pyrophosphate has been used to image acute myocardial infarctions due to its affinity for calcium deposits in infarcated myocardium[56]. The analogous paramagnetic metal salt ferric pyrophosphate has also been tested and shown to be efficacious at dosages of 350 mg/kg as an MR contrast enhancing agent of acute myocardial infarction[57]. However, significant respiratory toxicity was observed at dosages of 190 mg/kg and this precluded its further development.

The biodistribution and toxicity of naked lanthanide metal salts has been studied for many decades[58] and a variety of subchronic effects documented[59,60]. Chelating agents increase the

R_1	R_2	Acronym
-CO$_2$H	-CO$_2$H	EDTA
-CH$_2$N(CH$_2$CO$_2$H)$_2$	-CH$_2$N(CH$_2$CO$_2$H)$_2$	TTHA
(PO$_3$H$_2$ pyridine ring)	(PO$_3$H$_2$ pyridine ring)	DPDP

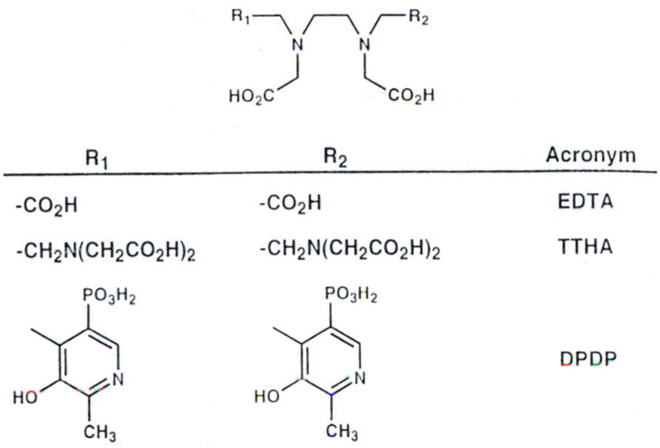

Figure 10-4. Schematic diagram of EDTA-based acyclic ligands EDTA, TTHA, and DPDP.

rate of elimination of lanthanides from the body[61]. The kinetics of distribution and clearance for a range of lanthanides[62] bound to weak (NTA) and stronger (EDTA) chelators [Figure 10-4] have been studied in detail; the strong chelate complexes were almost completely renally excreted while the weaker complexes deposited metal in liver spleen and bone (consistent with the distribution of uncomplexed lanthanide ions).

Metal Chelate Complexes

Metal ions are able to bind to a variety of donor atoms, resulting in metal complexes through the formation of coordinate covalent bonds between a metal cation and an electron donating ligand. Coordinate bonds consist of equally shared electron pairs donated to the metal ion by the ligand. The number of sites available around a metal ion for coordinate bonding by various ligands defines the coordination sphere and coordination number (typically six for transition metal ions and eight through twelve for lanthanide ions) of a given metal ion.

Relaxation parameters are often reduced when metal ions are chelated (lowering the number of bound water molecules), especially in the coordinatively saturated situation where there are no longer available open binding sites within the first coordination sphere (inner sphere) of the paramagnetic ion. However, where even a single water molecule is associated within the first coordination sphere, significant relaxation potency is retained[63]. The T2* relaxivity properties of gadolinium and dysprosium are largely unaffected by coordination of a metal ion with a chelating ligand, or by the presence of bound inner sphere water molecules. This T2* susceptibility contrast effect results from compartmentalization of the contrast agent within and without the vasculature, causing a (long-distance) loss of phase coherence of water protons in surrounding tissues which results in a reduction of signal intensity when used with a heavily T2 weighted pulse sequence.

The ability of paramagnetic transition and lanthanide metal ions (when chelated by a variety of ligands) to influence the proton relaxation times of protons in water molecules is well established[20]. Concerns that reduction of the number of water molecules bound within the first coordination sphere would dramatically reduce the ability of the resultant complexes to enhance proton relaxation processes on neighboring solvent water molecules were shown to be groundless[64]. A number of in vitro studies using GdEDTA and GdDTPA complexes demonstrated that while chelate formation did lower relaxation enhancement efficacy (as one might predict, due to fewer water molecules being available within the first coordination sphere), these complexes could still function as efficacious contrast agents.

The exclusion of water completely from the first coordination sphere of coordinatively saturated metal chelate complexes might have been predicted to eliminate completely the ability of such complexes to function as contrast agents. The mechanism by which these outer sphere relaxation agents operate is not well understood, but has been the subject of studies of manganese complexes of EDTA, EGTA, and NOTA [Figure 10-5]. The results of these studies[65,66] suggest that outer sphere interactions,

translational diffusion, and hydrogen bonding may all be important elements.

The design of metal chelate complexes as MR contrast enhancing agents has, however, focused much more on the use of coordinatively unsaturated metal complexes which function through conventional inner sphere relaxation mechanisms. The need for complexation arises, of course from the need both to modify the biodistribution and elimination of free metal ions from the body and the need to lower their toxicity. The required doses of such compounds (roughly 0.05–3 g of metal per patient) greatly exceed those of metal ions or complexes used in radioscintigraphy (Table 10-1). However, iodine-containing contrast agents are used in CT and other radiologic procedures at much higher doses than MR agents ($\sim$50–150 g iodine per patient). With the development of relatively nontoxic paramagnetic metal chelate complexes as MRI contrast agents, the contrast enhanced MRI procedure is likely to be safer than related CT procedures due to both the lower quantities of injectate used and the lack of ionizing radiation.

The synthesis of new contrast agents presently strikes a balance between sufficiently low

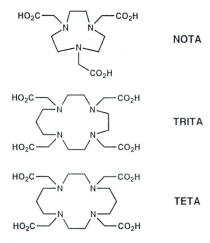

Figure 10-5. Schematic diagram of the macrocycles NOTA, TETA, and TRITA.

toxicity and adequate clinical efficacy (relaxivity). Knowledge of the chemical bonding and equilibrium processes involved in metal chelate formation and dissociation[35] is important to the development of new metal-based MRI contrast agents as well as providing an understanding of the safety and utility of existing agents.

Stability and Toxicity Metal chelate complexes arise from the formation of a complex between a single ligand that forms more than one coordinate bond to a metal ion. The multiple bonding of a single ligand is termed the chelate effect[67] and results in a significant increase in the stability of the metal complex formed. This leads to a thermodynamic concept termed the stability constant, a measure of how well a metal–ligand entity stays together.

Further, as a potential metal binding site within a ligand becomes more encapsulated, or preformed (for example through the use of a rigid macrocyclic structure), the reorganization entropy upon metal incorporation is decreased. This leads to a relatively higher stability constant for metal binding (evident, for example, in the greater stability of GdDOTA^{1-} relative to GdDTPA^{2-}, see below), and is termed the macrocyclic or clathrochelate effect[67].

The chelation of naked metal ions will markedly affect their relaxation properties, as well as the toxicity of the metal ions themselves described earlier. Solvent molecules have greatly restricted access to the metal ion nucleus (the inner coordination sphere), thus the transfer of unpaired electron spin information (magnetization) is less effective in chelate complexes than in free metal ion systems. On the other hand the solubility and in vivo toxicity properties of the free metal ions are also radically altered upon chelation, generally imparting beneficial characteristics for contrast media usage, through a lowering of toxicity and modification of biodistribution, plasma residues, and elimination routes.

Ideally, a specific localization of the paramagnetic chelate is desired to maximize its diagnostic value. For MR contrast enhancement agents, it is sufficient that the relaxation rates of the target tissue be enhanced relative to other tissues. The chemical structure of the metal chelate effectively determines its appropriate in vivo biodistribution and excretion routes. Complete clearance of the agent is desirable to reduce acute as well as chronic toxicological effects.

The in vivo metal chelate stability and toxicity are intimately related. Toxic effects from metal chelates can arise from the following.

> The presence of free metal ion due to chelate dissociation and possible transmetallation (the release of bound metal ion by a ligand in the presence of another metal ion for which the ligand has a much greater affinity).
> The presence of free ligand due to chelate dissociation.
> The intact metal chelate.
> Metabolites from the first three processes.

A balance needs to be struck between the requirement for a highly stable metal chelate complex, which results in part from the ability of a ligand to provide donor atoms to occupy most (if not all) coordination sites on a metal ion and the requirement that the high relaxivity of a paramagnetic ion be preserved as much as possible. Chelation can reduce relaxation processes but does not eliminate them, while still reducing the toxicity of a metal ion and providing desirable biodistribution characteristics to provide a useful agent for MRI contrast enhancement.

The lanthanide metals have no known mammalian function and, until their introduction as MRI contrast enhancement agents, biological studies were conducted for toxicologic reasons. Exposure to exogenous lanthanide complexes which are not stabilized in vivo results in transmetallation of free lanthanide to endogenous ligands (e.g., plasma proteins) with concomitant toxicity. Metal chelates have less avidity for binding to proteins, enzymes and membranes than do metal ions. Their in vivo calcium sequestering ability is greatly reduced, compared to that of free ligands. The effective in vivo stability of gadolinium chelates can be assessed by radiolabeling complexes with ^{153}Gd ($\gamma 97$ to $103\,keV$, $t_{1/2}$: $242\,d$) and studying the subsequent biodistribution over time of the radiolabeled tracer through well-counting or scintigraphic means[68]. Serial analysis of elimination, distribution and pharmacokinetic information provides results which can be extrapolated during the drug design and testing process to potential human applicability.

An understanding of the factors that affect the in vivo stability of a gadolinium complex is particularly important in predicting the degree of complex dissociation and subsequently in explaining its measured acute toxicity. This concept has also led to the development of formulations which minimize the amount of gadolinium released in vivo[35]. Ligands that exhibit enhanced selectivity for gadolinium over competing endogenous metal ions should yield highly stable and hence relatively nontoxic complexes.

A major consideration in determining the utility of a given complex with the ability to influence relaxation processes of nearby water molecules as a contrast enhancing agent is its in vivo toxicity and thus its in vivo stability. The simplistic approach towards evaluating stability, in which only published thermodynamic stability constant information is considered, has been shown to be inappropriate and even misleading. More thorough critical analyses of the importance of conditional stability data, and the competition in vivo for ligands by other metal ions in plasma (most notably Zn^{2+}, Cu^{2+}, Fe^{3+}, and Ca^{2+}) as well as competition for gadolinium by other biological ligands have recently appeared[35,69].

Linear Complexes

Chemistry   The utility of a variety of different ligands (especially EDTA) to detoxify naked metal ions was established as early as 1952[70]. This approach[64] suggested the application of EDTA and other linear polyaminopolycarboxylates such as DTPA and TTHA as chelates to reduce gadolinium metal ion toxicity, and formed the basis for the preparation of useful in vivo MR relaxation-based contrast agents. The ligand DTPA (diethylenetriaminepentaacetic acid) was first prepared in 1946[71] and its metal-binding properties were rapidly established[72].

The nonionic gadolinium MR contrast enhancing agent, GdDTPA-BMA, was prepared by combining gadolinium with the functionalized DTPA derivative DTPA-bis(methylamide), DTPA-BMA, which contains only three anionic carboxylate binding sites, to neutralize the cationic charge ($+3$) of the gadolinium ion. This neutral compound does not require the addition of sodium or NMG counterions, and is formulated as a low osmolar agent. A variety of different unsubstituted and hydroxyl substituted bisamide complexes have been evaluated, although none have yet shown sufficient improvement over GdDTPA-BMA to warrant clinical development.

Ranges of linear chelates have been utilized with metal ions such as manganese, dysprosium or ferric iron as well as gadolinium to impart specific properties to the resulting chelate complexes. Their utility lies in the degree of target specificity, beyond the extracellular fluid space, imparted by design of the ligand, or in their magnetic susceptibility (T2*) properties and other broader applications.

Examples of linear chelating agents that exhibit a degree of target specificity include the proposed hepatobiliary agents GdBOPTA and GdEOB-DTPA and the recently introduced Teslascan® (mangafodipir, MnDPDP). It has a molecular weight of 691.4 (as the free acid) and the structural formula illustrated in Figure 10-4. This complex is surprisingly stable to Mn(II) hydrolysis and has the highest known thermodynamic stability constant ($K_{therm} = 15.10$) of any Mn(II) chelate complex[73].

Gadolinium benzyloxypropionatotetraacetic acid, GdBOPTA, or gadobenate dimeglumine is a GdDTPA derivative[74] that contains a benzyloxy-methyl group in the backbone of the metal chelate [Figure 10-1]. It is believed this substituent group provides the required handle for the anionic hepatocyte receptor that also handles bromosulfophthalein[75,76]. The X-ray structure shows the gadolinium ion to be nine-coordinate, with the inclusion of a water molecule in the first coordination sphere.

The introduction of a lipophilic ethoxybenzyl (EOB) moiety onto the carbon backbone of GdDTPA provided the more lipophilic disodium GdEOB-DTPA [Figure 10-1]. The values of T1 relaxivity of GdEOB-DTPA were $5.3 \, \text{m}M^{-1} \text{s}^{-1}$ (20 MHz, 39 °C) in water, which dramatically increased to $16.6 \, \text{m}M^{-1} \text{s}^{-1}$ in the liver. Its high relaxivity in liver tissue is thought to be the result of confinement of the contrast agent to the intracellular space of the hepatocyte, wherein protein binding and increases in the microvisco-sity surrounding the agent lead to changes in the rotational correlation times, increasing T1 relax-ivity. Following intravenous administration GdEOB-DTPA is distributed principally into the extracellular fluid space but undergoes both renal and extrarenal elimination[77]. Comparative physicochemical and biological properties of these three contrast agents[78,79] are given in Table 10-4.

A more dramatic example of using protein binding to increase T1 relaxivity is demonstrated by the investigational MS-325. Also using a lipophilic moiety (a diphenylcyclohexyl group) attached to the gadolinium chelate backbone through a phosphodiester linkage, this agent exhibits one of the highest relaxivities observed for a gadolinium chelate, a ten-fold increase at 0.5 T. While the relaxivity is $6.6 \, \text{m}M^{-1} \text{s}^{-1}$ in buffered saline, when tested in human plasma, 96 percent of the agent binds protein, and relaxivity increases to $53.5 \, \text{m}M^{-1} \text{s}^{-1}$. The high degree of protein binding prevents rapid extravasation into the extravascular space, in vivo, allowing blood pool applications to be pursued with a 1–2 h imaging window[80,81].

Pharmacology Studies to determine the biodistribution and pharmacokinetics of metal complexes of EDTA and DTPA commenced as early as the 1950s[62]. EDTA at this time was commonly being used, as its calcium or sodium salt, for metal ion detoxification[70] and the uptake and renal clearance of its metal complexes were well documented. The use of DTPA to enhance renal excretion of the lanthanides, and applica-tions in nuclear medicine with Tc and Yb com-plexes resulted in a good understanding of their biodistribution. Detailed studies of the human biodistribution and clearance kinetics at clinically relevant dosages of GdDTPA[28], GdDOTA[29], GdDTPA-BMA[82,83], and GdHPDO3A[84] are described in Table 10-2.

All these agents behave as extracellular paramagnetic contrast agents exhibiting fast rapid renal clearance. Equilibration into the intersti-tium of both normal and pathological tissues can

Table 10-4

MRI Liver Agents

	MnDPDP	GdEOB–DTPA	GdBOPTA
Molecular weight g/mol	691	1064	1058
Charge	2^-	2^-	2^-
r_1, $\text{m}M^{-1} \text{s}^{-1}$ (20 MHz, 37 °C)	2.4	5.3	4.4
r_2, $\text{m}M^{-1} \text{s}^{-1}$ (20 MHz, 37 °C)	3.0	6.1	5.6
LD$_{50}$ (mice), mmol/kg	5.0	7.5	6
LD$_{50}$/effective dosage	500	≥ 75	≥ 60

result in the loss of contrast between the two tissues and this was recently demonstrated using a dynamic MR scanning technique[78]. Maximum tumor-to-liver contrast was observed 1–2 min after administration of the contrast agent, with complete loss of contrast in as little as 8 min. Hence, timing of the imaging protocol is critical with extracellular contrast agents to take advantage of the signal enhancing effect of the agent. This limited imaging window restricts the clinical use of nonspecific extracellular contrast agents in, for example, the liver.

Preclinical evaluation of the liver imaging agent MnDPDP consisted of imaging, pharmacology, toxicology, and drug metabolism studies[85]. MnDPDP administered intravenously at dosages of 0.01–0.05 mmol/kg enhanced the visualization of pathological conditions such as liver tumors and increased the signal-to-noise ratio (SNR) from the liver[86] by up to 200 percent. The complex distributes primarily to the liver and small intestine with less than 1 percent in the cecum, heart, lungs, spleen, brain, large intestine, and stomach 30 min after injection as $[^{54}Mn]DPDP$.

The pharmacokinetics of $GdBOPTA^{2-}$ in animals demonstrates rapid hepatocellular uptake and excretion of 2–50 percent of the administered dose into the bile[79]. The remainder of the drug undergoes urinary excretion. The extent of liver versus kidney excretion has recently been found to be strongly dependent on the species studied. In the rat, elimination takes place almost to the same extent (i.e., 50 percent in the first 8 h) through biliary and urinary excretion. In the rabbit[87] the cumulative urinary excretion is 64 percent while the biliary elimination is only 24 percent. In man GdBOPTA was excreted unchanged in the urine in amounts corresponding to 76–94 percent of the injected dose[88] with 2–4 percent eliminated fecally. GdBOPTA appears to be excreted primarily renally in an essentially unmetabolized form, but subchronic toxicity data and complete metabolism studies remain unreported. In animals the drug was highly efficacious, with marked T1 shortening and resultant increase in hepatic signal intensity. Since liver tumors show little or no uptake of the drug, liver-to-tumor image contrast was greatly increased on T1 weighted images.

The newest T1 based hepatobiliary contrast agent GdEOB-DTPA is chemically similar to GdBOPTA and has been reported to show greater biliary excretion in rats (70 percent versus 50 percent, respectively). GdEOB-DTPA is similar to other liver-specific paramagnetic compounds, a pronounced effect occurs in liver which may be due to GdEOB-DTPA binding to protein[89]. Its blood half-life is very short due to its renal excretion and rapid hepatocellular uptake. Unlike GdDTPA, GdEOB-DTPA is also specifically taken up by the hepatocytes and is excreted by the bile and feces. The hepatocyte specific uptake of GdEOB-DTPA is thought to be related to the low degree of protein binding (10–17 percent) in rats, dogs, and monkeys. The process of dose-dependent and species-dependent biliary excretion involves a capacity-limited step involving a transport mechanism (possibly the albumin binding organic anion transport system)[90].

With the exception of the liver, GdEOB-DTPA is distributed in the extravascular space and quantitatively eliminated, apparently unmetabolized. The excretion route of GdEOB-DTPA is primarily via the hepatocytes into the bile and feces. Hepatocyte uptake is accomplished by a specific carrier-mediated mechanism that is known to eliminate exogenous anionic molecules from the body[91].

Toxicity Preclinical pharmacology and toxicology studies carried out during the development of GdDTPA[92] have shown that in vivo demetalation of GdDTPA, with the deposition of free gadolinium in the liver and bone, poses a problem for applications of GdDTPA which require any significant residence time in the body beyond rapid clearance into the extracellular space and fast renal excretion.

A further drawback associated with the dimeglumine formulation of GdDTPA is its high osmolality in 500 mM solution of approximately 2000 mOsm/kg, compared with blood at approximately 300 mOsm/kg[93]. This osmolality is comparable to that of some iodinated contrast media, and raises the possibility that the adverse events associated with the use of hyperosmotic ionic media would also be observed in MRI (although the biological osmolar load is significantly less for MRI contrast media compared to that imposed by X-ray contrast media, as shown in Table 10-3)[36,37]. Additionally, while GdDTPA is extremely safe (assessed from LD$_{50}$ acute toxicity data in mice) at a dose range wherein a high signal intensity could be obtained using T1 weighted techniques (typically around 0.1 mmol/kg), there are a variety of applications for contrast enhancing agents above this dosage level for which GdDTPA is not optimal (based on osmolality and toxicity considerations).

The nonionic contrast enhancement agent GdDTPA-BMA behaves as a single particle in aqueous solution. It has an osmolarity of about 750 mOsm/kg at 500 mM concentration: while not isoosmolar with blood, this represents a major improvement when compared with 500 mM GdDTPA. This is reflected in the sixfold improvement in acute toxicity when assessed by intravenous administration, the LD$_{50}$ in mice is 34 mmol/kg, as gadodiamide injection (when formulated with 5 mol% of the calcium sodium form of the ligand DTPA-BMA) versus approximately 6.0 mmol/kg for formulated (dimeglumine) GdDTPA[9].

The LD$_{50}$ of MnDPDP was 5 mmol/kg (approximately 500 times the anticipated clinical dosage) when administered as an intravenous bolus injection in mice. The LD$_{50}$ of MnCl$_2$ in mice was 0.3 mmol/kg compared to 5.5–10 mmol/kg for GdDTPA and 10.6 mmol/kg for GdDOTA[9,94].

Other readily available acyclic polyaminopolycarboxylates such as EDTA, TTHA (Figure 10-5), and NTA have been evaluated (as their respective gadolinium complexes) as contrast enhancement agents. GdEDTA (LD$_{50}$ 0.3 mmol/kg in rats) has been shown to be even more toxic than GdCl$_3$ (LD$_{50}$ 0.5 mmol/kg in rats)[17] since it is able to labilize gadolinium (log $K_{stab} \sim 17$) for distribution to a wide variety of sites in vivo (primarily skeletal bone) while GdCl$_3$ rapidly forms insoluble hydroxide particles which aggregate in the liver and only slowly release gadolinium. GdTTHA, on the other hand, has an acceptable toxicity profile but with a nine-coordinate ligand (the three backbone amines and six carboxylates all act as donors) the complex is coordinatively saturated. Thus there are no water molecules in the first coordination sphere and the relaxivities are approximately half those of agents such as GdDTPA or GdDTPA-BMA. The complex GdNTA can theoretically exist with a 1:1 stoichiometry (although it has never been isolated) and significant in vivo metal exchange as well as ligand exchange can occur readily. This renders these compounds, as well as GdEDTA, much too toxic for clinical utility.

Cyclic Complexes

Chemistry It was recognized early in the development of gadolinium-based MR contrast enhancement agents that ligands with higher stability and lanthanide selectivity characteristics might provide improved contrast agents[95,96].

The superior properties of polyazapolycarboxylate macrocycles over acyclic ligands as lanthanide-specific chelates, which offered several desirable thermodynamic and kinetic stability properties over acyclic ligands, such as EDTA and DTPA, was long recognized[97]. The early studies[98,99] on DOTA and TETA (Figure 10-4) and on NOTA provided a good working knowledge of the pK_a, stability constants with lanthanides and physical properties of the gadolinium complexes of these ligands. The physical and metal-binding characteristics of GdDOTA made it the best choice from amongst this group of complexes due to the following.

Minimization of steric strain through the formation of eight five-membered rings upon metal complexation.

The macrocyclic effect[100], which is the primary cause of the four to eight orders of magnitude increase in stability over that of complexes containing acyclic ligands (see above).

DTPA takes up gadolinium extremely rapidly, rendering the metal ion kinetically labile in the presence of significant concentrations of competing metal ions and releasing gadolinium in vivo quite readily[101]. However in vitro studies, conducted over 7 days, may not be a good guide to the in vivo stability of these chelate complexes, in the context of plasma clearance half-lives of around 20 min. On the other hand DOTA, consistent with the other polyazacarboxylate macrocycles, is highly kinetically inert and takes up metal ions extremely slowly, consequently releasing them very slowly under competitive (in vivo) conditions. A half-life of 21 days for GdDOTA at pH 1.5 has been determined[102]. The log of the conditional stability constant of GdDOTA at pH 7.0 is 22.2, compared with 17.5 for GdDTPA, and, as discussed earlier, this is a more realistic determinant of complex stability.

GdDOTA has an r_1 of 3.4 mM^{-1}s^{-1} and an r_2 of 4.3 mM^{-1}s^{-1} (20 MHz, 37 °C) in aqueous solution[103]. These relaxivities are very close to those of GdDTPA and the effective clinical utilization of GdDOTA is expected to be similar at a comparable clinical dose (0.1 mmol/kg).

The more desirable characteristics of the nonionic acyclic gadolinium chelate complexes, compared with their ionic congeners, was not lost on contrast agent designers working with macrocyclic complexes, who promptly developed a range of nonionic DO3A (DOTA with three carboxylates) chelate complexes [Figure 10-3].

In attempting to achieve an optimal pharmacological profile with respect to charge balance, use was made of three anionic chelating groups, while the fourth carboxylate moiety was functionalized with a variety of amide, ester, and hydroxylated side chains[104]. The analogy to the newer generation of radiographic contrast is apparent, incorporating both nonionic properties and hydroxyl substituents to control solubility, osmolality, and viscosity in order to provide improvements in toxicity profile, patient comfort, and the freedom to utilize higher dosages safely.

GdDO3A has an osmolality of 400 mOsm/kg in aqueous solution, and an LD$_{50}$ (rats, intravenous) above 10 mmol/kg. The remaining physicochemical, metal binding, stability, and relaxivity properties of GdDO3A parallel very closely those of GdDOTA[105]. The first nonionic derivatized gadolinium macrocyclic complex approved for clinical use, GdHP-DO3A, has an improved biological tolerance profile compared with that of GdDO3A. A very similar new compound, GdDO3A-THB or gadobutrol [Figure 10-3], is also showing promise as a second-generation ECF contrast agent[106,107].

Pharmacology Preclinical development of GdDOTA followed a similar path to GdDTPA with comparative pharmacokinetic and acute toxicity studies[28,108] demonstrating a variety of analogous pharmacologic properties: no measurable accumulation in any organ, rapid clearance (distribution $t_{1/2}$ of 3 min and an elimination $t_{1/2}$ of 18 min, in rats), similar molecular weight, and hydrophilicity.

The foregoing makes it apparent that GdDOTA has been able to fulfill the same clinical needs as those met by GdDTPA[109]. A variety of cerebral and spinal lesions were detected, at the same dose levels, with comparable efficacy to GdDTPA contrast enhanced MRI[110,111]. The macrocyclic complex GdDOTA, gadoteric acid is marketed in Europe as Dotarem™. Recent studies demonstrated its efficacy in enhancing induced mammary tumors in rats, with three dosages studied (0.1, 0.2, and 0.5 mmol/kg) and optimal results observed at 0.2 mmol/kg. Clinical studies have recently demonstrated the efficacy of GdDOTA in the investigation of cardiac occlusion and reperfusion[112].

The 2′-hydroxypropyl derivative of GdDO3A, GdHP-DO3A, or gadoteridol (Figure 10-4) has received FDA approval and is sold in the United States under the brand name ProHance®[113–115]. This agent clears into the extracellular interstitium with a similar kinetic profile to the other ECF contrast enhancing paramagnetic chelates[84] GdDTPA, GdDTPA-BMA and GdDOTA.

Toxicity The superiority of GdDOTA over GdDTPA was shown by an 85 percent improvement in safety factor (the ratio of LD_{50} to the effective dose was 53 for GdDOTA versus 28 for GdDTPA), and by significantly higher stability in serum[116] based on metal retention (less than 2 percent gadolinium released after 150 h compared with 10 to 20 percent gadolinium released from GdDTPA under the same conditions.)

In addition to the battery of preclinical animal toxicology studies performed with GdHP-DO3A to obtain its FDA approval[117], extensive comparative studies evaluating the rates of metal release of a variety of linear and macrocyclic chelate complexes has recently been concluded. These studies reveal that, as expected, there is a greater degree of metal ion release after several weeks by the linear complexes, although the levels of metal released are so uniformly low as to have no perceived clinical significance[118]. The possibility of neurotoxicological phenomena specific to some macrocyclic complexes is also currently under investigation, due to the surprising post-clinical trial adverse event profile observed with ProHance®[119].

Clinical Applications

Since commercial introduction in the United States (1988), the use of ECF MR contrast agents has become commonplace. Currently, about 25 percent of the 13.4 million MRI procedures performed annually in the U.S. incorporate these agents[120]. The agents are used primarily in evaluations of the brain and spine, although additional applications continue to emerge.

Blood–Brain Barrier Defects The blood–brain barrier (BBB), at the level of the cerebral capillaries, limits the size and type of molecules that may pass from the blood stream, protecting the brain. When intact, the BBB prevents nonlipophilic (fat soluble) molecules including the hydrophilic ECF MRI contrast agents from entering the brain. Where disrupted, by tumors or other lesions, these agents accumulate in these regions, resulting in signal enhancement[121].

While contrast agents are currently used in nearly 40 percent of brain MRI scans, these agents are used in virtually all MRI evaluations of patients with actual or suspected neoplastic disease of the brain. Contrast enhanced MR can visualize lesions which would only be seen with difficulty without contrast use and can better delineate lesion extent[24]. The degree and rate of enhancement are used to suggest both type and grade of brain lesions. Extraaxial lesions such as meningiomas, neurinomas, and chrodomas generally enhance very rapidly following administration of ECF contrast agents. Intraaxial tumors such as glioma and astrocytoma demonstrate enhancement more as a function of malignancy. Low-grade glioma tends not to enhance as this tumor invades the brain without significantly disrupting the BBB, whereas the more aggressive glioblastoma and astrocytoma do enhance[122].

Metastatic lesions are not formed from brain cells and do not have a BBB, they frequently enhance intensely after contrast agent administration. This is most helpful in evaluation of patients with clinical signs of metastatic disease, but with negative unenhanced scans, in patients with metastatic lesions that appear treatable with surgery or radiation, and in patients enrolled in clinical cancer therapy trials.

Most contrast enhanced CNS imaging uses the standard 0.1 mmol/kg contrast dose. However, several of the ECF contrast agents have been shown safe at higher dosage, up to 0.3 mmol/kg. The use of higher dose is most helpful in characterizing suspected metastatic lesions. This finding can have a dramatic effect on treatment decision, as patients with only one or two lesions may be candidates for surgical resection, whereas patients with more, or diffuse metastatic disease, will generally be treated with radiation. Imaging protocols for high-dose neuroimaging generally call for following a 0.1 mmol/kg dose procedure with administration of an additional 0.2 mmol/kg contrast agent and repeating the scan[123–125].

The importance of obtaining both standard-dose (0.1 mmol/kg) and high-dose images was demonstrated in a series of 29 patients with known brain metastases. The addition of high-dose scans improved lesion contrast and significantly reduced the number of metastases identified (by ruling out suspected metastases). However, the high-dose scans suffered from flow artifacts, making the concurrent use of high- and standard-dose images necessary[126].

Multiple sclerosis is another CNS disease that exhibits BBB defects. The disruption of the BBB is a consistent early feature of new lesion development in relapsing-remitting and progressive multiple sclerosis. High-dose imaging is particularly useful in this application, and has been shown to increase the number of detectable lesions in relapse-remitting and progressive disease, but not in primary disease[127]. As these enhancing lesions demonstrate disease progression, both the presence and number of gadolinium ECF agent enhancing lesions are well correlated with clinical relapse, even in asymptomatic patients. Enhanced MRI imaging has become an integral part of clinical trials of mutiple sclerosis therapies, and is used as the primary endpoint for drug efficacy in investigational studies and as a secondary endpoint in definitive trials[128].

Extracellular paramagnetic agents, at standard and high doses, also play a role in the neuroimaging of infection and inflammation, for example in AIDS. High-dose scans have been shown to be useful for differentiating cerebritis from focal, mature lesions such as abscess or granuloma. These scans require the use of imaging at multiple time points before and after administration contrast media injections. For a given region of interest (ROI), signal intensity versus time curves demonstrate filling of the cavity (wash-in) and emptying or wash-out of the enhancement[25].

Contrast Enhanced MRA Fast scanning and the increasing temporal resolution of magnetic resonance scans are now positioning the imaging modality as a significant competitor to fluoroscopic angiography. The challenges to develop this technique have been significant, and so far are only partly resolved. Significant efforts have focused on developing this technique without contrast agents, using blood flow effects, phase contrast, and other innovative sequences. However, these images are not ideal, particularly in the abdomen, thorax, and periphery, and are not as familiar to practicing physicians as contrast based (X-ray) luminograms. Therefore, contrast based MRA techniques have been developed. As in the case of CT versus MRI, enhanced MRA compared to fluoroscopic angiography provides safety benefits including lower volumes of injectate, no ionizing radiation (to the patient or the medical personnel), and may be performed less invasively from an i.v. injection instead of arterial catheterization[129].

The greatest challenges in the development of these techniques have been the rapid extravasation of the ECF-contrast agents from the blood vessels, and the relatively low quantity of contrast material contained in small blood vessels, particularly as the material mixes with the blood pool and leaks into the extracellular fluid.

These related problems have been at least partially solved using first-pass imaging techniques. In these techniques, contrast agent is provided as a rapid bolus into the venous system and images are acquired as the material appears in the arteries (first) or veins (several seconds later) in the region of interest. While slower infusions of contrast material provide adequate visualization of larger vessels such as the aorta, the peak enhancement is too low to visualize smaller vessels. Rapid bolus administration provides a greater concentration of contrast agent in the vessel, allowing for a greater T1 reduction by timing the image acquisition to match the time when the central part of the *k*-space is read with the time of highest arterial concentration of agent. Combined with rapid bolus, three-dimensional techniques and breath-holding now allow high-resolution scanning of relatively small vessels.

Timing of the arrival of the contrast bolus is critical in this technique and a number of strategies for identifying the best acquisition time have been developed[130–132]. Contrast injectors are also frequently used to assure bolus rate and timing[133,134]. These systems also automatically follow the bolus injection with a rapid saline flush, a technique that significantly shortens time to first appearance of the signal and time to maximum signal intensity[135].

Contrast agent formulation may play a significant role in determination of the best agent for rapid bolus techniques. Factors to consider include safety, viscosity, and concentration. Safety is important as most contrast enhanced MRA techniques require high-dose contrast agent administration: typically at least 40 mL of a $0.5\,M$ solution[136]. Low viscosity facilitates rapid injection, and the viscosity of the available contrast agents may be lowered by warming them to body temperature. Gadobutrol, an investigational agent, has been tested at both the standard $0.5\,M$ and $1.0\,M$ concentrations. At the lower concentration this agent is a low-viscosity agent permitting rapid injection. At the higher concentration an equal dose of the agent may be administered in a lower volume to provide a greater peak signal intensity[137].

Cardiac and Cerebral Perfusion   Perfusion imaging is used to assess organ blood flow, volume, and function following an ischemic event: a myocardial infarction in the heart or stroke in the brain. Due to movement artifacts, the heart is the most technically challenging organ to image, requiring both a high level of spatial and contrast resolution together with ultrafast acquisition times. Ultrafast imaging techniques, including TurboFLASH and Echo Planar ima-

ging, have been used to follow the first pass of a bolus injection of contrast agent through the cardiac tissue with some success. However, with the currently available extracellular fluid gadolinium contrast agents, quantification of absolute values of myocardial perfusion has proved elusive. Two factors lead to this difficulty: first, the relationship between gadolinium-containing contrast agent concentration and signal intensity is nonlinear; second, the rapid diffusion of these agents into the interstitium limits obtainable signal/contrast enhancement[138].

Lacking the ability quantitatively to measure myocardial perfusion, researchers have focused on making better use of steady-state imaging, after the extracellular fluid agents have undergone diffusion. Contrast enhanced MRI may be used to identify and size myocardial infarcts and to distinguish between occlusive and reperfused myocardial infarcts. Furthermore, these agents appear useful for detection of areas of cell death in regions of reperfused infarction[139].

In the brain, perfusion imaging is desirable to improve visualization of cerebral blood flow, volume, and function, generally following some sort of known or suspected cerebral ischemic event. While the brain does not hinder MRI with motion artifacts, the blood–brain barrier, which is useful for the evaluation of lesions, hinders measurement of perfusion. The BBB limits the gadolinium chelates to the blood vessels and capillaries, a relatively small portion (2–3 percent) of the brain. This limits the number of gadolinium–water molecule interactions that can be made and the overall level of signal enhancement possible. This limitation has forced contrast agent researchers to search elsewhere for cerebral perfusion agents that might in the future include susceptibility agents or blood-pool agents[140].

Macromolecular Gadolinium-Based Agents

For a number of years contrast media researchers have sought to provide a contrast enhancing agent that would resist diffusion into the interstitium, remaining in the circulating blood pool. Such agents could, in theory, provide steady-stage enhancement for MRA and perfusion assessment. Furthermore, such agents might also provide superior enhancement in dynamic imaging techniques by reducing the amount of material extravasated during the first pass.

Extracellular agents diffuse into the interstitium because of their small size (the molecular weight of Gd-DTPA is 547 Da or 0.57 kDa). Techniques to keep these small chelates in circulation have focused mainly on increasing the overall size of the agent and have included a variety of soluble polymer-based systems, in vivo protein binding mechanisms and even ex vivo blood cell labeling. Other avenues of research have included particulate agents based on liposomes and iron oxide particles.

Through the mid-1990s, macromolecular approaches were greatly favored by contrast media researchers. These agents of interest typically had molecular weights in excess of 20,000 Da (20 kDa) with many investigational agents appearing in the 50–100 kDa range[141]. Gadolinium bearing chelates conjugated to albumin, dextran, and polylysine were studied in animal investigations but so far have not entered into human use.

In addition to offering increased plasma retention and the possibility of bioselectivity, macromolecular contrast agents may afford a more efficient means of affecting change in MR image contrast. First, each macromolecule carries a number, 30–60+, of signal altering moieties to the tissue of interest. Second, coupling of chelated paramagnetic ions to a macromolecule such as albumin-(GdDTPA)n is known, through the slowing of rotation tumbling, to result in a relaxivity (r_1) several times higher than that of the corresponding monomeric chelates GdDTPA and GdDOTA[142]. By taking advantage of these properties of macromolecular contrast agents a significant reduction in the molar dosage of agent administered to alter signal intensity may be achieved.

Gd-DTPA labeled albumin was the first macromolecular agent tested[143] and successfully demonstrated utility as a prototype macromolecular blood pool agent. However, concerns about the immunogenic potential of native albumin, the instability of albumin when undergoing heat sterilization and biodistribution studies, which showed prolonged retention of gadolinium in the liver and bone, precluded the clinical development of this agent[144].

In an attempt to circumvent the problems with labeled albumin, investigators turned to gadolinium labeled polylysine. These agents were somewhat smaller than the albumin based agents, permitting easier excretion, yet large enough to remain in the blood pool. One such formulation had an average weight of 48.7 kDa and was stable when heat sterilized. The material contained 60–70 Gd-DTPA moieties per molecule, providing T1 relaxivity of $13.1\,\mathrm{m}M^{-1}\mathrm{s}^{-1}$ compared to $3.67\,\mathrm{m}M^{-1}\mathrm{s}^{-1}$ for Gd-DTPA. This relaxivity increase was somewhat disappointing as the investigators had hoped for increased relaxivity based on both the number of gadolinium bearing moieties attached and the decreased rotational tumbling. The high degree of local segmental flexibility provided by the polylysine backbone appears to have minimized the reduction in rotation tumbling. From an acute toxicology standpoint the material was well tolerated: LD_{50} in mice of 17 mmol Gd/kg (compared with 7.5 mmol Gd/kg for Gd-DTPA). In animal models the agent had a relatively long plasma concentration half-life, yet was still renally excreted unmetabolized. However, like the albumin macromolecules, this agent also suffered from liver and bone retention and has not entered clinical development[145].

More recently, investigators have determined that molecular shape may also be used to keep macromolecules in the blood pool. Spherical or globular "starburst" dendrimers have been produced that match the blood pool retention of larger, linear polylysine based agents. Cascade-polymer, at 30 kDa is one such agent, with neither the anaphylactic potential of the albumin based agents nor the liver/bone retention of previous macromolecules[146–148]. The agent has been tested in a number of animal models and demonstrated utility for magnetic resonance angiography in both the arterial phase (first pass) and equilibrium phase and appears to be advancing toward clinical development[149].

While not formulated as a macromolecular contrast agent, the linear gadolinium chelate MS-325 is functionally similar. The chelate complex rapidly binds to serum albumin upon injection and then performs much like these agents. Once protein bound, MS-325 experiences a ten-fold increase in r_1 to around $50-60 \, \text{m}M^{-1} \text{s}^{-1}$. In addition MS-325 has further advantages in that unlike albumin-Gd-DTPA, there is no concern for immunogenic reactions and no albumin related sterilization issues[150]. Furthermore, the albumin binding is reversible allowing the agent to be renally eliminated. In the rat, MS-325 showed virtually no organ retention[80]. In early clinical trials the agent has been well tolerated and shown to provide vascular and arterial enhancement during both dynamic and steady-stage MR angiography[81,151].

As competitors to the extracellular fluid agents in vascular imaging, blood pool agents will provide a long steady-state imaging window. However, this steady state advantage has come at the price of creating a problem of distinguishing the arteries from the veins. Currently this is being accomplished using the same first-pass rapid bolus techniques used for the ECF agents (keeping track of which vessels enhanced in the arterial phase of the bolus) somewhat obviating the anticipated advantage steady-state imaging was intended to provide.

Tumor Perfusion and Vascular Permeability

Unlike normal tissue, tumor endothelium is known to be permeable to macromolecules and a variety of macromolecule based contrast agents have been tested as tumor permeability probes[152,153]. More recently, tumor epithelium permeability has been shown to be correlated to angiogenesis, the mechanism that allows tumors to grow new blood vessels[154]. Macromolecular contrast agents may find use in identification and in the angiogenic grading of tumors[155,156], in monitoring effectiveness of antiangiogenic therapies in tumors[157], and in estimating likely delivery of macromolecular based therapeutic products to tumors, with and without the use of pharmacologic hypertension[158].

Vascular permeability imaging may also have application in imaging inflammation and ischemia[141]. Furthermore, pro-angiogenic therapeutic strategies are being evaluated for the treatment of cardiovascular disease, and vessel permeability probes may have utility in monitoring these approaches.

Hepatobiliary Agents

As a frequent site of cancer metastases, the liver has received considerable attention from the imaging research community. Most liver imaging is performed to detect focal disease. This evaluation may for example help identify cancer patients who would benefit from partial liver resection.

Efforts to improve the utility of MRI for noninvasive liver evaluation have included developments in both imaging techniques and contrast agents. Imaging techniques have shortened acquisition times and motion artifacts. Several types of contrast agents have demonstrated utility in improving hepatic scans. These types include extracellular fluid, hepatobiliary, reticuloendothelial system and blood pool agents. These improvements have increased detection of focal liver lesions, including tiny lesions previously unseen. Current efforts now focus on differentiating hemangiomas and other small benign focal liver lesions from cancer, or to otherwise characterize the lesions[159].

Mangafodipir Trisodium

While extracellular fluid agents such as gadodiamide have demonstrated utility in enhancing hepatic images when combined with sophisticated dynamic imaging techniques, new tissue-targeted agents provide discriminatory enhancement over a wide imaging window. Hepatobiliary agents are taken up selectively by healthy liver hepatocytes, but not by metastases, cholangiocarcinomas and lymphomas that do not contain hepatocytes[160].

Mangafodipir (MnDPDP) is a chelate of manganese (II) and the ligand fodipir (DPDP). In vivo MR properties of mangafodipir are attributed to hepatocyte uptake of the manganese (II) ion. In vivo, mangafodipir rapidly dissociates into its two components. The manganese (II) ion is incorporated into the body store of manganese and eliminated through the urine and feces. The standard dose for mangafodipir trisodium is 5 µmol/kg. In clinical trials this dose has been provided as either a 10 µmol/ml 10–30 min infusion and as a 50 µmol/ml 1 min bolus injection. Steady-state signal enhancement is achieved about 10 min after administration, with enhancement detectable for up to 24 h[161].

Efficacy and safety has been evaluated through U.S. and European clinical trials. The European studies used the 10 µmol/ml infusion, the U.S. studies used the 50 µmol/ml bolus injection. In the European phase III studies, including patients with one to five liver lesions detected by any other imaging modality, significantly more lesions were found in mangafodipir enhanced scans than in unenhanced scans. The use of mangafodipir also increased confidence in identifying the presence of a lesion, quality of lesion delineation and lesion conspicuity. Of 624 patients evaluated for adverse events, 7 percent experienced one or more event. The most common adverse events were headache, vomiting, nausea, and feelings of warmth or flushing[162,163].

Similar efficacy was found in U.S. phase III trials. Adverse events were higher in the U.S. phase III trials, mainly due to injection site discomfort, with 67 percent of patients reporting some discomfort. Headache and gastrointestinal events were also experienced by this group at 5 and 12 percent rates respectively[161].

Clinical investigations of mangafodipir as a liver contrast enhancing agent also demonstrated contrast enhancement of the pancreas. Current research indicates that this agent might be used to detect and delineate small pancreatic tumors and when used with dynamic imaging techniques to differentiate pancreatitis[164].

Gadolinium Based Hepatobiliary Agents A number of gadolinium based hepatobiliary agents have been identified. Like mangafodipir, the gadolinium chelates are T1 shortening agents, providing enhancement on T1 weighted scans by increasing the signal intensity of normal liver.

Two agents have reached advanced clinical trials: gadobenate dimeglumine and gadoxetate disodium. In the scientific literature, gadobenate has been known as Gd-BOPTA and gadoxetate has been known as Gd-EOB-DTPA. Gadoxetate is rapidly taken up in the hepatocyte and excreted, intact, in the bile by organic anion carriers. Early clinical evaluation indicated that the agent provides enhanced lesion to liver contrast at a dose of 12.5 µmol/kg, with an imaging window at 20–45 min after administration[165].

Gadobenate is an acyclic gadolinium chelate with a distribution and elimination half life similar to that of gadopentetate. However, a small portion of the injected dose (about 4 percent) is taken up by the hepatocytes via the anionic transport mechanism and eliminated via the biliary route. Although the amount of gadobenate reaching the hepatocytes is small, the agent has a greater T1 shortening effect in the liver than that of gadopentetate because of protein binding to gadobenate, reducing rotational tumbling[159].

In clinical trials, gadobenate has been administered in doses of 50 and 100 µmol/kg. These trials suggest efficacy, particularly at the higher dose. The imaging window for gadobenate appears to be at 40–90 min, with greater contrast enhancement occurring later, after maximum renal excretion of the nontargeted agent, but before significant biliary excretion begins[166].

PARTICULATES

There has been a concerted effort to develop particulate contrast enhancing media for magnetic resonance imaging, since disease and dysfunction of the heart, lungs, liver, spleen, bone marrow lymphatics, and gastrointestinal tract have been demonstrated radiographically using particulates. The first particulate agents proposed for enhanced MR imaging have been adaptations of agents previously applied in conjunction with X-ray, ultrasound, and nuclear medicine studies[167–170].

Particulate Agents

The means by which particulate agents are able to alter MR signal intensity runs the entire gamut of contrast mechanisms through T1 enhancement, T2 enhancement, magnetic susceptibility, chemical shift, and diamagnetic effects. Consequently, particulate materials can be used to provide either positive or negative contrast enhancement. Negative contrast enhancement, a loss of signal intensity, is an effect shared by many superparamagnetic particles, clay particles, and perfluorochemical emulsions. However, the biophysical properties responsible for the effect are different for each agent. Positive contrast enhancement, an increase in signal intensity, is typically demonstrated by particulates incorporating paramagnetic metal ions. Representative vehicles for paramagnetic labels include macromolecules, emulsions, liposomes, and microspheres[169,171–173]. These substances act to reduce the T1 of water molecules which diffuse close to the paramagnetic metal ions. One possible drawback in the use of particulates of this type is that the access of water molecules to the paramagnetic metal ion might be restricted, resulting in a reduction in relaxivity. Other substances possessing an intrinsically short T1, such as oil emulsions, offer positive contrast enhancement without the concern for restricted water access.

In order to be effective, a particulate material must first provide a contrast differential by its distribution to, retention within, or elimination from normal and abnormal tissues. Once localized within a target organ, the agents must be able to affect a change in the MR signal intensity of those tissues. Distribution can be intracellular, due to phagocytosis; intravascular, due to entrapment within a vascular bed; or intracompartmental, due to the route of administration chosen[174]. The size, shape, chemical composition, charge, surface coatings, and hydrophobic or hydrophilic nature of a particulate agent all contribute to determining both its biodistribution and its magnetic resonance properties.

Of all these attributes, the size of the agent appears to be the single most important determinant of organ distribution. When administered intravenously, particles that are greater than 20 μm in diameter will become lodged within the capillary segments of the alveoli of the lungs. Nuclear medicine lung-scanning studies are routinely conducted using radiolabeled hydroxide aggregates, microspheres, and macroaggregated albumin particles in the size range 10–20 μm. However, a similar application in magnetic resonance imaging is yet to develop. Particulate agents for MRI are typically less than 5 μm in diameter in order to avoid entrapment within (and possible adverse effects to) the lungs. The mononuclear phagocytic cells of the reticuloendothelial system (RES) serve a scavenging function as they remove from the circulation particulate matter including contrast media. The liver and spleen contain 85–90 percent of these cells, with the remaining cells residing in the bone marrow and lymph nodes. The fixed macrophages of the liver and spleen demonstrate a preference for larger particles (50–500 nm) and those of the bone marrow and lymph nodes a preference for smaller particles (10–150 nm). This size preference may be circumvented, however, by administering materials that block or restrict the uptake of a particulate agent by a given organ.

Another means of restricting the distribution of a particulate agent to a desired body compartment is through direct instillation into the target

consequence of this more even distribution throughout the hepatic parenchyma, AMI-HS is effective in reducing the signal intensity of liver at one-fourth the dosage required for other magnetic particles. The status of a series of superparamagnetic-coated particulates currently in product development is described in Table 10-5.

It was hoped that receptor-targeted cell-specific iron oxides might allow detection and quantitation of metabolic disturbances. Studies in animal models of benign liver disease (e.g., fatty liver and hepatitis) show sustained liver uptake of particles despite hepatocellular dysfunction. This early work suggests that increased activity of macrophages sustains particle uptake in diseased liver[117]. Therefore it may be difficult to adapt receptor-targeted particulates to the diagnosis of diffuse liver disease.

Positive Contrast Applications of Superparamagnetic Agents In the mid 1990s investigators working with AMI-227 and other ultrasmall superparamagnetic iron oxide particles noted that while the T2 effects of the agent tended to predominate, the agents did provide some level of T1 shortening when used at low dose[189]. As AMI-227 has a long blood half-life, it was tested as a vascular enhancement (blood pool) contrast agent. In clinical studies the effect was most pronounced in hepatic vessels[190] but was seen in renal and coronary arteries[191].

A second iron oxide-based blood pool agent, PEG-Ferron or NC100150 [Clariscan[TM]], is currently in clinical trials. NC100150 particles consist of a single iron oxide crystal stabilized with a carbohydrate-polyethylene glycol (PEG) coat with an approximate particle diameter of 20 nm. The material has an exceptionally low $r_2 : r_1$ ratio, permitting potent T1 relaxation enhancement. The agent also has a long blood-pool half-life (more than 45 min)[192].

In animal imaging NC100150 demonstrated excellent contrast in blood vessels of the extremities, lungs[193] and liver. As a hepatobiliary agent, NC100150 provided a synergistic T2* parenchymal enhancement providing a "double-contrast" effect[194]. In early clinical investigations, NC100150 has indicated utility in MRA of abdominal arteries[195] and for imaging deep venous thrombosis[196]. Like the other blood-pool agents in development, differentiating arteries from veins in equilibrium phase imaging still remains the primary challenge.

Toxicity The major concerns relate to possible iron toxicity secondary to the breakdown of the particles and the release of absorbable iron species. In addition, carrier mediated toxic effects, either direct or indirect, such as immunogenic response, need to be considered. As prepared for oral administration, iron oxide particles are largely nonbiodegradable and nonreactive. In fact, there has been no compound related toxicity, either acute or subacute, reported in preclinical testing of Gastromark® and Abdoscan®. The incidence and potential for adverse effects, such as nausea,

Table 10-5

Superparamagnetic Contrast Agents

Name	Applications (Route of Administration)	Status (2000)
GastroMARK®	GI tract (oral, rectal)	Marketed in the U.S. and Europe
Abdoscan[TM]	GI tract (oral, rectal)	Marketed in Europe
Feridex®	Liver, spleen (intravenous)	Widely marketed
Combidex®	Liver, lymph (intravenous)	NDA filed in U.S. and Europe
Clariscan[TM]	Angiography (intravenous)	Phase II
AMI-7228	Oncology, cardiology (intravenous)	Completed Phase I

diarrhea, constipation, and mucosal irritation appears to be comparable to similar formulations used in the delivery of soluble iodinated or particulate barium agents for X-ray CT.

In contradistinction, iron oxide particles when administered intravenously are subject to degradation with the iron later appearing in the physiologic pool. In a pilot study, acute hemodynamic compromise (cause unknown) was observed in one patient after injection of a high dose of the Feridex iron oxide particles[183]. Toxicity studies of magnetite albumin microspheres have shown negligible adverse effects at dosages of 20 times the effective imaging dose. In theory, the use of these particles affords a safety margin as great as 250-fold before iron overload occurs. There have been no immunogenic responses and no intravascular coagulation effects detected in animals receiving these particles.

FUTURE DIRECTIONS

Extracellular MRI contrast agents have been commercially available in the U.S. since 1988. During that period, these agents have been validated in an expanding variety of applications, leading to the overall growth of contrast enhanced MRI. Procedure growth came from expanding the currently indicated uses of the agents in imaging the central nervous system and from establishing new uses outside the brain and spine. New regions have included the musculoskeletal imaging, magnetic resonance angiography (MRA), perfusion, functional brain and heart imaging, and fast abdominal imaging. Advances in imaging hardware and software have played a significant role in developing these new contrast agent uses, particularly with the development of fast imaging techniques.

The second decade of contrast enhanced MRI is bringing an increasing variety of contrast agents. These already include the hepatobiliary- and RES-specific agents, as well as materials for imaging the gastrointestinal tract. In the near future, blood-pool agents will be added to this list. Like the extracellular agents that came before them, these new agent classes will be evaluated in an expanding number of indications. In addition, like the extracellular agents, these agents will first be used in steady state applications, with dynamic applications to follow. Unlike the older agents, these newer products provide an additional level of development potential: contrast agent/hardware combination procedures[197,198].

Antibody Targeted Agents

The initial reports concerning the use of paramagnetically labeled monoclonal antibodies in MRI identified several important realities associated with the implementation of this technique. The low number of antigenic sites, limited antibody specificity, the relatively few paramagnetic chelates attached per antibody molecule, and the possible loss of binding specificity after conjugation were cited as practical hurdles to overcome. Iron oxide particles have been used with some degree of success to overcome these problems[199].

More recently, immunospecific agents based on liposomal and nanoparticulate systems carrying multiple gadolinium containing chelates have been investigated. In an effort to more directly depict the angiogenic process (as compared to the previously discussed capillary permeability measurements), two such systems have been directed to the $\alpha_v\beta_3$ integrin[200,201].

Hyperpolarized Noble Gases

The contrast media based imaging applications described here have all used contrast agents to modify the signal provided by protons (hydrogen atoms) stored in the tissues of the body. One significant area of the body, the airways, contains few protons and can only be imaged as a region lacking signal. Even proton-rich gases are not useful for imaging because of their low density compared to that of the surrounding tissues. Furthermore, tissues such as the parenchyma of the lungs are also difficult to image due to motion artifacts, short T2 and susceptibility artifacts.

Recently, researchers have pioneered a new imaging technique which uses hyperpolarized noble gases such as helium (^{3}He) and xenon (^{129}Xe) to provide positively enhanced contrast images of the lungs[202]. In conventional MRI, the hydrogen atoms in the body are polarized by placing the subject into the magnetic field. With hyperpolarized gas imaging, the gases are polarized ex vivo using lasers or strong magnetic fields. Polarization levels as high as 50 percent may be obtained; when stored under pressure in glass cells, such gases retain polarization for several days[203].

Using helium imaging, investigators have produced images that show normal and pathologic airway function in exquisite detail. Dynamic imaging of the inhalation and exhalation of hyperpolarized helium can sequentially delineate each segment of the airways. Helium is not absorbed by other body tissues so that just the airways are visualized. Promising clinical applications in development include the evaluation of emphysema and asthma patients. Unfortunately, the ^{3}He isotope (a uranium fission by-product) required for laser polarization is exceedingly rare. Researchers have been able to recover and reprocess some of the ^{3}He used in clinical evaluations and further development of "recycling" is expected to be critical to the commercial viability of helium imaging[204].

Hyperpolarization of the relatively abundant ^{129}Xe isotope has also been used and in this case there are no concerns about gas supply. However, xenon creates different challenges. Xenon is absorbed by the body, where it has pharmacologic activity as an anesthetic at a relatively low concentration. Ideally, contrast agents should not have pharmacologic activity. Furthermore, this absorption leads to some complexity in quantifying lung region volumes, although it may provide significant advantages. By imaging both the gas phase and the dissolved phase (absorbed by blood) of the ^{129}Xe, it may be possible to image ventilation and perfusion in the lung simultaneously. Furthermore, this technique may provide direct perfusion imaging of specific tissues such as the brain following hyperpolarized xenon inhalation.

REFERENCES

1. Watson AD, Rocklage SM, Carvlin MJ. In: Stark DD, Bradley WG, eds. *Magnetic Resonance Imaging*, Vol. 1, 2nd ed. St. Louis: Mosby Year Book, 372–437, 1992.
2. Lauffer RB. Magnetic resonance contrast media: Principles and progress. *Magn Reson Q* 6:65–84, 1990.
3. Mendonca Dias MH, Gaggelli E, Lauterbur PC. Paramagnetic contrast agents in nuclear magnetic resonance imaging. *Semin Nucl Med* XII:364, 1983.
4. Mendonca Dias MH, Lauterbur PC. Contrast agents for nuclear magnetic resonance. *Biol Trace Elt Res* 13:229, 1987.
5. Nelson KL, Runge VM. In: Runge VM, ed. *Enhanced Magnetic Resonance Imaging*. St. Louis: Mosby 57–74, 1989.
6. Bloch F. Nuclear induction. *Phys Rev* 70:460, 1946.
7. Lauterbur PC. Image formation by induced local interactions: Examples employing nuclear magnetic resonance. *Nature* 242:19, 1973.
8. Lauterbur PC, Mendonca Dias MH, Rudin AM. In: Dutton PC, ed. *Frontiers of Biological Energetics*. New York: Academic Press, 752–759, 1978.
9. Weinmann HJ, Brash RC, Press WR, et al. Characteristics of gadolinium-DTPA complex: A potential NMR contrast agent. *Am J Roentgenol* 142:619–624, 1984.
10. Carr DH, Brown J, Bydder GM, et al. Gadolinium-DTPA as a contrast agent in MRI: Initial clinical experience in 20 patients. *Am J Roentgenol* 143:215–224, 1984.
11. Laniado M, Weinmann HJ, Schorner W, et al. First use of GdDTPA/dimeglumine in man. *Physiol Chem Phys Med NMR* 16:157–165, 1984.
12. Bydder GM, Kingsley DPE, Brown J, et al. MR imaging of meningiomas including studies with and without gadolinium-DTPA. *J Comput Assist Tomogr* 9:690–697, 1985.
13. Claussen C, Laniado M, Schorner W, et al. Gadolinium-DTPA in MR imaging of glioblastomas and intracranial metastases. *Am J Neuroradiol* 6:669–674, 1985.
14. Komiyama M, Yagura H, Baba M, et al. MR imaging: possibility of tissue characterization of brain tumors using T1 and T2 values. *Am J Neuroradiol* 8:65–70, 1987. (Published erratum appears in *Am J Neuroradiol* 1987, 8:270.)
15. Frank H, Weissleder R, Brady TJ. Enhancement of MR angiography with iron oxide: Preliminary studies in whole-blood phantom and in animals. *Am J Roentgenol* 162:209–213, 1994.

16. Bertini I, Luchinat C. *NMR of Parmagnetic Molecules in Biological Systems.* Menlo Park CA: Benjamin Cummings, 47–83, 1986.

17. Bloembergen N. Proton relaxation times in paramagnetic solutions. *J Chem Phys* 27:572, 1957.

18. Solomon I, Relaxation processes in a system of two spins. *Phys Rev* 99:559, 1955.

19. Lauffer RB. Paramagnetic metal complexes as water proton relaxation agents for NMR imaging: theory and design. *Chem Rev* 87:901, 1987.

20. Gore JC, Physical factors in the design of contrast agents for MRI. *IEEE Eng Med Biol* Sept 1985, 39.

21. Grief WL, Buxton RB, Lauffer RB, et al. Pulse sequence optimization for MR imaging using a paramagnetic hepatobiliary contrast agent. *Radiology* 157:461–466, 1985.

22. Stark DD, Elizondo G, Fretz CJ. Liver-specific contrast agents for MRI. *Invest Radiol* 25(Suppl 1):S58, 1990.

23. Økesndal AN, Hals P-A. Biodistribution and toxicity of MR imaging contrast media. *J Magn Reson Imag* 3:157–165, 1993.

24. Muroff LR, Runge VM. The use of MR contrast in neoplastic disease of the brain. *Top Magn Reson Imag* 7:137–157, 1995.

25. Andreula CF, Recchia-Luciani AN. Rationale for the use of contrast media in MR imaging. *Neuroimaging Clin N Am* 7:461–498, 1997.

26. Hasso AN. Current status of enhanced magnetic resonance imaging in neuroradiology. *Invest Radiol* 28(Suppl 1):S3–S20, 1993.

27. Wedeking P, Tweedle M. Comparison of the biodistribution of ^{153}Gd-labeled Gd(DTPA)$^{2-}$, Gd(DOTA)$^{-}$, and Gd(acetate) in mice. *Int J Rad Appl Instrum (B).* 15:395–402, 1988.

28. Weinmann HJ, Laniado M, Mutzel W. Pharmacokinetics of GdDTPA/dimenglumine after intravenous injection into healthy volunteers. *Physiol Chem Phys Med NMR* 16:167, 1988.

29. Le Mignon MM, Chambon C, Warrington S, et al. Gd-DOTA. Pharmacokinetics and tolerability after intravenous injection into healthy volunteers. *Invest Radiol* 25:933–937, 1990.

30. Harpur ES, et al. Preclinical safety assessment and pharmacokinetics of gadodiamide injection, a new magnetic resonance imaging contrast agent. *Invest Radiol* 28(Suppl 1):S28–S43, 1993.

31. Brurok H, et al. Manganese dipyridoxyl diphosphate (MnDPDP): MRI contrast agent with antioxidant and cardioprotective properties? Abstract 1189 in *ISMRM*, Philadelphia, 1999.

32. Bhat KN, Arroyave CM, Crown R. Reaction to radiographic contrast agents: new developments in etiology. *Ann Allergy* 37:169–173, 1976.

33. Fareed J, Flammer R, Hoppensteadt D, et al. Molecular markers of contrast media-induced adverse reactions. *Semin Thromb Hemost* 10:306–328, 1984.

34. Spataro RF. Newer contrast agents for urography. *Radiol Clin North Am* 22:365–380, 1984.

35. Cacheris WP, Quay SC, Rocklage SM. The relationship between thermodynamics and the toxicity of gadolinium complexes. *Magn Reson Imaging* 8:467–481, 1990.

36. Thrall JH. In: Swanson DP, Chilton HM, Thrall JH, eds. *Pharmaceuticals in Medical Imaging.* New York: Macmillan, 253, 1990.

37. Katayama H, Yamaguchi K, Kozuka T, et al. Adverse reactions to ionic and nonionic contrast media. A report from the Japanese Committee on the Safety of Contrast Media. *Radiology* 175:621–628, 1990.

38. Ansel G, Tweedie MCK, West CR, et al. The current status of reactions to intravenous contrast media. *Invest Radiol* 15:S32–S39, 1980.

39. Hartman GW, Hattery RR, Witten DM, et al. Mortality during excretory urography: Mayo Clinic experience. *Am J Roentgenol* 139:919–922, 1982.

40. Murphy KJ, Brunberg JA, Cohan RH. Adverse reactions to gadolinium contrast media: a review of 36 cases. *Am J Roentgenol* 167:847–849, 1996.

41. Meuli RA, Maeder P. Life-threatening anaphylactoid reaction after iv injection of gadoterate meglumine. *Am J Roentgenol* 166:729, 1996.

42. Baxter AB, Melinkoff S, Stites DP, et al. Immunogenicity of gadolinium-based contrast agents for magnetic resonance imaging. Induction and characterization of antibodies in animals. *Invest Radiol* 26:1035–1040, 1991.

43. Lauterbur PC. Progress in NMR zeugmatographic imaging. *Philos Trans R Soc Lond (Biol)* 289:483–487, 1980.

44. Young IR, Clarke GJ, Bailes DR, et al. Enhancement of relaxation rate with paramagnetic contrast agents in NMR imaging. *J Comput Tomogr* 5:543–547, 1981.

45. Carr DH, Brown J, Bydder GM, et al. Intravenous chelated gadolinium as a contrast agent in NMR imaging of cerebral tumours. *Lancet* 1:484–486, 1984.

46. Runge VM, Clanton JA, Lukehart CM, et al. Paramagnetic agents for contrast-enhanced NMR imaging: a review. *Am J Roentgenol* 141:1209–1215, 1983.

47. Lauterbur PC, Jacobson MJ, Rudin AM. Water proton relaxation by manganous ion in tissues. In: *Proceedings of the Nineteenth Experimental NMR Conference*, Blacksburg VA, 1978.

48. Goldman MR, Brady TJ, Pykett IL, et al. Quantification of experimental myocardial infarction using nuclear magnetic resonance imaging and paramagnetic ion contrast enhancement in excised canine hearts. *Circulation* 66:1012–1016, 1982.

49. Caillé JM, Lemanceau B, Bonnemain B. Gadolinium as a contrast agent for NMR. *Am J Neuroradiol* 4:1041–1042, 1983.

50. Pitt GC, Martell AK. The design of chelating agents for the treatment of iron overload. *Inorg Chem Biol Med* 279, 1980.

51. Atkins HL, Som P, Fairchild RG, et al. Myocardial positron tomography with manganese-52 m. *Radiology* 133:769–774, 1979.

52. Chauncey DM, Schelbert HR, Halpern SE, et al. Tissue distribution studies with radioactive manganese: a potential agent for myocardial imaging. *J Nucl Med* 18:933–936, 1977.

53. Cotzias GC. Manganese in health and disease. *Physiol Rev* 38: 503, 1958.

54. Maynard LS, Fink S. The influence of chelation on radiomanganese excretion in man and mouse. *J Clin Invest* 35:831, 1956.

55. Cotzias GC, Borg DC, Bertinchamps AJ. In: Seven MJ, ed. *Metal-binding in Medicine*. Philadelphia: JB Lippincott, 50–58, 1960.

56. Corbett JR, Lewis M, Willerson JT, et al. ^{99m}Tc-pyrophosphate imaging in patients with acute myocardial infarction: comparison of planar imaging with single-photon tomography with and without blood pool overlay. *Circulation* 69:1120–1128, 1984.

57. Maurer AH, Knight LC, Siegel JA, et al. Paramagnetic pyrophosphate. Preliminary studies on magnetic resonance contrast enhancement of acute myocardial infarction. *Invest Radiol* 25:153–163, 1990.

58. Arvela P. Toxicity of rare-earths. *Prog Pharmacol* 2:69, 1979.

59. Durbin PW, Williams MH, Gee M. et al. Metabolism of the lanthanons in the rat. *Proc Soc Exp Biol* 91:78, 1956.

60. Haley TJ. In: Gschweider KA, Eyring L, eds. *Handbook on the Physics and Chemistry of Rare Earths*. New York: Elsevier/North Holland, 1979.

61. Laszlo D, Ekstein D, Lewin R. Biological studies on stable and radioactive rare earth compounds. I. On the distribution of lanthanum in the mammalian organism. *J Natl Cancer Inst* 13:559, 1952.

62. Rosoff B, Siegel E, Williams GL, et al. Distribution and excretion or radioactive rare earth compounds in mice. *Intl J Appl Radiat Isot* 14:129, 1983.

63. Bloch J, Navon G. A nuclear magnetic resonance relaxation study of iron(III) EDTA in aqueous solution. *J Inorg Nucl Chem* 42:693, 1980.

64. Dobson CM, Williams RJP, Xavier AV. Ethylenediaminteraacetatolanthanite(III), -prasodimate(III), europate(III), and -gadolinate(III) complexes as nuclear magnetic resonance probes of the molecular conformation of adenosine 5′-monophosphate and cytidine 5′-monophosphate in solution. *J Chem Soc Dalton Trans* 1762, 1974.

65. Geraldes CF, Sherry AD, Brown RD, et al. Magnetic field dependence of solvent proton relaxation rates induced by Gd^{3+} and Mn^{2+} complexes of various polyaza macrocyclic ligands: implications for NMR imaging. *Magn Reson Med* 3:242–250, 1986.

66. Oakes J, Smith KG. Structure of Mn − EDTA^{2-} complex in aqueous solution by relaxation nuclear magnetic resonace. *J Chem Soc Faraday Trans 2* 77:299, 1981.

67. Martell AE. In: Martell AE, Anderson WF, Badman DG, eds. *Development of Iron Chelates for Clinical Use*. New York: Elsevier/North Holland, 1981.

68. Engelstad BL, White DL, Huberty JP, et al. Hepatobiliary magnetic resonance contrast agents assessed by gadolinium-153 scintigraphy. *Invest Radiol* 22:232–238, 1987.

69. Tweedle MF, Gaughan GT, Haglan J, et al. Considerations involving paramagnetic coordination compounds as useful NMR contrast agents. *Int J Rad Appl Instrum (B)* 15:31–36, 1988.

70. Belknap EL. EDTA in the treatment of lead poisoning. *Ind Med Surg* 21:305, 1952.

71. Bersworth FC. Aliphatic polycarboxylic amino acids and methods for making them. US Patent 2,407,645. Sept 17, 1946 (Martin Dennis Co.).

72. Harder R, Chaberek S. The interaction of rare earth ions with diethylenetriaminepentaacetic acid. *J Inorg Nucl Chem* 11:197, 1959.

73. Rocklage SM, Cacheris WP, Quay SC. Manganese(II) N,N'-dipyridoxylethylenediamine-N-N'diacetate-5,5′-bis(phosphate). Synthesis and characterization of a paramagnetic chelate for magnetic resonance imaging enhancement. *Inorg Chem* 28:477, 1989.

74. Pavone P, Patrizio G, Buoni C, et al. Comparison of Gd-BOPTA with Gd-DTPA in MR imaging of rat liver. *Radiology* 176:61–64, 1990.

75. Cavagna F, Tirone P, Felder E. In: Ferrucci JT, Stark DD, eds. *Liver Imaging: Current Trends and New Techniques*. Boston: Andover Medical, 384–393, 1990.

76. Vittadini G, Felder E, Tirone P, et al. B-19036, a potential new hepatobiliary contrast agent for MR proton imaging. *Invest Radiol* 23(Suppl 1):S246–S248, 1988.

77. Schuhmann-Giampieri G. Nonlinear pharmacokinetic modeling of a gadolinium chelate used as a liver-specific contrast agent for magnetic resonance imaging. *Arzneimittelforschung* 43:1020–1024, 1993.

78. Saini S, Stark DD, Brady TJ, et al. Dynamic spin-echo MRI of liver cancer using gadolinium-DTPA: animal investigation. *Am J Roentgenol* 147:357–362, 1986.

79. Patrizio G, Pietroletti R, Pavone P. Gd-BOPTA: efficacy of a new hepatobiliary contrast agent in the case of acute and chronic jaundice, as compared to Gd-DTPA. In: European Congress of NMR in Medicine and Biology, Strasbourg, 1990.

80. Parmelee DJ, et al. Preclinical evaluation of the pharmacokinetics, biodistribution, and elimination of MS-325, a blood pool agent for magnetic resonance imaging. *Invest Radiol* 32:741–747, 1997.

81. Lauffer RB, et al. MS-325: albumin-targeted contrast agent for MR angiography. *Radiology* 207:529–538, 1998.

82. Van Wagoner M, Worah D. Gadodiamide injection. First human experience with the nonionic magnetic resonance imaging enhancement agent. *Invest Radiol* 28:(Suppl 1):S44–S48, 1993.

83. Van Wagoner M, O'Toole M, Worah D, et al. A phase I clinical trial with gadodiamide injection, a nonionic magnetic resonance imaging enhancement agent. *Invest Radiol* 26:980–986, 1991.

84. McLachlan SJ, Eaton S, De Simone DN. Pharmacokinetic behavior of gadoteridol injection. *Invest Radiol* 27(Suppl 1):S12–S15, 1992.

85. Rocklage SM, Van Wagoner M. In: Ferrucci JT, Stark DD, eds. *Liver Imaging: Current Trends and New Techniques.* Boston: Andover Medical, 374–383, 1990.

86. Elizondo G, Fretz CJ, Stark DD, et al. Preclinical evaluation of MnDPDP: new paramagnetic hepatobiliary contrast agent for MR imaging. *Radiology* 178:73–78, 1991.

87. Cavagna F. Biliary agents: new formulations. In: Liver Imaging: Current Trends in MRI, CT & US, International Symposium and Course, Boston, 1990.

88. Pirovano G, Lorusso V, Tirone P. Tolerance and pharmacokinetic evaluation of Gd-BOPTA/Dimeg at high doses in healthy volunteers. *J Magn Reson Imag* 3(Suppl P):155, 1993.

89. Weinmann HJ, Schuhmann-Gampieri G, Schmitt-Willich H, et al. A new lipophilic gadolinium chelate as a tissue-specific contrast medium for MRI. *Magn Reson Med* 22:233–237, discussion 242, 1991.

90. Schuhmann-Giampieri G, Schmitt-Willich H, Press WR, et al. Preclinical evaluation of Gd-EOB-DTPA as a contrast agent in MR imaging of the hepatobiliary system. *Radiology* 183:59–64, 1992.

91. Schuhmann-Giampieri G. Liver contrast media for magnetic resonance imaging. Interrelations between pharmacokinetics and imaging. *Invest Radiol* 28:753–761, 1993.

92. Tauber U, Weinemann HJ, Panzer M, et al. Body autoradiographic studies in rats with gadolinium-diethylenetriaminepentaacetic acid, a new contrast agent for magnetic resonance imaging. *Arzneimittelforschung* 36:1089–1091, 1986.

93. Runge VM. Gd-DTPA: an i.v. contrast agent for clinical MRI. *Int J Rad Appl Instrum (B)* 15:37–44, 1988.

94. Bousquet JC, Saini S, Stark DD, et al. Gd-DOTA: characterization of a new paramagnetic complex. *Radiology* 166:693–698, 1988.

95. Desreux JF. Nuclear magnetic resonance spectroscopy of lanthanide complexes with a tetraacetic tetraaza macrocycle: unusual conformation properties. *Inorg Chem* 19:1319, 1980.

96. Desreux JF, Merciny E, Loncin MF. Nuclear magnetic resonance and potentiometric studies of the protonation scheme of two tetraaza tetraacetic macrocycles. *Inorg Chem* 20:987, 1981.

97. Stetter HS, Frank W. Complex formation with tetraaza-cycloalkane-N,N',N'',N'''-tetraacetic acids as a function of ring size. *Angew Chem Int Ed Eng* 15:686, 1976.

98. Loncin MF, Desreux JF, Merciny E. Coordination of lanthanides by two polyamino polycarboxylic macrocycles: formation of highly stable lanthanide complexes. *Inorg Chem* 25:2646, 1986.

99. Geraldes CFGC, Alpoim MC, Marques MPM. Nuclear magnetic resonance and potentiometric studies of the protonation scheme of a triaza triacetic macrocycle and its complexes with lanthanum and lutetium. *Inorg Chem* 24:3876, 1985.

100. Clay RM, Corr S, Micheloni M. Noncyclic reference ligands for tetraaza macrocycles. Synthesis and thermodynamic properties of a series of alpha, omega-di-N-methylated tetraaza ligands and their copper(II) complexes. *Inorg Chem* 24:3330, 1985.

101. Tweedle MF, Eaton SM, Eckelmann WC, et al. Comparative chemical and structure and pharmacokinetics of MRI contrast agents. *Invest Radiol* 23(Suppl 1):S236–S239, 1988.

102. Knop RH, Frank JA, Dwyer AJ, et al. Gadolinium cryptelates as MR contrast agents. *J Comput Assist Tomogr* 11:35–42, 1987.

103. Doucet D, Meyer M, Bonnemain B. In: Runge VM, ed. *Enhanced Magnetic Resonance Imaging.* St. Louis: Mosby, 87–104, 1989.

104. Gries H, Frenzel T, Niedballa U. Polyhydroxylated macrocyclic contrast agents for MRI. In: *Society of Magnetic Resonance in Medicine.* Annual Scientific Meeting, San Francisco, 1991.

105. Gaughan G. In: Runge VM, ed. *Enhanced Magnetic Resonance Imaging.* St. Louis: Mosby, 105–116, 1989.

106. Lemke AJ, et al. Safety and use of gadobutrol in patients with brain tumors (phase III trial). *Rofo Fortschr Geb Rontgenstr Neuen Bildgeb Verfahr* 167:591–598, 1997.

107. Vogler H, et al. Pre-clinical evaluation of gadobutrol: a new, neutral, extracellular contrast agent for magnetic resonance imaging. *Eur J Radiol* 21:1–10, 1995.

108. Allard M, Doucet D, Kien P, et al. Experimental study of DOTA-gadolinium. Pharmacokinetics and pharmacologic properties. *Invest Radiol* 23(Suppl 1):S271–S274, 1988.

109. Parizel PM, Degryse HR, Gheuens J, et al. Gadolinium-DOTA enhanced MR imaging of intracranial lesions. *J Comput Assist Tomogr* 13:378–385, 1989.

110. Oudkerk M, et al. Safety and efficacy of dotarem (Gd–DOTA) versus magnevist (Gd–DTPA) in magnetic resonance imaging of the central nervous system. *Invest Radiol* 30:75–78, 1995.

111. Brugieres P, et al. Randomised double blind trial of the safety and efficacy of two gadolinium complexes (Gd–DTPA and Gd–DOTA). *Neuroradiology* 36:27–30, 1994.

112. Revel D, et al. Contrast-enhanced magnetic resonance tomoangiography: a new imaging technique for studying thoracic great vessels. *Magn Reson Imaging* 11:1101–1105, 1993.

113. Runge VM, et al. Clinical safety and efficacy of gadoteridol: a study in 411 patients with suspected intracranial and spinal disease. *Radiology* 181:701–709, 1991.

114. Carvlin MJ, De Simone DN, Meeks MJ. Phase II clinical trial of gadoteridol injection, a low-osmolal magnetic resonance imaging contrast agent. *Invest Radiol* 27(Suppl 1):S16–S21, 1992.

115. DeSimone D, et al. Evaluation of the safety and efficacy of gadoteridol injection (a low osmolal magnetic resonance contrast agent). Clinical trials report. *Invest Radiol* 26(Suppl 1):S212–S216, discussion S232–S235, 1991.

116. Magerstadt M, Gansow O, Brechbiel MW, et al. Gd(DOTA): an alternative to Gd(DTPA) as a T1,2 relaxation agent for NMR imaging or spectroscopy. *Magn Reson Med* 3:808–812, 1986.

117. Soltys RA. Summary of preclinical safety evaluation of gadoteridol injection. *Invest Radiol* 27(Suppl 1):S7–S11, 1992.

118. Tweedle MF. Physicochemical properties of gadoteridol and other magnetic resonance contrast agents. *Invest Radiol* 27(Suppl 1):S2–S6, 1992.

119. Shellock FG, Hahn HP, Mink JH, et al. Adverse reaction to intravenous gadoteridol. *Radiology* 189:151–152, 1993.

120. Arlington Medical Resources. *The Imaging Market Guide; United States Edition; Book One: Procedure Reports.* Arlington Medical Resources, Valley Forge, 1999.

121. Sage MR, Wilson AJ, Scroop R. Contrast media and the brain. The basis of CT and MR imaging enhancement. *Neuroimaging Clin N Am* 8:695–707, 1998.

122. Mathur-De Vre R, Lemort M. Invited review: biophysical properties and clinical applications of magnetic resonance imaging contrast agents. *Br J Radiol* 68:225–247, 1995.

123. Sze G, et al. Comparison of single- and triple-dose contrast material in the MR screening of brain metastases. *Am J Neuroradiol* 19:821–828, 1998.

124. Yuh WT, Parker JR, Carvlin MJ. Indication-related dosing for magnetic resonance contrast media. *Eur Radiol* 7(Suppl 5):269–275, 1997.

125. Yuh WT, Maley JE. Contrast dosage in the neuroimaging of brain tumors. Principles and indications. *Magn Reson Imaging Clin N Am* 6:113–124, 1998.

126. Fellner F, et al. Experiences with gadodiamide, a non-ionic contrast agent, in MRI of brain metastases. *Rontgenpraxis* 51:203–211, 1998.

127. Filippi M, et al. Comparison of triple dose versus standard dose gadolinium–DTPA for detection of MRI enhancing lesions in patients with MS. *Neurology* 46:379–384, 1996.

128. Miller DH, et al. The role of magnetic resonance techniques in understanding and managing multiple sclerosis. *Brain* 121(Pt 1): 3–24, 1998.

129. Prince MR. Why inject contrast for magnetic resonance angiography? Editorial. *Invest Radiol* 33:483–484, 1998.

130. Schoenberg SO, et al. Arterial-phase three-dimensional gadolinium magnetic resonance angiography of the renal arteries. Strategies for timing and contrast media injection: original investigation. *Invest Radiol* 33:506–514, 1998.

131. Prince MR, et al. Contrast-enhanced abdominal MR angiography: optimization of imaging delay time by automating the detection of contrast material arrival in the aorta. *Radiology* 203:109–114, 1997.

132. Ho VB, Foo TK. Optimization of gadolinium-enhanced magnetic resonance angiography. *Invest Radiol* 33:515–523, 1998.

133. Earls JP, et al. Hepatic arterial-phase dynamic gadolinium-enhanced MR imaging: optimization with a test examination and a power injector. *Radiology* 202:268–273, 1998.

134. Earls JP, et al. Breath-hold single-dose gadolinium-enhanced three-dimensional MR aortography: usefulness of a timing examination and MR power injector. *Radiology* 201:705–710, 1996.

135. Hany TF, et al. Optimization of contrast timing for breath-hold three-dimensional MR angiography. *J Magn Reson Imaging* 7:551–556, 1997.

136. Runge VM, Wells JW. Update: safety, new applications, new MR agents. *Top Magn Reson Imaging* 7:181–195, 1995.

137. Heiland S, et al. Perfusion-weighted MRI using gadobutrol as a contrast agent in a rat stroke model. *J Magn Reson Imaging* 7:1109–1115, 1997.

138. Passariello R, De Santis M. Magnetic resonance imaging evaluation of myocardial perfusion. *Am J Cardiol* 81:68G–73G, 1998.

139. Saeed M, Wendland MF, Higgins CB. Contrast media for MR imaging of the heart. *J Magn Reson Imaging* 4:269–279, 1994.

140. Unger EC, Ugurbil K, Latchaw RE. Contrast agents for cerebral perfusion MR imaging. *J Magn Reson Imaging* 4:235–242, 1994.

141. Brasch RC. Rationale and applications for macromolecular Gd-based contrast agents. *Magn Reson Med* 22:282–287, discussion 300–303, 1991.

142. Marchal G, Bosmans H, Van Hecke P, et al. MR angiography with gadopentetate dimeglumine-polylysine: evaluation in rabbits. *Am J Roentgenol* 155:407–411, 1990.

143. Schmiedl U, et al. Comparison of the contrast-enhancing properties of albumin-(Gd–DTPA) and Gd–DTPA at 2.0 T: an experimental study in rats. *Am J Roentgenol* 147:1263–1270, 1986.

144. Schmiedl U, et al. Albumin labeled with Gd–DTPA as an intravascular, blood pool-enhancing agent for MR imaging: biodistribution and imaging studies. *Radiology* 162: 205–210, 1987.

145. Schuhmann-Giampieri G, et al. In vivo and in vitro evaluation of Gd–DTPA-polylysine as a macromolecular contrast agent for magnetic resonance imaging. *Invest Radiol* 26:969–974, 1991.

146. Adam G, et al. Dynamic contrast-enhanced MR imaging of the upper abdomen: enhancement properties of gadobutrol, gadolinium–DTPA–polylysine, and gadolinium–DTPA–cascade-polymer. *Magn Reson Med* 32:622–628, 1994.

147. Adam G, et al. Gd–DTPA-cascade-polymer: potential blood pool contrast agent for MR imaging. *J Magn Reson Imaging* 4:462–466, 1994.

148. Wiener EC, et al. Dendrimer-based metal chelates: a new class of magnetic resonance imaging contrast agents. *Magn Reson Med* 31:1–8, 1994.

149. Dong Q, et al. Magnetic resonance angiography with gadomer-17; an animal study original investigation. *Invest Radiol* 33:699–708, 1998.

150. Lauffer RB, et al. MS-325: a small-molecule vascular imaging agent for magnetic resonance imaging. *Acad Radiol* 3(Suppl 2):S356–S358, 1996.

151. Grist TM, et al. Steady-state and dynamic MR angiography with MS-325: initial experience in humans. *Radiology* 207:539–544, 1998.

152. Shames D, et al. Measurement of capillary permeability to macromolecules by dynamic magnetic resonance imaging: a quantitative non-invasive technique. *Magn Reson Med* 29:616–622, 1993.

153. Opsahl LR, Uzgiris EE, Vera DR. Tumor imaging with a macromolecular paramagnetic contrast agent: gadopentetate dimeglumine-polylysine. *Acad Radiol* 2:762–767, 1995.

154. Brasch R, et al. Assessing tumor angiogenesis using macromolecular MR imaging contrast media. *J Magn Reson Imaging* 7:68–74, 1997.

155. Brasch RC. What is angiogenesis and why image it? *Diagnostic Imaging* 73–75, June 1996.

156. Su MY, et al. Tumor characterization with dynamic contrast-enhanced MRI using MR contrast agents of various molecular weights. *Magn Reson Med* 39:259–269, 1998.

157. Muhler A. The future of contrast-enhanced magnetic resonance angiography; Are blood pool agents needed? Editorial. *Invest Radiol* 33:709–714, 1998.

158. Su M-Y, Nalcioglu O. Investigation of the enhanced delivery of small and macromolecular agents into tumors under hypertension condition induced by a vasoconstrictor. Abstract 1331 in *ISMRM*, Philadelphia, 1999.

159. Hahn PF, Saini S. Liver-specific MR imaging contrast agents. *Radiol Clin North Am* 36:287–297, 1998.

160. Mahfouz AE, Hamm B. MR imaging of the liver. Contrast agents. *Magn Reson Imaging Clin N Am* 5:223–240, 1997.

161. Nycomed, 50 μmol/mL (mangafodipir trisodium) injection, package insert, 1997.

162. Rummeny EJ, et al. MnDPDP for MR imaging of the liver. Results of an independent image evaluation of the European phase III studies. *Acta Radiol* 38:638–642, 1997.

163. Torres CG, et al. MnDPDP for MR imaging of the liver. Results from the European phase III studies. *Acta Radiol* 38:631–637, 1997.

164. Ahlstrom H, Gehl HB. Overview of MnDPDP as a pancreas-specific contrast agent for MR imaging. *Acta Radiol* 38:660–664, 1997.

165. Reimer P, et al. Phase II clinical evaluation of Gd-EOB-DTPA: dose, safety aspects, and pulse sequence. *Radiology* 199:177–183, 1996.

166. Caudana R, et al. Focal malignant hepatic lesions: MR imaging enhanced with gadolinium benzyloxypropionictetra-acetate (BOPTA)–preliminary results of phase II clinical application. *Radiology* 199:513–520, 1996.

167. Davis SS, Frier M, Illum L. In: Guinot P, Couvreur P, eds. *Polymeric Nanoparticles and Microspheres.* Boca Raton FL: CRC Press, 1990.

168. Jendrasiak GL, Frey GD, Heim RC. Liposomes as carriers of iodolipid radiocontrast agents for CT scanning of the liver. *Invest Radiol* 20:995–1002, 1985.

169. Klaveness J. In: Runge VM, ed. *Enhanced Magnetic Resonance Imaging.* St. Louis: Mosby, 117–128, 1989.

170. Mattrey RF, Nemcek AA, Shelton R, et al. In vivo estimation of perfluorooctylbromide concentration in tissues. *Invest Radiol* 25:915–921, 1990.

171. Eisenberg AD, Conturo TE, Mitchell MR, et al. Enhancement of red blood cell proton relaxation with chromium labeling. *Invest Radiol* 21:137–143, 1986.

172. Moseley ME, White DL, Wang S, et al. Vascular mapping using albumin-(Gd-DTPA), an intravascular MR contrast agent, and projection MR imaging. *J Comput Assist Tomogr* 13:215–221, 1989.

173. Seltzer SE. The role of liposomes in diagnostic imaging. *Radiology* 171:19–21, 1989.

174. Hahn PF, Stark DD, Saini S, et al. Ferrite particles for bowel contrast in MR imaging: design issues and feasibility studies. *Radiology* 164:37–41, 1987.

175. Kent TA, Quast MJ, Kaplan BJ, et al. Assessment of a superparamagnetic iron oxide (AMI-25) as a brain contrast agent. *Magn Reson Med* 13:434–443, 1990.

176. Hahn PF, Stark DD, Weissleder R, et al. Clinical application of superparamagnetic iron oxide to MR

imaging of tissue perfusion in vascular liver tumors. *Radiology* 174:361–366, 1990.

177. Listinsky JJ, Bryant RG. Gastrointestinal contrast agents: a diamagnetic approach. *Magn Reson Med* 8:285–292, 1988.

178. Gillis P, Koenig SH. Transverse relaxation of solvent protons induced by magnetized spheres: application to ferritin, erythrocytes, and magnetite. *Magn Reson Med* 5:323–345, 1987.

179. Josephson L, Lewis J, Jacobs P, et al. The effects of iron oxides on proton relaxivity. *Magn Reson Imaging* 6:647–653, 1988.

180. Majumdar S, Zoghbi SS, Gore JC. Pharmacokinetics of superparamagnetic iron-oxide MR contrast agents in the rat. *Invest Radiol* 25:771–777, 1990.

181. Saini S, Stark DD, Hahn PF, et al. Ferrite particles: a superparamagnetic MR contrast agent for the reticulo-endothelial system. *Radiology* 162:211–216, 1987.

182. Saini S, Stark DD, Hahn PF, et al. Ferrite particles: a superparamagnetic MR contrast agent for enhanced detection of liver carcinoma. *Radiology* 162:217–222, 1987.

183. Stark DD, Weissleder R, Elizondo G, et al. Superparamagnetic iron oxide: clinical application as a contrast agent for MR imaging of the liver. *Radiology* 168:297–301, 1988.

184. Weissleder R, Elizondo G, Wittenberg J, et al. Ultrasmall superparamagnetic iron oxide: characterization of a new class of contrast agents for MR imaging. *Radiology* 175:489–493, 1990.

185. Weissleder R, Elizondo G, Wittenberg J, et al. Ultrasmall superparamagnetic iron oxide: an intravenous contrast agent for assessing lymph nodes with MR imaging. *Radiology* 175:494–498, 1990.

186. Weissleder R, Reimer P, Lee AS, et al. MR receptor imaging: ultrasmall iron oxide particles targeted to asialoglycoprotein receptors. *Am J Roentgenol* 155:1161–1167, 1990.

187. Reimer P, et al. Asialoglycoprotein receptor function in benign liver disease: evaluation with MR imaging. *Radiology* 178:769–774, 1991.

188. Reimer P, et al. Dynamic signal intensity changes in liver with superparamagnetic MR contrast agents. *J Magn Reson Imaging* 2:177–181, 1992.

189. Chambon C, et al. Superparamagnetic iron oxides as positive MR contrast agents: in vitro and in vivo evidence. *Magn Reson Imaging* 11:509–519, 1993.

190. Mayo-Smith WW, et al. MR contrast material for vascular enhancement: value of superparamagnetic iron oxide. *Am J Roentgenol* 166:73–77, 1996.

191. Stillman AE, et al. Ultrasmall superparamagnetic iron oxide to enhance MRA of the renal and coronary arteries: studies in human patients. *J Comput Assist Tomogr* 20:51–55, 1996.

192. Saeed M, et al. Value of blood pool contrast agents in magnetic resonance angiography of the pelvis and lower extremities. *Eur Radiol* 8:1047–1053, 1998.

193. Nolte-Ernsting C, et al. Experimental evaluation of superparamagnetic iron oxide particles in pulmonary MR angiography. *Rofo Fortschr Geb Rontgenstr Neuen Bildgeb Verfahr* 168:508–513, 1998.

194. Nolte-Ernsting C, et al. Abdominal MR angiography performed using blood pool contrast agents: comparison of a new superparamagnetic iron oxide nanoparticle and a linear gadolinium ploymer. *Am J Roentgenol* 171:107–113, 1998.

195. Schmidt M, et al. MRA of the aorta, renal and pelvic arteries: extracelluar vs. intravascular contrast agents. Abstract 356 in *ISMRM*, Philadelphia, 1999.

196. Sunden P, et al. 3D Turbo MRA, with a new blood pool contrast agent NC 100150 – a single diagnostic method for deep venous thrombosis and pulmonary embolism. Abstract 1906 in *ISMRM*, Philadelphia, 1999.

197. Low RN, et al. Peritoneal tumor: MR imaging with dilute oral barium and intravenous gadolinium-containing contrast agents compared with unenhanced MR imaging and CT. *Radiology* 204:513–520, 1997.

198. Low RN, Francis IR. MR imaging of the gastrointestinal tract with i.v. gadolinium and diluted barium oral contrast media compared with unenhanced MR imaging and CT. *Am J Roentgenol* 169:1051–1059, 1997.

199. Gupta H, Weissleder R. Targeted contrast agents in MR imaging. *Magn Reson Imaging Clin N Am* 4:171–184, 1996.

200. Spins DA, et al. Detection of tumor angiogenesis in vivo by alphaVbeta3-targeted magnetic resonance imaging. *Nat Med* 4:623–626, 1998.

201. Anderson SA, et al. Rapid, one-step antibody-targeted magnetic resonance contrast enhancement of neovascular $\alpha V \beta 3$ epitopes using a nanoparticulate emulsion. Abstract 144 in *ISMRM*, Philadelphia, 1999.

202. Saam BT. Magnetic resonance imaging with laser-polarized noble gases. *Nat Med* 2:358–359, 1996.

203. Kauczor H, Surkau R, Roberts T. MRI using hyper-polarized noble gases. *Eur Radiol* 8:820–827, 1998.

204. Schad LR, et al. Hyperpolarized gases – a new type of MR contrast agents? *Acta Radiol* 412(Suppl 1):43–46, 1997.

CHAPTER 11

MR Imaging of the Breast

Luann J. Culbreth

The potential for magnetic resonance imaging (MRI) to play a role in the detection and staging of breast cancer was recognized as early as four years before the first commercial nuclear magnetic resonance (NMR) scanner became available in 1982. Yet by the late 1980s, MRI was thought to have no significant role in breast imaging due in part to the limitations of the current imaging techniques and the more widely available, less expensive mammographic and sonographic techniques. Other deficiencies with MR imaging included the lack of sufficient resolution to identify small lesions, inferior signal-to-noise ratio, and the inherently poor contrast in the breast tissue. However, when the contrast agent gadolinium DTPA was introduced in Europe, renewed research showed that breast cancer was consistently enhanced with the gadolinium agent and that benign and malignant lesions could be differentiated. This revelation boosted the efforts of many investigators into what has become one of today's most pursued applications of MRI. The ensuing controversy over silicone breast implants has also made breast MRI the modality of choice for identifying associated implant complications in the body.

Currently, breast cancer ranks second to lung cancer as the leading cause of death from cancer among women. However, breast cancer is the most commonly detected cancer in women worldwide and accounts for more premature deaths. The incidence of breast cancer increases with age and is rarely diagnosed before age 25 yet begins to increase significantly afterwards. Recent increases in the incidence of breast cancer have received considerable attention. Researchers feel this dramatic increase is due not only to a true increase in the rate of the disease but partly to a coincidence with the dramatic increase in public awareness of the need for breast self-examination and mammographic screening. The American Cancer Society recommends a baseline mammogram at age 35 and an annual or semiannual mammogram after age 40. In the Netherlands, public health authorities recommend all women aged between 50 and 70 to have a mammogram each year. Unfortunately, women in all parts of the world continue to ignore the importance of breast self-examination and mammographic screening. Only 20–25 percent of the women in the United States for whom screening is recommended actually follow the established guidelines.

Breast cancer screening is the evaluation of a population of women with no obvious indications of breast cancer in an effort to detect signs of cancer at an earlier stage than without screening. Mammography has been established as the method of choice for breast cancer screening and its objective is to detect cancer before clinical symptoms develop and before it metastasizes to areas outside the breast. Mammography is capable of detecting cancers before they can be palpated; yet even very large masses may not be demonstrated by mammography. The Breast Cancer Detection Demonstration Project (BCDDP) revealed that approximately 9 percent of palpable cancers will not be seen with mammography. Although mammography is known to be a very sensitive technique for breast cancer detection, it has a high rate of false-positive results, approximately 80 percent. A new imaging technique capable of detecting breast cancer and diagnosing the lesion as benign or malignant could potentially reduce the large number of invasive procedures performed, i.e., biopsy. The ability to characterize breast tumors has been the driving force in the search for an in vivo MRI "biopsy" technique. Another potential role for MR imaging is in the preoperative staging of breast cancer to help define possible multicentric disease, whose presence is important in choosing between the surgical approaches, lumpectomy, and mastectomy. The accurate depiction of carcinomas on MR images may also be used to document the response to radiation or chemotherapy.

BREAST ANATOMY

Development

The breast, or mammary gland, is a gland of the skin whose essential function is milk secretion: lactation. Breast development begins in the embryo during the fifth week of gestation. During the second trimester the lactiferous ducts are formed and by full term the breast is a network of branching ducts. At puberty, an increased output of estrogen by the ovaries stimulates the elongation of the mammary ducts and there is an increase in fat deposits and connective tissue. The areola and nipple grow and become pigmented during this time. During adolescence, the formation of the lobules and continued fat deposition occurs with associated estrogen and progesterone secretion by the ovaries. Maturation of the breast may take many years and may not actually be complete until after a full-term pregnancy. During pregnancy, the lobules increase in size and structure to prepare for lactation. After lactation, and after menopause, the breast undergoes a degree of atrophy and involution.

Structure

The breast [Figure 11-1] lies on the pectoralis major muscle and generally extends from the second to the seventh rib. A network of fibrous connective tissue runs between the skin and the deep superficial fascia giving structure and support to the breast. These ligaments are known as the *suspensory ligaments of Cooper*. The Cooper ligaments traverse through the fat that surrounds the parenchymal tissue. The fat is of variable thickness and does not completely isolate the mammary glands, as epithelial tissue extends beneath the skin and traverses through the breast. The fatty tissue gives the breast its smooth shape and contributes to its size. Breast size, however, does not contribute to the amount of milk produced during lactation. Between the breast parenchyma and the pectoralis major muscle is a layer of fat known as the retromammary space. The deep fascia projects through this space and into the muscle. This incomplete isolation of the breast makes the assured elimination of breast cancer by mastectomy virtually impossible.

The breast parenchyma consists of 15 to 20 lobes, or segments. In each segment there are

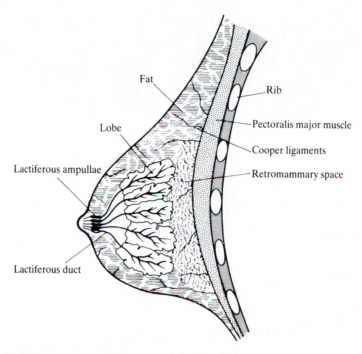

Figure 11-1. Sagittal drawing of the female breast structure.

several lobules. The lobule [Figure 11-2] is composed of the intralobular terminal duct and the alveoli: the milk-secreting cells. From the lobule extends the extralobular terminal duct. Histologists have defined the extralobular terminal duct and the lobule as the terminal duct lobular unit (TDLU). Not only is the TDLU important physiologically due to milk production, it is also believed to be the site where most lesions are developed.

During lactation, milk is conveyed from the TDLU into the lactiferous, or mammary, ducts. As the ducts approach the nipple, expanded sinuses, or ampullae, are present where milk may be stored. Approximately eight lactiferous ducts originate in or empty into the nipple. The nipple is the center of the areola. The areola contains smooth muscle, sebaceous glands, and hair follicles, giving it a bumpy appearance.

Vascular supply to and drainage from the breast is provided by the axillary, intercostal, and internal mammary arteries and veins. Nerves supplying the breast primarily come from the thoracic intercostal nerves with some supply from the cervical plexus. Lymphatic drainage from the breast is primarily to the axillary lymph nodes; there is also some drainage to the internal mammary chain.

TECHNICAL CONSIDERATIONS

For MR imaging to play a principal role in breast cancer management, providing vastly improved specificity and sensitivity over conventional imaging techniques, it must meet several major technologic considerations.

1. It must have high resolution (approximately 1 mm in all three planes) for improved delineation of tumor margins and for the detection of small lesions that may or may not be seen by mammography.

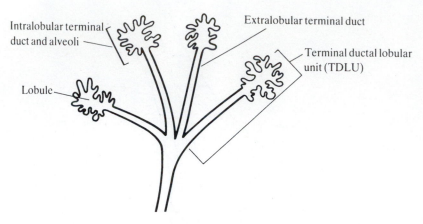

Figure 11-2.   Terminal ductal lobular unit.

If insufficient resolution fails to identify these lesions, the MR images will be falsely reported as negative for malignancy.

2. It should employ fat suppression for differentiation of enhancing tumors from fat.

3. Acquisition time should be rapid (preferably about 5 min) to differentiate enhancing tumors from normal breast parenchyma that will show delayed enhancement.

4. All of the breast should be imaged, including breast tissue near the sternum (far medial) and into the axillary tail (lateral).

Patient Setup

A marker that can be identified on the MR image, such as an oil bead, should be placed over the nipple and on any palpable areas of concern on the affected breast. Before imaging, an intravenous drip should be started to facilitate the infusion of the contrast agent. The patient should remain on the table, positioned in the coil between the pre- and postcontrast images. Every effort must be made to make the patient as comfortable as possible to prevent even the slightest patient movement during and in between the scanning sequences.

The patient should be in the prone position, with the breasts positioned in a dedicated breast coil [Figure 11-3]. Today, many MR manufacturers have breast coils available. Whether the coil configuration is linear, quadrature, or phased array, dedicated breast coils allow for better 3D acquisitions, improved SNR, and reduced aliasing motion artifacts from the rest of the body. Some breast coils will allow for either unilateral or bilateral acquisitions. Since MR imaging is not a breast screening test, a unilateral exam may be typically performed in only the diseased breast.

Resolution

For *specificity*, a lesion that is identified by mammography must also be able to be identified by MR imaging. The objective of adequate resolution to visualize mammographically detected lesions can be achieved with relatively low-resolution gradient echo methods that are commonly available. Current literature indicates the potential is low for a false-negative finding at MR when a lesion has been identified on mammography. However, two-dimensional imaging, which may require relatively thick sections with interslice gaps, is limited in the demonstration of small lesions because of volume averaging effects and the interslice gaps. The reduced resolution in the slice direction limits the quality of the image reformations. Results of some studies indicate that dynamic imaging with

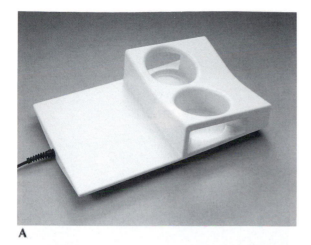

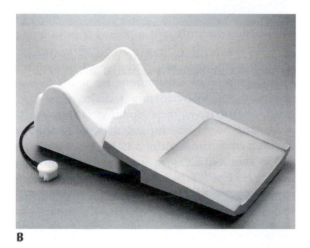

Figure 11-3. **A** Dedicated quadrature breast coil (Courtesy MRI Devices Corporation.) **B** Bilateral receive-only breast coil. (Courtesy Picker International.)

low-resolution 2D methods without fat suppression is helpful in enabling distinction of benign fibroadenomas (which often enhance) from malignancy, suggesting that cancers enhance more quickly than fibroadenomas. Yet overlap exists in this group, making biopsy necessary to exclude malignancy. For this reason, the uncertain gain in specificity obtained with dynamic imaging does not appear to justify the reduced resolution required to achieve dynamic images.

For *sensitivity*, improvements in MR pulse sequences can provide the spatial and contrast resolution needed to greatly enhance lesion conspicuity. New high-definition MRI methods have potential for supplementing conventional diagnostic imaging methods for breast diagnosis in some clinical situations. Three-dimensional acquisitions are capable of producing high-resolution thin sections without intersection gaps, and SNR with 3D is improved by a factor of the square root of the number of sections compared to 2D studies with the same number of signal averages. Nearly isotropic 3D acquisitions also allow for workstation multiplanar reconstructions of the volume data to produce mediolateral and craniocaudal mammographic projections of the breast. Coronal and oblique views [Figure 11-4] are also available from the same 3D acquisition. An acquisition matrix of $128 \times 256 \times 1024$ (slice, phase, frequency) converted to a display matrix of $128 \times 256 \times 256$, with section thicknesses of 1.4–1.6 mm and unilateral FOVs of 20–22 cm, produces final voxel sizes of $1.4 \text{ mm} \times 0.8 \text{ mm} \times 0.8 \text{ mm}$ to $1.6 \text{ mm} \times 0.9 \text{ mm} \times 0.9 \text{ mm}$. 3D imaging not only improves image resolution but also facilitates image processing methods. 3D image data can be transferred to an independent console for image reformations and maximum intensity projection (MIP) ray tracing. Multiple-angle, fast reformations allow the radiologist to follow questionable lesions to determine their identity, whether vessel or mass, and the relationship of the defect to other structures. The hyperintense breast nodules within the entire volume can be demonstrated without overlying soft tissue with the use of MIP ray tracing [Figure 11-5].

Contrast Enhancement

Early research with gadolinium-DTPA revealed that breast cancer consistently enhanced and that these enhancing lesions could often be differentiated from some benign lesions. Most tumors demonstrate rapid contrast enhancement within the first 5 min. Because of this, tumors could be

the silicone is still contained within the fibrous capsule. Although intracapsular tears do not necessarily lead to silicone leakage, the Food and Drug Administration (FDA) has recommended removal of torn implants. Since intracapsular tears cannot be reliably seen with ultrasound, MRI has become the method of choice for evaluating this complication. The tear is confirmed by the free portions of the capsule that are seen suspended within the implant. This appearance of the capsule within the implant has been termed the linguine sign or free-floating loose thread sign [Figure 11-11]. A number of conventional MR techniques can be used to illustrate intracapsular tears. Low resolution body coil imaging can be utilized. Fat suppression or silicone specific sequences are not needed.

An extracapsular tear is one in which the silicone is outside the fibrous capsule and within the breast parenchyma. Extracapsular rupture constitutes approximately 10 percent of all silicone gel-filled breast implant failures. Most frequently extravasated silicone is confined to the original area in which the implant was placed. Not infrequently, however, the extravasated silicone may result in "islands" of involvement, sometimes extending to a variable distance of more than 20 cm. Studies indicate that almost all silicone implants have at least small amounts of extracapsular free silicone that can be attributed to a microscopic silicone gel bleed. However, in patients with silicone implants and a palpable mass or image peculiarity, the question of free silicone or tumor arises. The dense appearance of silicone on a mammogram can oftentimes resemble a mass. This distinction is of vital importance and cannot always be made by conventional imaging methods [Figure 11-12]. The prolonged T1 and T2 of silicone and its frequency difference from fat and water allows several options for imaging. Similar to fat suppression techniques, silicone-specific sequences may be used to characterize the silicone collection on the basis of either the chemical shift of the silicone or its T1. STIR sequences are commonly used, as well as T2-weighted sequences.

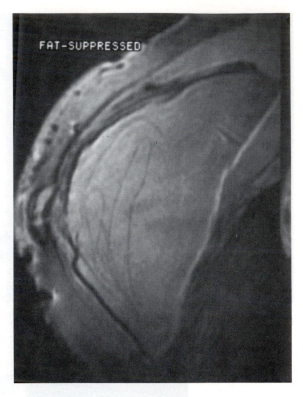

Figure 11-11.   Intracapsular tear with the linguine sign.

FUTURE OF BREAST MR

The utilization of MRI in the breast is still in its infancy. As it becomes more widely accepted, MRI's potential uses may include the following.

1. Its improved sensitivity may be used to determine whether lumpectomy candidates with presumed solitary nodules actually have multifocal disease.
2. Its ability to distinguish silicone from enhancing tumor may be used to examine patients with silicone injections and implants who cannot be adequately examined with conventional imaging methods.
3. Evaluation of implants for identifying ruptures and locating free silicone.
4. Its lack of contrast enhancement from fat and scar could be used in the evaluation of

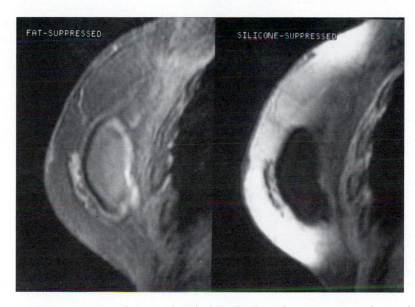

Figure 11-12. Extracapsular tear identified by the free silicon anterior to the implant.

mammographically suspect lesions that may be radial scar, postoperative scar, or fat necrosis.

5. Three-dimensional MR imaging may be used in patients when breast cancer is strongly suspected and conventional imaging studies, such as mammography and ultrasound, fail to demonstrate a lesion.

The use of MRI for reducing the number of breast biopsies is less likely at facilities where the core needle biopsy is well accepted. Mammographically guided stereotactic and sonographically directed core needle biopsies of suspicious masses are easily obtained, are much less expensive, and provide true histology. MRI cannot effectively compete with this approach if specificity is the only goal. At these centers, the main role of MRI involves improved definition and sensitivity of the detection of breast lesions. However, the higher sensitivity of MRI could result in the demonstration of a large number of questionable lesions that would not be seen with conventional imaging. The clinician is then faced with a situation in which a tumor may be present but tissue cannot be obtained to confirm malignancy. If the clinician decides to observe the

lesion over time, it may become incurable; on the other hand, in an attempt to cure, the surgeon may remove a breast in which the lesion is benign. Considering this dilemma, in order for MRI to achieve true clinical value, a method for MRI stereotactic localization and biopsy is required.

The current surgical approach to lumpectomy is to localize and remove the tissue of concern. If the pathologist determines that inadequate margins are obtained, the patient is reexcised. In a recent study this was shown to occur in 50 percent of lumpectomy cases. Studies have shown that MRI combined with laser treatment may provide an alternative to the surgical approach. MRI could show the extent of laser treatment by identifying the areas of heating and tumor margins. The future of breast conservation treatment may be improved by MRI.

CONCLUSIONS

MR imaging of the breast is a rapidly evolving application that could improve the detection and evaluation of breast anomalies. Its application could improve clinical efficiency and become a cost-effective method for treatment of various based on years of experience, the diagnosis of breast disease with MR imaging still poses questions for researchers.

SUGGESTED READING

Harms SE, Flamig DP. MR imaging of the breast. *J Mag Res Imag* 3:277–283, 1993.

Harms SE, Flamig DP, Helsey KL, et al. Magnetic resonance imaging of the breast. *Mag Res Q* 8: 139–155, 1992.

Harms SE, Flamig DP, Helsey KL, et al. Fat-suppressed three-dimensional MR imaging of the breast. *RadioGraphics* 13:247–267, 1993.

Kopans DB. *Breast Imaging*. Philadelphia: Lippincott, 1989.

McNamara MP, Middleton MS. Mapping of extravasated silicone following breast implant rupture. *RSNA Scientific Program*, Vol. 209, 1998.

Pierce WB, Harms SE, Flamig DP, et al. Three-dimensional gadolinium-enhanced MR imaging of the breast. *Radiology* 181:757–763, 1991.

CHAPTER 12

Fundamentals of Image Interpretation

Bartram J. Pierce

INTRODUCTION

As the field of magnetic resonance imaging has flourished in the past decade the importance of the technologist has increased dramatically. The radiologist, in order to remain competitive in the community and keep up with the ever increasing workload, has come to rely more than ever on the abilities of the MR technologist. Patient screening, patient interview, protocol optimization, and image filming routinely fall to the technologist, many times without direct contact or communication with the radiologist. The technologist is expected to be able to operate independently; to make decisions depending on the clinical history, patient symptoms, and what is visualized on the monitor. It is the responsibility of the technologist to equip him/herself with the knowledge and tools necessary to shoulder this independence. The ability to interpret, on a clinical basis, what one sees on the monitor is a major step in allowing the technologist to perform independently.

This chapter aims to give both the experienced technologist and the novice a fundamental understanding of how to approach clinical image interpretation from the technologist's perspective: what it takes to develop a good basic knowledge of recognition; and a cursory look at some normal anatomy and some of the most commonly encountered abnormalities and disease processes. It is not intended to be an exhaustive compilation of all the technologist may encounter; there are many excellent definitive texts for that. By giving the technologist a good foundation we can foster confidence and independence, which in turn will lead to a better exam for the patient and a more complete and appropriate exam for the radiologist.

The ability to correctly interpret what you see on the monitor is the end result of a process that contains many steps. This process can be likened to construction of a five-level pyramid starting with a strong wide foundation for the base and continuing up to the apex. The five levels that prepare the technologist for image interpretation are as follows.

Normal anatomy—structure and function.
Abnormal anatomy.
Accurate and complete patient history.

Pathology.

Accurate clinical interpretation.

The base of the pyramid, where all good clinical interpretation must start, is a good working knowledge of the normal anatomy of the area of interest. Technologists need to be familiar with the normal structures of the regions they examine. They need to comprehend where those structures lie in relation to each other and be able to visualize them in three different planes. They should be familiar with anatomic and positional variants. Because MRI allows us to change the tissue contrast depending on the pulse sequence technologists need to be able to identify these structures under a variety of pulse sequences (T1 weighted, T2 weighted, gradient echo, proton density, and inversion recovery). In addition the technologist needs to be well versed in the physiology of each structure; how they function on their own and in relation to other structures. Familiarity with the circulatory distribution is often helpful, especially in the brain.

MRI has its own set of artifacts; some caused by machine, some produced by physiology. Technologists need to be aware of these artifacts, their causes, and their solutions, and to be able to differentiate an artifact from anatomic or pathologic structures.

This wealth of information, although necessary for good clinical interpretation, cannot be learned overnight or even prior to scanning patients. It must be learned a little at a time. Knowing where to look if you run into questions, where to find good reference material, as well as the will to learn and hands-on experience are all invaluable in this learning process. Having laid this solid foundation it is time to take the next step.

It is very difficult to tell which of the next two levels comes first or is more important. They are both crucial to the correct interpretation of images. These two levels are as follows.

Knowledge of disease processes.

Obtaining a complete and accurate history from the patient and/or referring physician.

First, let us discuss the significance of being familiar with the disease processes the technologist is likely to encounter on a daily basis. As patients are referred to the MR suite for an exam, the technologist is not always given complete information regarding the patient's condition. This can be frustrating because it is the responsibility of the technologist to make sure the correct exam is performed on the patient. For example, the requisition slip requests a brain MRI. Under diagnosis, the physician (or receptionist) has merely written "sensorineural hearing loss on Lt." This should be an indication that the exam ordered (i.e., routine brain) may not be the best way to approach this patient's problem; an exam that focuses on the VIIth and VIIIth cranial nerves might be more appropriate. The technologist can then consult with the radiologist or the referring physician to make sure the correct exam is performed. In this particular case, if the technologist had not been aware of the major area in the brain responsible for hearing loss, a routine exam might have been performed and pathology missed. As the technologist learns which areas of the brain are affected by particular pathological processes then he/she will have an idea where the lesion might be located that is causing the patient's symptoms. Knowing where to look for a problem gives the technologist an edge in tailoring the exam.

An accurate and complete patient history is not an optional item, it is a necessity. Unfortunately the referring physician does not always provide the radiologist and/or technologist with a great amount of medical history. Magnetic resonance imaging is very sensitive but frequently is not very specific. The more comprehensive the history you obtain from the patient or the referring physician, the better you will be able to tailor the exam to the patient's problem. As you become more and more familiar with the pathological processes, it becomes easier to obtain a much more detailed and accurate patient history. This is because you now have some insight into what you are looking for and what symptoms or conditions match what the patient is telling you. You are able to ask more pointed, pertinent questions.

This patient history and the knowledge of disease processes will be very instrumental in helping the technologist clinically evaluate the images seen on the monitor. For example, a patient presents with symptoms that include acute onset, weakness of the right side, and slurred speech with some resolving of these symptoms since their onset. The technologist sees an area of high intensity signal on the T2 weighted axials and intermediate to low signal on the T1 images. The area is wedge-shaped and is contained within one vascular territory. By putting these facts together the technologist can feel comfortable that what he/she is seeing is probably a stroke or cerebral vascular accident (CVA) which will not require intravenous contrast. Given slightly different symptoms and appearance the technologist might come up with a different conclusion and consult with the radiologist about the possibility of a tumor. When talking with the radiologist about what is seen on the monitor, the radiologist will most likely ask about the patient's symptoms and use the same logic as you did to decide how to proceed. The more information you can give them the better they are able to make a definitive diagnosis.

Once you are knowledgeable regarding normal anatomy, disease processes, and the patient's symptoms you can begin to consider how the various abnormalities present themselves on the monitor. An excellent learning tool is to review each MRI report daily. Read the radiologist's report. See whether your visual observation matches the radiologist's verbal description. Did the radiologist's interpretation seem to concur with what you saw on the monitor? Did they see something you didn't? Did you see something they didn't? Don't be afraid to pull cases and ask questions of your radiologist. On interesting cases contact the referring physician to obtain more information such as the pathology report or the status of the patient.

CLINICAL INFORMATION AND PATIENT HISTORY

It is the technologist's responsibility to furnish the radiologist with as much information about the patient's symptoms as possible. This assures that the correct exam has been ordered and performed, assists the technologist in correct clinical interpretation of the images, and assists the radiologist in making a more accurate differential diagnosis. Most of the time the referring physician supplies neither the MRI facility or the radiologist with adequate information concerning the reason for the exam. During the patient screening process it is important for the technologist to acquire correct, detailed clinical information about the patient and his/her symptoms. It is helpful if the technologist has some idea of the type of questions to ask. With time, the technologist will get better at deciphering the explanations of the patient and at giving the proper information to the radiologist.

Although different exams may call for different types of questioning, many questions are global in nature. Frequently the patient may not understand or be able to answer a particular question. The technologist needs to become skilled at rephrasing or rewording questions, for example,

> Original question: What type of exam are you here for?
> Rephrased question: Why did you go to see the doctor?

Here is a list of common questions asked about the patient and his/her symptoms. You won't need to ask them all each time; it's intended to get you thinking.

> What type of problems (symptoms) are you having?
> > Weakness, pain, parathesia (numbness), vertigo, tinnitus, speech difficulty, hearing loss, etc.
> Where is the location of your problem? Can you point to it?

Onset of symptoms

Acute, if so when?

Chronic, if so how long?

Gradual onset

Rapid onset

Have you ever had these symptoms before?

Are your laboratory tests abnormal?

Any history of trauma to the affected area? If so when?

Any history of recent illnesses? If so when?

Any history of major medical problems? If so what?

Any history of surgery to the area being imaged?

If so why?

What type of surgery and where?

Any other medical treatment to the area to be imaged?

Radiation therapy (can change T1 and T2 signal characteristics)

Chemotherapy

Have you ever had prior studies for this problem?

Have you ever had an injury to this part of your body?

If so, when and what happened?

Once you feel certain that you know what exam the patient is to have and why the patient has been referred, you can start developing a more detailed list of pertinent questions. This is where the questions become more pointed and more exam specific.

In exams where the primary complaint is pain, that is the spine (cervical, thoracic, lumbar) and the musculoskeletal system (knee, hip, wrist, shoulder, etc.), there are five questions the technologist should ask.

1. What is the quality of the pain? Is it sharp, dull, stabbing, constant, intermittent, or cramping?

2. What is the location of the pain? Is it front, back, side, all over?

3. Does the pain radiate or stay in one place? If so, where and when?

4. What makes the pain better?

5. What makes the pain worse?

The more information you can obtain from your patient and/or referring physician, the more effective the MRI study will be in helping to make a diagnosis, for two reasons. First, it allows you to tailor the exam to the specific complaint of the patient, thereby making the MRI exam much more sensitive. Secondly, the radiologist will be able to prioritize the list of differential diagnoses thereby helping to make the MRI exam more specific. The patient receives a more complete exam and the referring physician receives the information he/she needs to improve the patient's care.

You have now reached the apex of the pyramid. You have acquired the necessary knowledge of normal anatomy and disease processes. You have gained the ability to obtain an accurate and complete medical history from the patient. You have become familiar with normal tissue characteristics and some common abnormal structures. Along with all this comes the ability to interpret those images. As you are exposed to more and more images and clinical situations your knowledge will grow, the pyramid will become wider at the base and taller at the apex, and your ability to assist the radiologist will improve. You will be able to make independent decisions based on the clinical interpretation of the images you produce.

CLINICAL IMAGING

Introduction

Through the miracle of modern technology, both in computed tomography (CT) and magnetic resonance imaging (MRI), we are now able to visualize internal anatomical structures that have remained hidden for decades due to superimposition. No longer are we bound by the two-dimensional cell of the radiograph.

MRI gives us the capability of imaging directly in any and all planes or orientations we choose. Although this is a tremendous advantage for discerning pathology it can sometimes get quite confusing to those viewing the images. The technologist learning cross-sectional anatomy needs to recognize structures in all three dimensions and their relationships to other structures. He/she needs to be able to visualize a structure so clearly that it can be mentally sliced or viewed from different directions.

There are three basic orthogonal planes used in MRI; axial (transverse), sagittal, and coronal [Figure 12-1]. Axial (transverse) orientation splits the body into superior (top) and inferior (bottom) portions. This is the orientation most commonly seen in computed tomography. Sagittal orientation divides the body into left and right sections. If the portions are equal then it is termed the mid sagittal plane. Coronal orientation divides the body into front (anterior) and back (posterior) sections. In addition to the above three planes, which by definition are perpendicular to each other, the MRI system allows us to image in any oblique orientation. The ability to image directly in any plane without loss of resolution is one of the strong points of MRI. It gives the technologist and/or the radiologist the capacity to orient the direction of imaging to best visualize the anatomical structures in question. This can be done without moving the patient into an uncomfortable or compromising position.

The technologist needs to interpret each structure as it appears on the monitor. The section or slice of anatomy is just a small piece of a larger structure. It is important to be able to know what lies behind or in front of; above or below; to the right or left; an example of this is shown in Figure 12-2. As you slice through the cone from right to left the resulting image grows larger revealing the hollow middle. If the same cone is sliced from top to bottom the image still reveals the hollow middle but looks very different; this can be seen by viewing the lateral

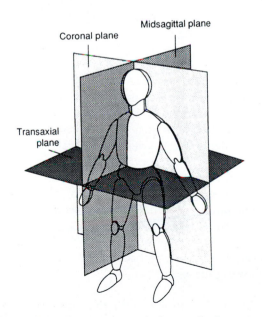

Figure 12-1. Commonly used planes of reference through the body.

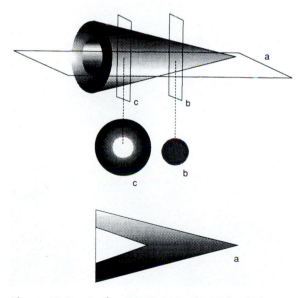

Figure 12-2. As the cone is imaged or "sliced" in various locations the resulting images reveal the hollow middle (a and c) or the solid upper portion (b).

ventricles of the brain in each orientation. Look at representative coronal, sagittal, and axial images [Figure 12-3] from a routine brain scan; the lateral ventricles appear different in each image. As you become familiar with the anatomical structures and their orientation, you'll find it easier to know which image plane gives the best view of the structure. Once you are relatively comfortable with the idea of seeing the same structure in different planes, you can commit its name and function to memory.

It is beyond the scope of this text to give a comprehensive review of the normal anatomy and pathology the technologist will encounter. There are many excellent texts available which present the normal anatomy and associated pathology in all orientations. Some will even show matching cadaver sections of the actual anatomy. Texts such as these are a necessity in all MRI departments. What the technologist must do is develop a system to systematically learn and review the anatomy as the images are seen on the

screen. The best way to approach this is to pick a region of the body that you scan routinely and learn the major structures first, then work your way down to smaller and smaller areas. It is a daunting task, and to attempt to do it all at once is futile, not to mention frustrating. Those of you involved mainly in neuro MRI will of course wish to concentrate on neuroanatomy then branch out into musculoskeletal as time allows. And there will be those of you who perform predominately musculoskeletal exams who'll wish to learn about that region first.

Whatever your need, start with a good anatomy text and as you view the images make a mental note of the structures and their names. Pick a few structures each time you view the images and review the ones you learned previously. Learn to read or study the images, not just stare blankly at them. Think about how that structure would look in a different plane. It is sometimes helpful to pull routine cases and go over the anatomy with a marking pencil and your anatomy book. Don't be afraid to question your radiologists. The better you know the anatomy the better you can help them. Don't rush. Learn a few structures each day. Before long, you will be able to recognize all the major structures in a particular area of interest. As you learn each structure begins to be cognizant of its function, how it relates to or affects other functions of the body, and what problems occur if that structure or area is damaged. Which area of the brain controls speech? Which area controls balance? If the patient is experiencing visual difficulties where might you expect to find a lesion? Which lumbar nerves give rise to anterior thigh pain? Medical imaging is like trying to solve a giant jigsaw puzzle. You have all the pieces if you can just fit them together properly.

Every technologist should strive to build a strong foundation by becoming familiar with the following ideas.

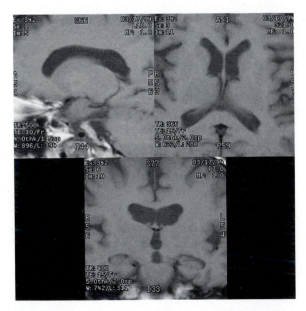

Figure 12-3. T1 weighted images demonstrating the different appearances of the lateral ventricles when sliced or imaged in sagittal, axial, and coronal planes.

Normal anatomy of all the major structures of the area being imaged including the innervation and vasculature anatomy.

Functions of each major structure.

Relationships between major structures.

As an MRI technologist you have probably noticed the images on the monitor can vary considerably in their appearance depending on the acquisition pulse sequence. In computed tomography (CT) the technologist always had a standard to fall back on. Bone, having the greatest electron density (i.e., the most dense), was always white, showing the highest intensity. Air, having the least electron density (i.e., the least dense), was always black, showing the lowest intensity. Everything else was in between. The technologist had little control over the physics of acquiring the image and the resultant image showed nothing of the biological properties of the object being scanned. The computer-generated image was merely a map of the attenuated X-ray beam as it passed through different densities of tissue.

With the advent of MRI, the technologist now has the ability to image biological functions not merely electron density. Simply by selecting the pulse sequence, the technologist has the ability to change how the images will be acquired and what factors will influence that image. The technologist controls whether the image will represent a T1 weighted image, a T2 weighted image, or a proton density weighted image. Each selection can change the appearance of the resultant image. The anatomy is still in the same place but it appears differently on the monitor. Fortunately

for the technologist and the radiologist, MR imaging is not a giant guessing game. There are rules and standards which hold true for each of the differently weighted sequences. These rules must be learned in order to successfully identify the structure in question by the appropriate selection of the acquisition sequence.

Routine spin echo pulse sequences use parameters listed in Table 12-1 to acquire information weighted as T1, T2, or proton density. As long as the images are acquired as specified, each will have certain characteristic signal intensities. For the purposes of grasping the fundamentals of how particular structures appear on differently weighted images, we shall stay in the realm of spin echo imaging and discuss the appearance of T1, T2, and proton density images. Once you have become familiar and comfortable with these images you can move on to the subtle nuances in the appearance of gradient echo, fast spin echo, and inversion recovery images.

The signal intensities of anatomical structures and substances will be the same regardless of where they are found in the body. For example, cerebrospinal fluid (CSF) found in the brain will show similar signal intensity as that found in the spinal column using the same pulse sequence. We will focus on the signal intensities of anatomical structures and substances found in the following regions: brain, spinal cord, and musculoskeletal system. If the technologist can master the basic anatomical structures of these three regions, using T1, T2, and proton density imaging

Table 12-1

Spin Echo Pulse Sequence Parameters: Echo Time, TE, and Repetition Time, TR

TE/TR Parameters	Weighted Image
Short TE (< 30 ms) Short TR (< 800 ms)	T1 weighted images
Short TE (< 30 ms) Long TR (> 2000 ms)	Proton density images
Long TE (> 60 ms) Long TR (> 2000 ms)	T2 weighted images

parameters along with an understanding of some common pathology, then the ability of clinical interpretation will follow.

Brain Imaging

The signal intensities of different tissues found in the brain will vary with the pulse sequence used to acquire the image. In most departments, routine head or brain scan protocols call for imaging in the axial, coronal, and sagittal planes using both T1 and T2 weighted images.

Cerebrospinal fluid (CSF) has a very high water concentration giving it very long T1 and T2 relaxation times. On T1 weighted images it will have very little signal and thus appear dark [Figure 12-4A]. On T2 weighted images this same CSF will have a very high signal and appear bright [Figure 12-4B]. This can be a very useful benchmark in recognizing T1 and T2 weighted images if you do not know the parameters of the scan. Simply check the signal intensity of the CSF.

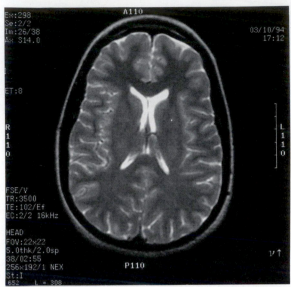

B

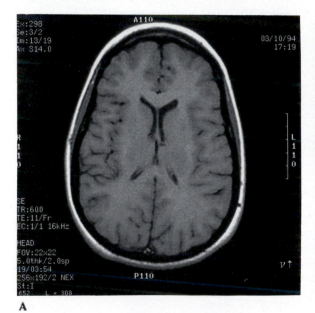

A

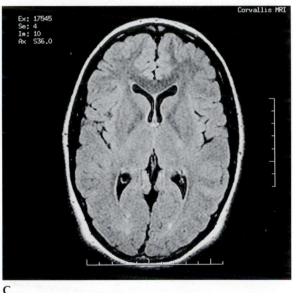

C

Figure 12-4. **A** T1 weighted (600/11) axial image through the lateral ventricles demonstrating the dark signal intensity of the CSF and intermediate signal intensity of the gray matter and higher signal white matter. **B** T2 weighted (3500/102Ef) axial image at the same level of **A** illustrating the now bright signal intensity of CSF and the reversed roles of the gray/white matter compared to the T1 weighted images. **C** A FLAIR (10000/102/2000) image at the same level of **A** and **B** illustrating the dark CSF. Notice that the gray/white matter signal intensities are the same as in the T2 weighted image **B**.

The exception to this benchmark is the recent introduction of a new and very versatile pulse sequence called FLAIR (fluid attenuated inversion recovery). The sequence has been extremely helpful in visualizing lesions near the ventricles and in situations where it is important to differentiate CSF from edema. In the past it has been difficult to see periventricular pathology because of the inherent bright signal of the existing CSF on T2 weighted images. FLAIR is an inversion recovery pulse sequence that is heavily T2 weighted combined with an inversion time that nulls out, or voids, signal from CSF without affecting interparenchymal fluid. In short, when performing a FLAIR sequence you obtain a T2 weighted image with black, or very dark, CSF. The majority of periventricular or interparenchymal lesions will continue to exhibit bright signal intensity against the backdrop of black CSF.

The fact that water has a very long T2 relaxation time is extremely helpful when it comes to recognizing pathological processes in the brain. Almost all pathological processes will involve an increase in the water content of the cells and surrounding area due to edema (cytotoxic, vasogenic, or interstitial). Due to the long T2 of water and the sensitivity of MRI to these changes, the T2 weighted images will be extraordinarily sensitive to edema. Edema will appear as low signal or dark/gray on T1 weighted images and as a high signal or bright on T2 weighted images very similar to CSF. In fact, edema can be so bright on T2 weighted images the underlying pathology can be obscured.

Bone, such as the temporal bone, will appear black or dark on T1 and T2 weighted images of the brain. We no longer have to experience the beam-hardening artifact of CT when imaging through the petreous region. This gives MRI a great advantage over CT in the posterior fossa and the area of the internal auditory canal [Figure 12-5]. Calcifications within the brain itself such as calcified choroid plexus or basal ganglia calcifications appear to be dark to intermediate on T1 weighted images and dark

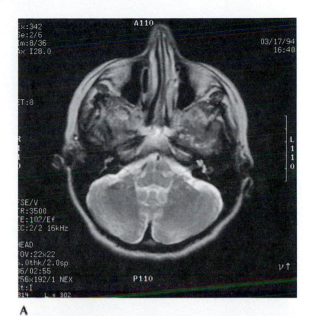

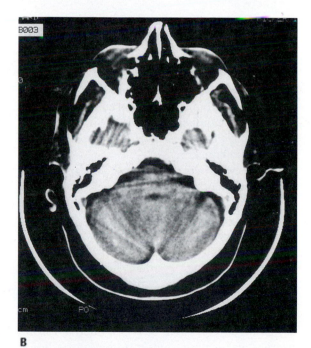

Figure 12-5. **A** T2 weighted (3500/102Ef) axial image through the petreous bones showing the absence of the beam-hardening or Hounsfield artifact seen. **B** A CT at approximately the same level showing the Hounsfield artifact.

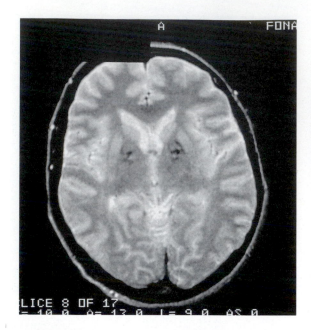

Figure 12-6. Basal ganglia calcifications as seen on a T2 weighted (2500/85) image showing the lack of signal.

Figure 12-7. T1 weighted (600/11) axial image at the level of the internal carotid arteries demonstrating the lack of signal caused by fast-flowing blood.

or black on T2 images [Figure 12-6]. Because there are some limitations in imaging calcium it is advisable to compare the MRI with computed tomography in cases where the presence of calcium is a concern.

Another structure that will appear dark or black on T1 and T2 weighted spin echo images of the brain is fast-flowing blood [Figure 12-7]. Non-invasive arterial and venous flow studies can be performed by MR angiography in departments equipped with the specialized apparatus. But even during routine head scans, the technologist should be sufficiently familiar with the observed vascular structures to accomplish effective visualizations. This includes the vertebral/basilar artery, circle of Willis, internal carotid arteries, and venous sinuses. Often an occlusion of the internal carotid artery or an arteriovenous malformation (AVM) is seen during routine scanning [Figure 12-8].

Fat is another substance that can be helpful as a benchmark. It has a very short T1 relaxation

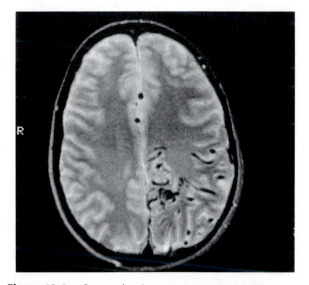

Figure 12-8. Surgery/angio proven arteriovenous malformation (AVM) left occipital parietal region. Notice the plethora of arteries indicated by the lack of signal.

time, therefore will always be bright on T1 weighted images. It has an intermediate T2 relaxation time and will appear gray on T2 weighted images. The appearance of fat on T1 weighted images can sometimes prove to be a problem in postgadolinium contrast studies if precontrast studies are not performed first. This can be especially critical in the pituitary fossa and the skull base where both the fat-containing areas and the enhancing areas will appear identical on the T1 weighted images. The advent of fat saturation pulse sequences has helped remedy this situation by suppressing the fat signal and allowing the enhancing region to be the only high signal intensity or bright area seen.

We have talked about the CSF, bone, blood, and fat in the head. What about the actual brain tissues, the gray and white matter?

Gray matter of the brain is formed by multiple neuron cell bodies supported by layers of glial cells. There are no significant extracellular spaces except for perivascular spaces. It is composed of 80 percent water, 10 percent protein, and 9 percent phospholipids. White matter is composed predominantly of myelinated nerve fibers which form tracts that interconnect the gray matter regions. Compared to gray matter, the concentration of water is less (70 percent) and phospholipids higher (20 percent).

Due to the lower water content of white matter, it will have a shorter T1 and T2 relaxation time than gray matter. On T1 weighted images the gray matter will appear as an intermediate density (gray) somewhat darker than white matter. On T2 weighted images the signal intensities tend to be reversed; the white matter appears as a darker gray than the higher signal gray matter [Figure 12-4].

Gadolinium is a T1 shortening contrast agent currently in widespread use in MRI departments. It is advantageous for the technologist to be familiar with the normal enhancing structures so that a mistake will not be made as to whether or not you are looking at a pathological abnormality. Table 12-2 lists those structures normally enhanced by gadolinium.

Table 12-2

Commonly Enhancing Structures with the Administration of Gadolinium

Dural sinuses
   Superior sagittal sinus
   Transverse sinuses
Nasopharynx mucosa
Choroid plexus
Pituitary gland
Infundibulum
Cavernous sinuses

You should now be familiar with the normal anatomical structures and signal intensities found within the brain. A compilation of these can be found in Table 12-3. While looking at the images on the monitor begin to recognize any areas that look peculiar or show abnormal or out of place signal intensities. With MRI this is sometimes easier than you might think. It has been said that anybody shown a grossly abnormal MRI would be able to say it wasn't normal. Three rules of thumb may help you to begin the search for abnormal areas.

Are the right and left halves of the brain symmetrical?

The body has done a wonderful engineering job. In the brain the two hemispheres should appear roughly identical. If there is an area of concern on one side does it exist on the other? If not, there's a good chance it's an abnormality.

Are there areas that exhibit any signs of mass effect?

Pathological processes such as tumors usually take up more space than the original structure, either by destroying it or pushing it out of the way. Look at the ventricles; are they effaced? Look at the sulci and gyri; are they still crisp and clear, not swollen or distorted?

Table 12-3

Summary of MRI Tissue Characteristics of Brain Structures

	Relaxation Time		Image Contrast		
	T1	T2	PD	T1	T2
CSF	long	long	gray	dark	bright
Gray matter	intermediate	intermediate	isointense	gray	gray
White matter	short	short	gray/dark	bright	dark
Fat	short	intermediate	bright	bright	gray
Cortical bone	long	short	dark	dark	dark
Air	long	short	dark	dark	dark
Blood (fast flow)	long	short	dark	dark	dark
Edema	long	long	bright/gray	gray/dark	bright
Protein	short	long	bright/gray	bright	bright

When looking at the T2 weighted images are there any bright signal intensities other than the CSF spaces and venous structures?

Remember that edema will be of high signal and that most pathological processes will result in increased edema. The only high signal you should see on T2 weighted images should be in the areas where you would expect CSF or ocular vitreous. If an area of high signal intensity is seen, compare it to the same area on the T1 weighted images. Does it reflect CSF or edema?

Depending upon answers to these questions, you must decide whether to terminate the exam, do additional pulse sequences, or have the radiologist review the images and do additional pulse sequences after the administration of intravenous (IV) contrast media.

There are several abnormal findings you will see often during day to day scanning. Among them are these.

Demyelinating/white matter disease.
Stroke, ischemia, or infarction.
Tumor/metastatic disease.

These entities will most probably make up the majority of the abnormal scans you will see, so you should be well versed in their appearance. Keep in mind that all the above conditions can have variable presentations on MRI depending on type, location, and age of onset. Some typical features will be discussed here.

MRI has proven to be the modality of choice for imaging white matter/demyelinating disease due to its extreme sensitivity to subtle changes in the water content of white matter and myelin. Although there is a plethora of different diseases that affect the white matter, multiple sclerosis (MS) is one the technologist will see very often. The appearance of MS on MRI is very characteristic. High signal or bright lesions of varying sizes and shapes on T2 weighted images found in the periventricular white matter (especially in the centrum semiovale), cerebellum, brain stem and corpus callosum [Figure 12-9]. These lesions may or may not be visible on T1 and proton density weighted images. The appearance of these high signal lesions, however characteristic of MS, are not specific for this diagnosis without the accompanying clinical picture. This is one case where an accurate and detailed patient history will prove invaluable to the radiologist during diagnosis.

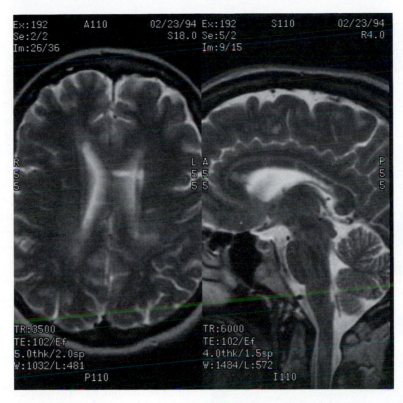

Figure 12-9.   Typical high signal lesions on T2 weighted images seen in patients presenting clinically with multiple sclerosis. Notice the diagnostic longitudinal lesions seen in the corpus callosum.

Stroke may be defined as a sudden focal neurologic deficit lasting longer than 24 hours and is the expressed clinical manifestation of cerebrovascular disease. The patient usually presents with an acute onset of some neurologic deficit (usually lateralized) that may have resolved over time. The stroke will result in the appearance of edema which will appear as a high intensity signal (bright) on T2 weighted images. T1 weighted images will reflect an intermediate to dark signal depending on the age of the event. Often the area involved is wedge-shaped and lies within one vascular territory. Unless the infarcted area is very large, one will not see any mass effect. Figure 12-10 demonstrates a typical stroke as seen on T1 and T2 weighted images.

The introduction of echo planar imaging capabilities with such pulse sequences as diffusion and perfusion have increased our ability to image ischemic changes such as stroke and to see abnormal results much more quickly. It takes a certain amount of time from the onset of symptoms to see changes in signal intensity on the T1 and T2 weighted images. The use of diffusion imaging in patients with suspected infarcts will show changes in signal intensity much sooner than the T1 and T2 weighted images. As is illustrated in Figure 12-11(A–D) the routine T1, T2 and FLAIR images are normal or slightly abnormal and the diffusion images are grossly abnormal. Diffusion sequences image the random movement of water throughout the brain and gives the referring physician

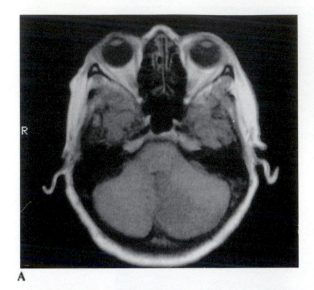

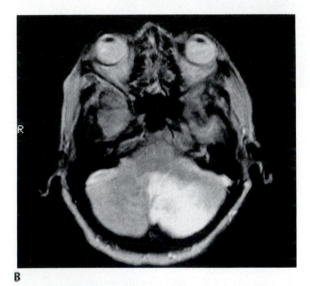

Figure 12-10. T1 weighted (500/16) and T2 weighted (2500/85) axial images depicting the typical appearance of stroke or infarct. Low signal intensity on T1 and high signal intensity on T2 represents edema. The wedge-shaped area lies within one vascular territory with minimal mass effect. No enhancement was seen with administration of gadolinium.

information on the actual area of the brain damaged by the stroke. After a certain period of time the diffusion images will cease to reflect acute events. This helps age the infarction as acute or sub-acute.

Perfusion imaging, another fast imaging technique, along with the rapid injection of contrast material allows for the imaging of the cerebral blood flow. This allows calculation of the stroke penumbra or the area at risk. This is the area of the brain not destroyed by the acute event and potentially salvageable by rapid intervention. As advances are made with immediate stroke treatment and intervention such as thrombolytics these pulse sequences will become more important in determining the course of treatment and the eventual outcome.

Many of the patients that will be seen in the MRI department will be there to rule out tumor or mass lesion. They might present with rather bizarre neuro findings or simply just a headache that won't go away. They may have been recently diagnosed with a primary tumor somewhere in their body that has the propensity to metastasize to the brain and are being staged for treatment; or they have had a cancer in the past and are now presenting with a symptom that could be attributable to metastatic brain disease. Most facilities have typical protocols for tumor and metastatic studies always involving the use of the intravenous contrast material. Although the appearance of tumors on MRI is quite variable depending on location, size, tumor type and age, there are some typical findings the technologist can look for. Tumors may exhibit the presence of edema, sometimes massive amounts; this results in a very bright signal on T2 weighted images and intermediate to dark signal on T1 images. Where the appearance of stroke is somewhat wedge-shaped, the tumor edema will vary in size and shape, frequently crossing vascular boundaries and presenting with a ragged edge. Most tumors produce some mass effect on adjacent structures. The use of a T1 shortening contrast agent such as gadolinium will produce enhancement of the tumor body and a high

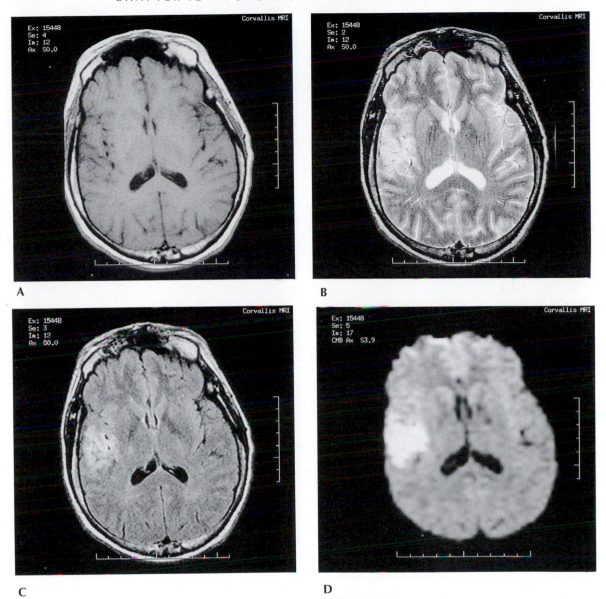

Figure 12-11.   Images illustrating an acute right middle cerebral artery distribution infarct. **A** T1 weighted (650/13) image showing minimal signal intensity change; **B** T2 weighted (3500/102) image and **C** FLAIR (9700/102/2000) image showing a slight increase in signal intensity due to increased intracellular fluid; **D** diffusion weighted echo planar imaging sequence illustrating the grossly positive nature of diffusion imaging in acute infarcts.

intensity or bright signal on the T1 weighted images. The use of this contrast agent is sometimes necessary to delineate tumor mass from edema. Figures 12-12 through 12-14 demonstrate three tumor types commonly encountered in the brain: a meningioma, a glioma, and a metastatic lung cancer. By comparing certain characteristics, such as formation of edema, location, mass effect, and enhancement qualities, a more definitive differential diagnosis can be made. Although they all appear similar, through the judicious use of the proper pulse sequences, imaging planes, and gadolinium contrast agent, the technologist can give the radiologist a more complete diagnostic exam.

Spine Imaging

The spinal cord and other neural tissues are imaged very nicely on MRI, which has several advantages over other imaging modalities.

Intrathecal contrast is not necessary to assess cord size and the shape or extent of a tumor

Ability to see above and/or below a tumor blockage

No beam-hardening artifacts

In patients where symptomology or clinical evaluation make it difficult to point to a specific nerve root or disk space, a larger area can be surveyed well on sagittal images

The spinal cord and other neural tissues, such as exiting nerve roots, will appear as intermediate gray signal intensity on all pulse sequences. The acquisition of either T1 or T2 weighted images allow the technologist to change the surrounding CSF contrast to either dark (T1) or bright (T2) thereby further accentuating the cord. The spinal cord should be nearly homogeneous in signal intensity and nearly symmetrical in shape. In a normal cord there should be no dark or bright signals. The appearance of any dark or bright signals or the bulging of an area should tip the

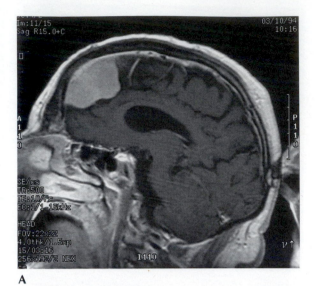

A

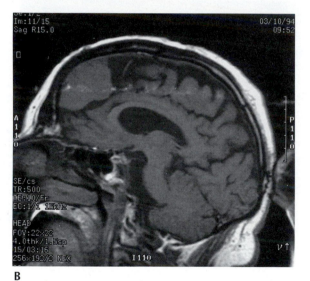

B

Figure 12-12. T1 weighted (500/10) sagittal images of the classic presentation of a frontal lobe meningioma before **A** and after **B** the administration of gadolinium. Notice the intense enhancement, extra axial midline location, and lack of edema.

technologist to investigate further. As we saw in the brain, almost all pathological processes will exhibit an increase in signal on T2 weighted

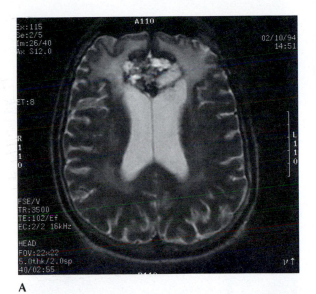

A

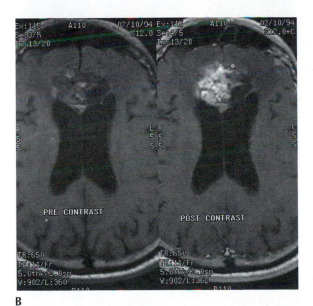

B

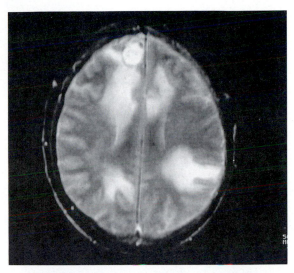

A

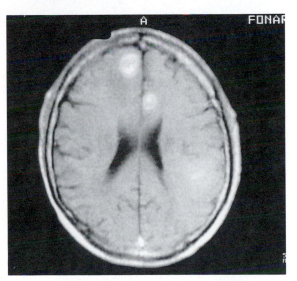

B

Figure 12-13.   Biopsy proven glioblastoma multiforme. **A** The T2 weighted (3500/102Ef) images demonstrate a lesion with a very heterogeneous signal intensity that crosses the midline. Notice the bright signal in the white matter typical of edema. **B** Pregadolinium and **C** postgadolinium T1 weighted (650/11) images showing heterogeneous enhancement of the tumor. Surrounding white matter edema appears low in signal.

Figure 12-14.   Multiple lesions of metastatic lung cancer. **A** T2 weighted (2500/85) images illustrating the massive edema typically associated with metastatic lesions. **B** Postgadolinium image showing the typical ring lesion.

images. Therefore the technologist should be sure to obtain both T1 and T2 weighted images. If the clinical picture strongly suggests a cord lesion, as in severe myelopathy, it is strongly advisable to administer contrast and to obtain pre- and postcontrast T1 images. In Figures 12-15 and 12-16 we see two common cord lesions, an ependymoma imaged in the sagittal plane and a multiple sclerosis (MS) plaque imaged in the coronal and sagittal planes.

The CSF found in the spinal column will appear just as it appeared in the brain, low signal or dark on the T1 weighted images and relatively high signal or bright on T2 weighted images [Figure 12-17]. The spinal cord will appear intermediate gray, or of higher signal intensity than CSF on T1 weighted images and of lower intensity than CSF on T2 images. Imaging the spinal cord using heavily T2 weighted images

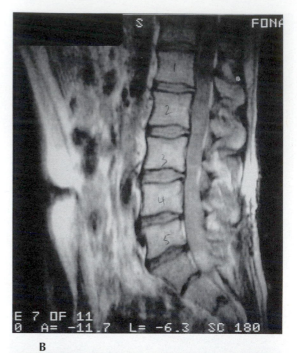

B

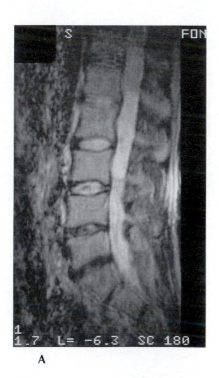

A

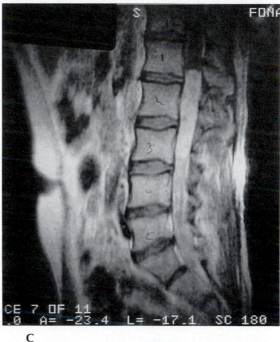

C

Figure 12-15. Cord ependymoma extending from L1 to L3. **A** T2 weighted (2000/85) sagittal image showing the bright signal of the mass, **B** pregadolinium, and **C** postgadolinium T1 weighted (700/30) images illustrating the intense enhancement of the tumor and the ability to delineate the actual extent of the tumor mass compared to noncontrast images.

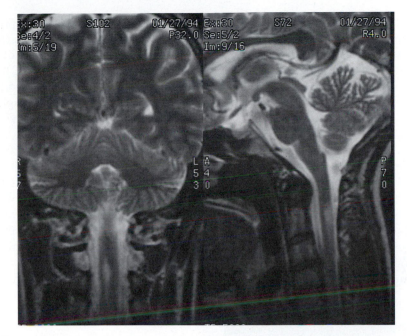

Figure 12-16. T2 weighted coronal and sagittal images of the upper cervical cord illustrating a typical MS plaque.

gives the so-called myelographic effect [Figure 12-17]. The ability to image in the sagittal plane is a great advantage in MRI in screening for any cord-related pathology, for example, disc protrusion, cord compression, intradural lesions, and extradural lesions. The capability of MRI to image above a blockage in the cord obviates the need for myelograms, which are difficult and often impossible to accomplish on patients with a blockage. In addition, MRI can see lesions inside the spinal cord. All these capabilities have revolutionized diagnosis and treatment of spinal cord disease and injuries.

The bony vertebral column is a common area of MR imaging. Due to the tremendous ability of MRI to visualize the bone marrow, it is the modality of choice for imaging marrow-destroying processes such as metastatic disease and hematopoetic disorders. On T1 weighted images the vertebral bodies should be very homogeneous and of intermediate to higher signal intensity [Figure 12-18A] relative to the adjacent disc.

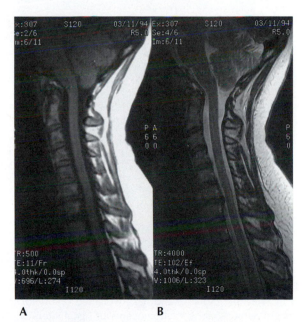

A   B

Figure 12-17. **A** T1 weighted (500/11) sagittal images of the cervical spine illustrating the low signal intensity of CSF. **B** T2 weighted (4000/102Ef) sagittal images of the cervical spine demonstrating the myelographic effect of bright CSF against the darker cord.

Commonly encountered pathology, such as fractures, replacement of the marrow by infective processes, or metastatic disease, will usually cause a decrease in signal intensity resulting in a darker appearance [Figure 12-19] of the vertebral body on T1 weighted images. It is important to remember the injection of paramagnetic contrast material can mask this change in vertebral body signal intensity. When imaging patients with suspected metastatic disease, always obtain T1 weighted images before administration of contrast material. When viewing T2 weighted images, expect to see the same homogeneous signal intensity as on the T1 images although somewhat less intense [Figure 12-18B]. Whenever the technologist sees vertebral bodies that are not homogeneous in signal intensity, they

should suspect some abnormal process. Loss of the cortical endplates of the vertebral body is seen frequently with discitis or some other infectious process [Figure 12-20]. A commonly encountered, usually benign condition, seen in vertebral bodies is a bone hemangioma. This will usually yield a high signal on T1 weighted images [Figure 12-21].

Intervertebral discs consist of two distinct components. The nucleus pulposus is a richly hydrated, incompressible, gelatinous substance surrounded by a tougher ring of fibrous collagen, called the annulus fibrosis. Discs in young, healthy individuals are usually well hydrated (85 to 90 percent water content). The relatively high content of the nucleus pulposus will produce a low signal intensity on T1 weighted images and a high signal intensity on T2 weighted images and proton density images [Figure 12-18]. The

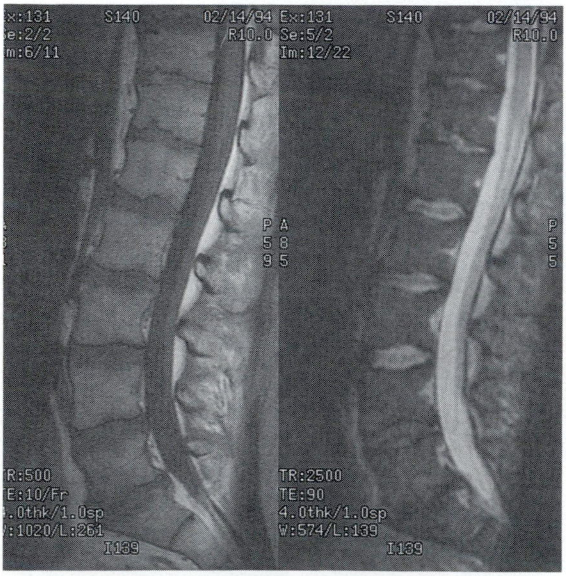

Figure 12-18. Sagittal images of the lumbar spine. **A** T1 weighted (500/10) and **B** T2 weighted (2500/90) images demonstrating the homogeneous signal intensity of the vertebral bodies. Notice the bright signal intensity of the disc spaces on the T2 images signifying disc hydration. At L45 and L5S1 the signal intensity on the T2 images has decreased due to loss of water, i.e., disc degeneration.

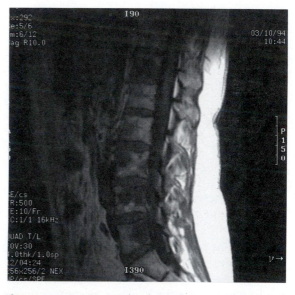

Figure 12-19. T1 weighted (500/10) sagittal image of the lumbar spine illustrating the mottled low signal vertebral bodies typically seen in metastatic disease. Compare the heterogeneous signal of the vertebral bodies with those of a normal spine, as seen in Fig. 12-18*A*.

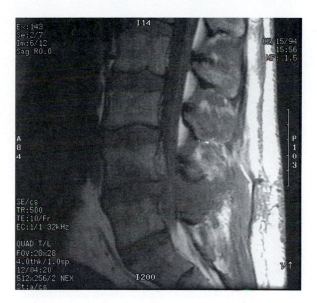

Figure 12-20. Biopsy proven postoperative disc infection. Notice the loss of the cortical endplates at L45.

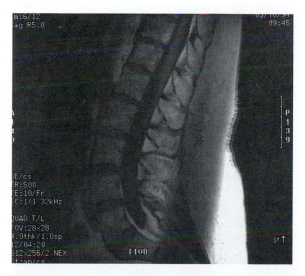

Figure 12-21. T1 weighted (500/10) sagittal lumbar spine illustrating the high intensity signal of a typical benign bony hemangioma at T11, T12, and L5.

fibrous annulus ring functions rather like a ligament and will appear as a thin dark ring of low signal on all techniques. On sagittal T2 weighted images a thin dark line appears at the anterior portion of the intervertebral disc. This is the normal intervertebral cleft.

With normal aging there is loss of water from the disc (70 percent water content), resulting in loss of disc height and desiccation of the disc. This loss of water contributes to a loss of signal on both T1 and T2 weighted images. Degeneration of the disc is best appreciated on T2 weighted images [Figure 12-18B]. The ability of MRI to evaluate the status of the disc, before actually bulging or herniation, gives the referring physician important information for the continued management of the patient with chronic back pain.

Other than degenerative disc disease, the most common disorder the technologist is likely to encounter when performing MRI of the spine is the herniated disc. This is where a good clinical history can point to the problem area before viewing any images. It will also allow the technologist to focus the effort of the exam at the proper disc levels. The differentiation of disc herniation versus disc bulging can sometimes cause the radiologist some anxiety, although the technologist should be able to recognize a frank disc herniation. Look for the disc material to push through the annulus creating some obvious mass effect on the CSF space in the sagittal projection [Figure 12-22] on either T1 or T2 weighted images. On normal T1 weighted axial images the exiting nerve roots should appear as dark signal structures surrounded by the brighter signal of epidural fat [Figure 12-23A]. In a suspected disc herniation the disc material can be seen encroaching and sometimes obliterating this relationship [Figure 12-23B].

Magnetic resonance imaging to delineate post-operative scar, or fibrosis formation from recurrent disc herniation, is a request frequently made by referring orthopedists, neurologists, and neurosurgeons. Although each department has its own protocol for this exam, it usually involves

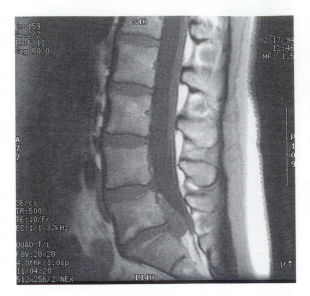

Figure 12-22. T1 weighted (500/10) sagittal lumbar spine depicting a large herniation at the L5S1 level. Note the obvious mass effect on the thecal sac and the matching signal intensities and continuation of the disc space and the extruded material.

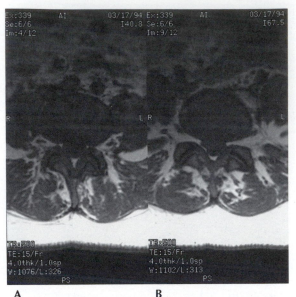

A   B

Figure 12-23. **A** Normal T1 weighted (500/15) axial lumbar spine image. **B** Extruded disc shown deforming the thecal sac in a midline herniation.

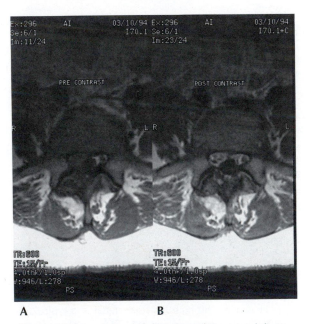

A   B

Figure 12-24. **A** Pregadolinium and **B** postgadolinium axial T1 weighted (600/15) images. In **A** notice the low signal intensity "mass" on obliterating the right nerve root. In **B** the administration of gadolinium enhances the majority of the mass, typical of postoperative fibrosis.

acquisition of precontrast images, the administration of contrast (gadolinium) and subsequent postcontrast images using the same pulse sequence at the same location. Scar tissue, with its increased vascularity compared to disc material, and the addition of a T1 shortening contrast agent should show an increased signal intensity compared to the disc material [Figure 12-24].

As you view more and more images, you will become increasingly familiar with the many variations of normal and abnormal spiral anatomy. A summary of the MRI characteristics of spinal column structures can be found in Table 12-4. Some common pathological entities and their signal characteristics are found in Table 12-5.

Musculoskeletal Imaging

MRI is used to perform imaging studies on bone and soft tissue due to its superior soft tissue

Table 12-4

MRI Tissue Characteristics of Spinal Column Structures

Feature	T1 Weighted Image	Proton Density Image	T2 Weighted Image
Spinal cord	intermediate/gray	intermediate/gray	gray
CSF	dark	intermediate/gray	bright
Vertical body	intermediate/gray	intermediate/gray	intermediate/gray
Intervertebral disc	gray	light gray	bright
Fat	bright	light gray	gray
Cortical bone	black	black	black

Table 12-5

Common Pathological Entities of the Spine

Pathological Process	T1 Signal	T2 Signal
Disk herniation	heterogeneous	increased
Postoperative scar		
acute	increased	very increased
chronic	heterogeneous	decreased
Osteophytes (spurs)	heterogeneous	decreased
Metastatis	decreased	increased

contrast. In fact, MRI is the modality of choice in imaging disorders of the bone marrow and soft tissue. Its use in the musculoskeletal system has risen dramatically over the past few years. Structures commonly evaluated are the temporomandibular joint, shoulder, elbow, wrist, ankle, hip, and knee along with the associated soft tissue areas.

Depending on your facility's exam mix you may not see a lot of musculoskeletal cases. Remember that MRI of the joints is very demanding, due to the small structures and subtle soft tissue changes, and requires specialized surface coils, small fields of view, and exact protocols.

Most of the contrast in the musculoskeletal system is due to the presence of high signal fat highlighted against the lower signals of muscle and bone. T1 and proton density weighted images, due to their high signal to noise, illustrate the anatomy quite well. As we have seen in other areas of the body the use of T2 weighted images allows us to be sensitive to fluid collections. In the musculoskeletal system they are likely to be abscess formations, neoplasms, joint effusions, and cysts. Both T1 weighted and T2 weighted images are necessary when imaging the musculoskeletal system.

It is important to get a good clinical history from the patient in order to adequately cover the region of interest. A good procedure to follow is to have the patient point to the area that hurts with *one finger* then place a marker (vitamin E capsules work well) on the skin at that point. Center your scanning over this area.

If the patient presents with a mass, palpate it and note its characteristics for the radiologist.

Is the mass firm, soft, hard?

Is it painful to the touch?

Approximately how big is it?

Has it grown slowly or quickly?

One of the most important characteristics the radiologist and the referring physician will want to know is whether or not the mass is invading the cortical bone and is there more than one muscle group involved. The best way to represent cortical invasion is to acquire images in the axial plane. Figure 12-25 illustrates just how well the cortical bone–muscle interface is seen using an axial acquisition.

One of the most commonly examined areas of the musculoskeletal system is the knee. The ability to rule out meniscal tears without the injection or invasiveness of an arthrogram and clearly visualize the supporting structures of the knee gives MRI a distinct advantage over other procedures. Commonly visualized structures of the knee are listed in Table 12-6.

When examining the knee, images are always obtained in multiple planes even though most structures can be visualized best in one particular plane. Coronal images are needed to define the collateral ligaments and posterior femoral condyles. The anterior and posterior cruciate ligaments are best visualized in the sagittal plane, as are the medial and lateral menisci and the

insertion of the various muscle groups. Sagittal images are also best for the articular hyaline cartilage of the femur and tibia. Axial images best demonstrate the patellar facets and articular cartilage of the patellofemoral joint.

The most common cause of knee pain and disability is due to the tearing or rupturing of the

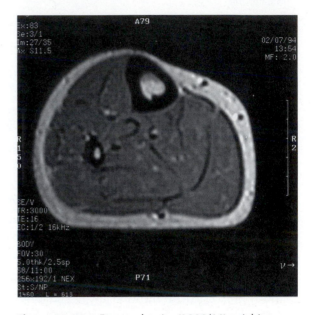

Figure 12-25. Proton density (3000/16) axial image through the lower leg demonstrating the normal cortical bone–soft tissue interface. Notice the delineation of the muscle bundles as well as the arteries and veins.

Table 12-6

MR Characteristics of Structures in the Knee

Structure	T1 Weighted Image	T2 Weighted Image
Meniscus (medial/lateral)	dark/black	dark/black
Posterior cruciate ligament	dark/black	dark/black
Anterior cruciate ligament	intermediate/gray	intermediate/gray
Hyaline cartilage	bright	gray
Cortical bone	dark/black	dark/black

menisci. The menisci are two C-shaped fibro-cartilaginous structures that sit both medially and laterally between the femoral condyles and the tibial plateaus. The menisci serve several functions.

Distribution of torsional and compressive forces during mechanical loading.

Distribution of synovial fluid over the articular cartilages.

Shock absorption.

Prevention of synovial impingement.

Facilitation of complex movement.

Limitation of abnormal movement.

Intact menisci are of uniform low signal (black) on both T1 and T2 weighted images and appear as triangular-shaped structures when imaged in the sagittal plane [Figure 12-26]. A frank tear of the meniscus can be readily seen on sagittal T1, proton density, and T2 weighted images as seen in Figure 12-27.

Other structures commonly injured are the anterior and posterior cruciate ligaments. The posterior cruciate ligament (PCL) arises from the lateral aspect of the medial femoral condyle, crosses the anterior cruciate ligament, and attaches to the posterior intercondyloid fossa of the tibia. In the sagittal plane the normal PCL is visualized as a single, uniform, solid, dark band on both the T1 and T2 images [Figure 12-28]. If the patient is positioned properly (15-degree external rotation) the entire PCL can be seen in one image. Any increase in signal on either the T1 or T2 images should be construed as abnormal, denoting hemorrhage possibly related to a partial tear or strain [Figure 12-29]. In the event of a complete disruption of the ligament you might see a gap or loss of continuity of the ligament and the presence of edema. The anterior cruciate ligament (ACL) extends from its tibial attachment, anterior to the intercondyloid eminence, to the medial aspect of the lateral femoral condyle. Unlike the PCL, the ACL is composed of several distinct fibrous bands. It normally appears as a dark, low intensity signal

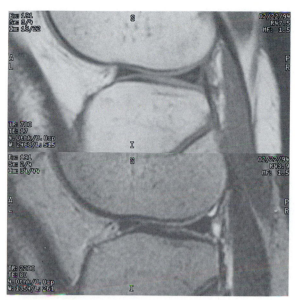

Figure 12-26. Normal-appearing meniscus on T1 weighted (700/17) and T2 weighted (2200/80) sagittal images. Notice the triangular shape and the dark almost black signal intensity.

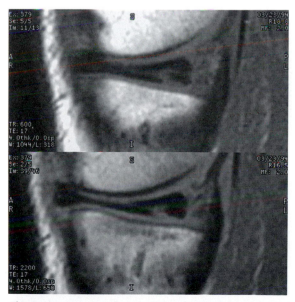

Figure 12-27. Frank tear of the posterior horn medial meniscus on both T1 weighted (600/17) and proton density (2200/17) sagittal images. Notice how you can follow the bright signal line (tear) all the way to the articular surface.

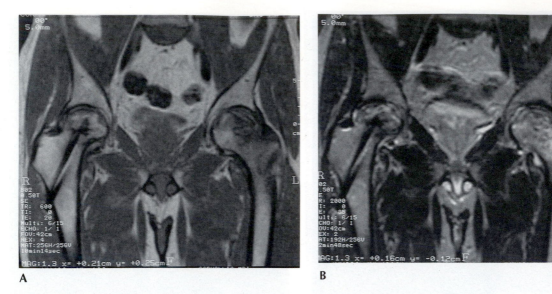

A   B

Figure 12-34. Abnormal appearing hips on **A** T1 weighted (600/17) coronal and **B** T2 weighted coronal images. On the right hip notice the placement of two metallic pins for femoral neck fracture. On the left, notice the typical low heterogeneous signal intensity on T1 and bright heterogeneous signal intensity on T2.

Table 12-7

MR Characteristics of Musculoskeletal Structures

Structure	T1 Weighted Image	Proton Density Image	T2 Weighted Image
Fat	bright	bright	gray
Muscle	intermediate	intermediate	dark/gray
Bone marrow	intermediate	intermediate	intermediate
Cortical bone	dark	dark	dark
Hyaline cartilage	bright	bright	gray
Ligament/tendon	dark	dark	dark
Fibrous tissue	dark	dark	dark
Edema	dark	bright	bright
Solid organs	variable	variable	variable

with the signal characteristics and capabilities it grants you. It is not a modality that can be learned overnight but one that takes effort and perseverance.

The magnetic resonance imaging technologist needs to take the responsibility and make the effort to learn enough to be able to clinically interpret what is seen on the monitor. Then and only then, will the technologist be rewarded by becoming an extension of the radiologist and an integral part of the imaging team.

SUGGESTED READING

Brant-Zawadski M, Norman D, eds. *Magnetic Resonance Imaging of the Central Nervous System.* New York: Raven Press, 1987.

Bushong SC. *Magnetic Resonance Imaging – Physical and Biological Principles.* St Louis: Mosby, 1988.

Hesselink JR, Edelman RR, eds. *Clinical Magnetic Resonance Imaging.* Philadelphia: Saunders, 1990.

Mink JH, Reicher MA, Crues JV. *Magnetic Resonance Imaging of the Knee.* New York: Raven Press, 1987.

Pomeranz SJ. *Craniospinal Magnetic Resonance Imaging.* Philadelphia: Saunders, 1989.

Schmalbrock P, Chakeres DW. *Fundamentals of Magnetic Resonance Imaging.* Baltimore: Williams and Wilkins, 1992.

Stoller DW, ed. *Magnetic Resonance Imaging in Orthopaedics and Rheumatology.* Philadelphia: Lippincott, 1989.

CHAPTER 13

Protocol Development Strategies

William Faulkner, Jr.

MR is an imaging modality with limitless possibilities for imaging planes and tissue contrasts. A patient could lie within an MR imager, be imaged for hours on end, and never have the exact same acquisition repeated. Often the pulse sequence and/or plane that best demonstrates the pathology is the one you should have done. In 1985, most systems offered the user only two choices in pulse sequences: spin echo (SE) and inversion recovery (IR). Few people in clinical practice understood the tissue contrast controls with IR, so SE was used almost exclusively. For T1 weighting, TR = 500 ms and TE = 20 ms (or the shortest TE available on the system) were used. A T2 sequence was obtained using TR = 2000 ms with TE = 40 ms and 80 ms. Early on, it was not possible to choose the two echo times independently of each other so the later echo was chosen by virtue of the early echo. TR = 2000 ms was the longest TR selected because of time constraints.

Since it was not uncommon for a T2 weighted sequence to last over 17 min, using TR > 2000 ms was not even a serious consideration. Total exam times could easily last over 1 h and still not consist of more than three separate series or scans.

Current systems now come with a plethora of sequences and imaging options. Popular types of data acquisition methods, such as fast gradient echo sequences (GRE), fast or turbo spin echo (FSE), 3D acquisitions, vascular sequences, and magnetization transfer, make it seem impossible to choose the right acquisition sequence and method. The purpose of this chapter is to give some suggestions for making MR protocol development as painless as possible. Refer to Chapter 6 for additional information on scan parameter selection.

OPTIMIZATION

Scan Time

Optimizing protocols means different things to different people. To some, it means shortening the exam time to increase throughput; to others, it means putting together a series of sequences to maximize the amount of information produced. But maximize and optimize do not mean the same thing. Figure 13.1 shows the relationships between the parameters that directly affect the overall scan time. The important point here is

255

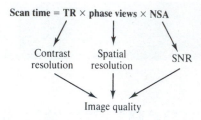

Figure 13-1. Relationships between parameters that affect the overall scan time.

that all three parameters contributing to scan time affect what could be termed image quality. Increasing any one of these three elements will cause the scan time to increase and the overall throughput to decrease. Working *with* the radiologist becomes important very quickly when trying to devise a protocol which seeks to strike a compromise between image quality (amount of information) and scan time (throughput). In this chapter I use the terms *image quality* and *amount of information* interchangeably.

Contrast Resolution

A radiologist's ability to provide the referring physician with diagnostic information is largely related to the amount of information represented on the images. The three elements of the scan time formula, contrast resolution, spatial resolution, and signal-to-noise (SNR), are the main components of image quality. Perhaps the most important of these is contrast resolution. We can have an image with superior SNR and outstanding spatial resolution, 512×512 imaging matrix, 14-cm field of view (FOV), and 1-mm slice thickness, for example. But if the MR signal intensity between the abnormal and the normal tissues is identical, and the anatomy has not changed, then no pathology will be seen. I realize this may be somewhat oversimplified, but first to catch the eye are often large differences in signal intensity, areas of high contrast. Increasing the contrast between structures increases the ability to differentiate between the structures.

The first step in working with the radiologist to develop a scan protocol is to determine the desired type of contrast. In other words, how does the radiologist want the image to look. If a fatty tumor is suspected then it may be best to include a T1 weighted sequence where fat will be seen as high signal intensity. If it is desirable to have bright fluid-filled structures, or bright CSF then perhaps a sequence with heavy T2 weighting would be appropriate. It has been my experience that if protocols are implemented without *specific goals or expectations*, then no one will like the resultant images. This is certainly true when dealing with contrast. Figure 13-2A and B is acquired with a fast spin echo (turbo spin echo) pulse sequence. The difference is that Figure 13-2A is acquired with TR = 2200 ms, TE = 13 ms, and ETL = 4; whereas Figure 13-2B is acquired with TR = 6000 ms, TE = 91 ms, and ETL = 16. One of the major benefits of using FSE sequences is that a longer TR is now possible without long scan times. While the image on the right is certainly more T2 weighted, and has higher contrasts between structures, the signal from the CSF is so intense that visualizing small MS plaques in the periventricular white matter would be difficult.

When determining the best contrast necessary for the clinical indication, consider also the type of pulse sequence to use. The two main types of pulse sequences are spin echo and gradient echo. Spin echo pulse sequences can be acquired using conventional spin echo (CSE) or "fast spin echo" (FSE). FSE sequences collect multiple lines of *k*-space in a single TR period. The number of lines filled in each TR is determined by the echo train length (ETL). The higher the ETL, the faster the scan time but the greater the image blurring. Image blurring with FSE sequences can be minimized by decreasing the space or time between echoes. This is usually accomplished by increasing the receiver bandwidth.

The major advantage of FSE sequences is the ability to use long TR times without a huge penalty in acquisition time. For T1 weighted images, FSE sequences can be used, however it is

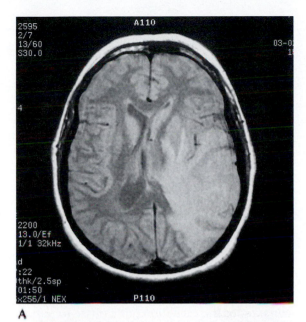

Figure 13-2. Images acquired with a fast spin echo (turbo spin echo) pulse sequence. **A** TR = 2200 ms, TE = 13 ms, ETL = 4. **B** TR = 6000 ms, TE = 91 ms, ETL = 16.

advisable to keep the ETL to 4 or less. When acquiring T2 weighted images, it is desirable to reduce the T1 contrast as much as possible. Since the TR controls the amount of T1 weighting seen in an image, the TR should be increased to 4000 ms or higher. ETLs of 16 or higher can be used when acquiring T2 weighted FSE. It is important to remember, however, that increasing the ETL does increase image blurring and use of higher receiver bandwidths should be considered.

If one desires to use FSE sequences to acquire proton density (PD) weighted images, there are some things that should be kept in mind. First is the selection of the TR. When imaging the brain, most radiologists are used to seeing PD images with TRs of between 2000 and 2500. The main reason is, as previously stated, longer TR times would cause the CSF to have such high signal that visualization of periventricular abnormalities may be difficult. In order to acquire PD weighted FSE images with contrast similar to that seen with conventional spin echo, try to match the TR as closely as possible. Secondly, PD weighted images require the use of a short TE. FSE sequences using short TEs are more susceptible to image blurring than those acquired with longer TE times. To minimize image blurring, use an ETL on the order of 4. Systems with faster gradients (i.e., slew rates of 50 or higher) may be able to use a slightly higher ETL, but greater than 8 is not recommended. Again, increasing the receiver bandwidth can help reduce the image blurring.

In some instances, an extremely long ETL is desired. Sequences using a high ETL (i.e., 128 or greater) in combination with half Fourier reconstruction, can produce a single image in one TR. This type of acquisition may be known as "single shot fast spin echo" (SS-FSE) or "half Fourier RARE". With such a sequence, the effective TE may be greater than 1000 ms. In this case, the only spins contributing to the MR signal are from fluids obviating the need for "fat sat". This type of technique has been termed "static fluid imaging" and can be used to acquire "MR cholangiograms" (MRCP) or "MR myelograms."

Inversion recovery (IR) spin echo sequences begin with a 180-degree RF pulse, followed by a 90-degree excitation pulse and a 180-degree refocusing pulse. The time between the initializing 180 and the 90 is referred to as the "time of inversion" or TI. Selecting a TI that is 69 percent of a tissue's T1 time will produce an image in which the signal from that specific tissue is zero or nulled. Because longitudinal magnetization is inverted with the initializing 180-degree pulse, the TR for IR sequences is often rather long (2000–10,000 ms). The adaptation of FSE sequences to IR sequences has allowed for reasonable scan times. There are two main types of fast inversion sequences in use today, STIR and FLAIR.

The STIR sequence (short TI inversion recovery) uses a relatively short TI to null the signal from fat. The exact TI time will vary depending on the field strength as T1 times are field strength dependent. STIR sequences are very useful in musculoskeletal MR at both high and low field. With either field strength, however, one should remember that STIR sequences are not the same as so-called "fat sat" sequences. STIR suppresses fat based on its T1 time and can therefore suppress other short T1 substances such as fat and blood. Additionally, they are not particularly compatible with contrast enhancement, due to the paramagnetics T1 shortening.

FLAIR (fluid attenuated inversion recovery) sequences use a much longer TR and TE to produce a base sequence that is T2 weighted. A relatively long inversion time is also selected so as to null the signal from CSF. FLAIR sequences have been shown to be very useful when imaging the brain for pathology such as demyelinating diseases, stroke, abscess, and hemorrhage. Because of FLAIR's ability to demonstrate numerous pathologic conditions, many sites have replaced the proton density weighted sequence in the brain with FLAIR.

Gradient recalled echo (GRE) sequences are also a useful tool when certain contrasts are desired. GRE sequences do not employ a 180-degree refocusing pulse and therefore have increased sensitivity to magnetic susceptibility and chemical shift. This can give GRE sequences certain advantages over spin echo sequences. Small areas of chronic hemorrhage are more easily seen because of increases in local field inhomogeneities. Since GRE sequences can be acquired very rapidly, they can be used to acquire images in a breath-hold. Increased gradient performance can allow for more slices in a 2D multislice sequence and/or reduced scan times.

There are two main types of GRE sequences, steady state and spoiled. The steady state sequences (FISP and GRASS are a couple of examples) can be used to acquire images with bright fluid for T2-like contrasts. This can be useful in imaging the cervical spine and joints. Spoiled sequences, such as FLASH and SPGR use either an extra gradient application or an alteration of the excitation pulse phase to remove signal contribution from long T2 spins. This allows for increased T1 contrasts. Spoiled sequences are more useful in the brain and for breath-hold body imaging but in general, spoiled sequences have slightly lower SNR than steady state sequences.

Selection of the TE with GRE sequences can produce images with fat and water either in-phase, or out-of-phase. At 1.5 T, fat and water are in and out of phase every 2.2 ms. At 0.2 T, fat and water are in and out of phase every 16.5 ms. Selecting an out-of-phase TE will cause a reduction or even cancellation of signal in voxels containing both fat and water. In body imaging, use of in- and out-of-phase imaging is useful when looking for fatty infiltration in the liver, characterization of adrenal masses, and visualization of the pancreas, as well as for other applications.

Gradient echo sequences do have their disadvantages. When metal implants and/or areas of air–tissue interface are present, magnetic susceptibilities can cause severe artifacts. As GRE sequences do not use RF refocusing pulses prior to the echo, field inhomogeneities (due to susceptibility of the main field) are not corrected for. While SE sequences cannot totally correct for inhomogeneities, such as those with metal implants, they are certainly less susceptible than GRE sequences. These artifacts can be reduced in GRE sequences by using small voxels and a short TE.

Another technique used for altering tissue contrast is magnetization transfer (MT or MTC). MT sequences use a presaturation RF pulse to excite the tightly bound spins in molecules such as proteins. These large molecules have an extremely short T2 and usually do not contribute to MR contrast. Because of the manner in which the RF pulse is applied, the bound spins "transfer" some of their magnetization to the free spins thereby reducing their contribution to the MR signal. The reduction in signal is primarily due to the amount of magnetization transfer to the free spins in various tissues. In the brain, the use of MT can reduce the signal from gray and white matter 30–40 percent. Following the administration of gadolinium, the use of MT may increase the conspicuity of gadolinium enhancing lesions. MTC can also be useful with 3D TOF intracranial MRA sequences to reduce the signal from proteinaceous "background" tissue.

Echo planar imaging (EPI) has begun to find utility in routine clinical MR imaging. Initially, EPI was useful for acquiring "snap shot" images to eliminate the effects of patient motion. "Snap shot," or "single shot" EPI collect all the desired lines of k-space in a single excitation. EPI collects data by generating a train of gradient echoes produced by continuously alternating the polarity of the read-out (frequency encoding) gradient. A slight alteration of the phase encoding gradient between read-out periods shifts the phase of the data to the next line in k-space. There are two major types of EPI sequences: spin echo and gradient echo. As the name implies, spin echo EPI uses a 90- and 180-degree RF pulse prior to the generation of the gradient echo train. A gradient echo EPI would not employ a 180-degree refocusing pulse. Regardless of the type of EPI acquisition performed, EPI sequences are essentially a gradient echo acquisition and the image contrast is so reflected. It is important to note, however, that since the

gradient echo EPI sequence does not employ a 180-degree refocusing pulse, the contrast has more susceptibility weighting than does the spin echo EPI.

EPI sequences are very useful in acquiring diffusion and susceptibility weighted sequences. Diffusion refers to the diffusion of water molecules. In normal brain tissue, water moves freely through the cell membranes. In the event of a stroke, water diffusion slows greatly in the area of infarction. By applying additional gradients to either side of the 180-degree RF pulse in a heavily T2 weighted spin echo based sequence, signal from normally diffusing water is dephased and yields little or no signal. Spins in water molecules with restricted diffusion, however, are unaffected by the diffusion gradients and are refocused yielding high signal. The amplitude of the diffusion gradient is an option that may be set by the operator. Increasing the gradient amplitude, or "b-value" will increase the diffusion weighting. In other words, the higher the b-value, the greater the contrast between the areas of normal and abnormal diffusion. Since diffusion weighted imaging (DWI) is highly sensitive to motion, bulk patient motion would severely degrade the image. Although any spin echo based sequences can be modified to acquire diffusion weighted images (DWI), EPI is well suited because of its ability to acquire images so quickly that effects of patient motion are essentially eliminated.

Perfusion imaging can be performed by several techniques. The most widely available uses an EPI acquisition to "track" a bolus of contrast in the first pass through the brain. Data acquired in this fashion can be used to derive information relating to cerebral blood volume, mean transit time, and cerebral blood flow. This type of data can be particularly useful when staging acute strokes. The contrast mechanism is derived from the increased susceptibility cause by the high concentration of gadolinium as it passes through cerebral circulation immediately following a rapid bolus injection. Again, EPI is useful because of its ability to rapidly acquire image data and its increased susceptibility compared to other sequences.

Both spin echo EPI and gradient echo EPI can be used to acquire perfusion studies of the brain. Spin echo EPI has less susceptibility than gradient echo EPI and will provide greater contrast based on small vessel perfusion. In order to obtain sufficient drop in signal intensity during the first pass however, it may be necessary to use a double dose of gadolinium. Gradient echo based EPI, however, will demonstrate a significant drop in signal intensity during the first pass with a single dose of gadolinium. The increased susceptibility will cause a reduction in overall image quality (compared to spin echo EPI) and the image contrast will be more related to large vessel perfusion.

No one pulse sequence or combination of parameters will always show pathology. MR is not a modality where pathological tissues *have* to show themselves. Contrast, as seen on an MR image is a function of the tissue relaxation times (T1 and T2), spin density, and flow characteristics in conjunction with the selected pulse sequence timing parameters. When determining the optimum contrast, consider the types of pathological conditions you might be looking for and work to change the sequence timing parameters to bring out the contrast desired. Only as a starting point should you try protocols from other centers. They were developed by other people to meet their needs. Unless your goals and/or expectations are identical to theirs, the protocols may not be acceptable. Two other factors must also be kept in mind. First, all MR systems do not have the same sequences and imaging options. In fact, many of the published articles and papers are written by people working on systems using nonproduct hardware and/or software. Secondly, T1 relaxation time depends on field strength. A sequence done with $TR = 500 \, ms$ on a $0.5 \, T$ system will not have the same image contrast as the same sequence performed with $TR = 500 \, ms$ on a $1.5 \, T$ system.

Signal-to-Noise Ratio

Signal-to-noise ratio (SNR) is the ratio of MR signal to noise. Our intent is to produce images with sufficient MR signal to override the noise. When the MR signal is reduced, the noise becomes more apparent. This may produce images that appear noisy or grainy. The following formula shows the relationship between SNR and scanning parameters.

$$SNR \propto \sqrt{\text{total sampling time}} \\ \times \text{voxel volume} \times \text{signal intensity}$$

Signal intensity is determined by the T1, T2, spin density, and flow characteristics of the tissue, and the pulse sequence timing parameters we select (TR, TE, flip angle, etc.). As an example, a sequence with $TE = 80 \, ms$ will produce less transverse magnetization during the time the echo is sampled than a sequence with $TE = 20 \, ms$, and will thus produce a lower SNR image. Since the timing parameters also control the image contrast, we seldom use them as a direct control of SNR. We should, however, remain aware of their effect on SNR. Table 13.1 shows the effect on SNR of various pulse sequence timing parameters.

SNR vs Spatial Resolution vs Scan Time

The voxel volume is determined by the field-of-view (FOV), imaging matrix selection, and the slice thickness. These parameters also affect our spatial resolution. As demonstrated by the previously described SNR formula, decreasing the voxel volume increases the spatial resolution,

Table 13-1

Scan Timing Parameters, SNR Table

Increasing TR increases SNR
Increasing TE decreases SNR
Increasing flip angle generally increases SNR

but it directly reduces the SNR. Of all the spatial resolution parameters, it is FOV that affects SNR the most. If we reduce the FOV by a factor of 2, we reduce the SNR by a factor of 4, since FOV controls the voxel volume in two dimensions. In selecting the spatial resolution, we must constantly weigh our choice against the available SNR. *Every time we decrease the size of the voxel, we reduce our available MR signal.* MR does not give us unlimited amounts of signal. We determine how much signal will be present by our selection of scan parameters. High spatial resolution does not do us any good unless we have enough SNR to support it.

Total Sampling Time

Another way to think of sampling time, is as the time spent listening to the signal. The scan parameter that most of us choose on a day-to-day basis goes by several names. Some of these names include number of excitations (NEX), number of signals averaged (NSA), number of acquisitions (NA or NAQ), or simply signal averages. Whatever the name, this parameter is usually selected according to the total time of the scan and whether we desire additional signal. Using two signal averages is analogous to putting two coats of paint on a fence. The scan is simply done twice and the signals averaged together. There are two important points to remember about signal averages. Doubling averages doubles the scan time, but *does not* double the SNR, because we are sampling noise as well. The overall result is that if we double the number of signals averaged (NSA), we increase the SNR by the square root of 2, a value of 1.41, or 41 percent.

In working with the radiologist to establish protocols, we must first look at getting the contrast desired. After that, we must look to providing the necessary SNR to bring the MR signal far enough above the noise to enable us to see the contrasts between tissues. In general, the higher the contrast between two structures, the

lower the SNR needed to visualize them. A train traveling with its light on is much easier to see if you are standing in the middle of the tracks at midnight than if you are standing on the tracks at noon. Tissues with low contrasts generally require more SNR to be visualized adequately. Increasing the spatial resolution reduces the SNR and therefore reduces our ability to differentiate structures of low contrast. Figure 13-1 shows the relationships between spatial resolution, contrast, and SNR.

GOAL-ORIENTED SCANNING

The relationships in Figure 13-3 mean that a change in one parameter causes a change in another. Setting a protocol involves compromising on the elements that determine the quality of our image. I once heard a presentation by a knowledgeable technologist describing this as goal-oriented scanning. While we do need routine protocols to guide us in our day-to-day scanning endeavors, certain studies must be tailored to clinical needs. As an example, we may desire all our T2 weighted sagittal lumbar spines to be acquired using a spin echo sequence, 256×256 imaging matrix, 4-mm slice thickness, and two signal averages. Depending on our system, this scan could last over 17 min. If our patient presents with metastatic disease to the lumbar vertebral bodies, we can expect them to be in a considerable amount of pain and unable

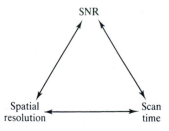

Figure 13-3. Relationships between SNR, scan time, and spatial resolution.

to tolerate the entire series of scans, let alone one 17-min acquisition. That's when we need to evaluate our goal. Using Figure 13-1 we see that if scan time becomes our goal, we decrease it at the cost of SNR (reducing the number of averages) or at the cost of spatial resolution (using fewer phase encoding views). This is where together the technologist and the radiologist must objectively look at the protocol, set a goal, and decide how best to obtain it.

Signal-to-noise ratio can be looked upon as money in the bank. If we want to increase the spatial resolution of the sequence, we do so at the cost of SNR and scan time. We can improve the spatial resolution as long as we have the SNR to pay for it, and as long as we don't mind spending the time. Remember, we have done no good if we increase the spatial resolution beyond where we have enough MR signal to adequately visualize the structures over the noise level.

If we have a noisy image and we want to improve it, we have two choices: we can increase the voxel size at the cost of spatial resolution. The voxel size is controlled by three factors: slice thickness, acquisition matrix, and FOV. If we increase the slice thickness by 30 percent (e.g., 3 mm to 4 mm) then we only increase the SNR by 30 percent. If we change from a 256×256 acquisition matrix to a 256×128 matrix, we increase the SNR by a factor of 2. But if we increase the FOV, we find that we make the greatest increase in the SNR for the amount of change in the FOV. The FOV controls our pixel size in both the x and the y direction, so a change of 20 percent in FOV (e.g., 20 cm to 24 cm) will yield a 40 percent increase in SNR.

The second way to increase the SNR is to increase the NSA. From the relationship SNR $\propto$ $\sqrt{NSA}$ we see that doubling the NSA yields only a 41 percent increase in SNR. In order to double the SNR on any sequence, we need to increase the NSA by a factor of 4. But this increases the scan time by a factor of 4; a 5-min scan now takes 20 min. Or we could increase the FOV by 50 percent (e.g., 14 cm to 21 cm) without affecting the scan time.

MR is a modality of compromises, so we must approach protocol development with goals in mind. I think it is routine protocols that are the most difficult to develop. Routine protocols are the ones you use when there is no specific area or abnormality suspected. In this case, we want to try and cover the maximum number of possibilities and keep the scan time to a reasonable duration. If we are going to perform three different sequences, why not obtain three orthogonal (or at least different) planes? MR is unique in its ability to provide us with orthogonal, even oblique, imaging. Why not take advantage of it? Next, if we are going to obtain three sequences, why not obtain three different pulse sequences and/or contrasts? Again, MR is unique in this ability. Another reason for using a different pulse sequence in another plane, is that we don't always know what pathology will be present, so we can't be sure which pulse sequence will best demonstrate the potential disease process.

Lastly, I believe that if radiologists and technologists work together to establish goals and expectations, the radiologists will get the information they desire and expect, and the technologists will get the satisfaction of working as an important part of a team utilizing the most incredible medical imaging technology of the century to improve the quality of patient care.

CHAPTER 14

Artifacts

Gregory L. Wheeler

Magnetic resonance is an imaging modality that introduces radiowaves into the patient via radiofrequency (RF) coils. The radiowaves returned are collected by a receive coil to be translated into an image. As the radiowaves return to the imaging coil they have been modulated and altered by local magnetic fields within the tissues and vessels in the body carrying information used to represent the patient's area of interest. The return signal is translated into a two-dimensional image based on the three-dimensional area of interest. The signal also carries false information that is not representative of the patient's anatomy. When this information appears on the image it can often obliterate the true signal from the tissue and can mimic pathology. This false information is called an *artifact*.

In this chapter, different categories and types of artifacts that are a part of MR imaging will be discussed. As MR technologists it is important to be familiar with artifacts. It is the responsibility of the technologist to understand the principles behind the various types of artifacts and how to reduce their effects. The radiologist will then have available the best possible representation of the area of interest with which to make a diagnosis. The artifacts are grouped into three categories: inherent physiology, physics, and hardware or mechanics. The artifacts in these categories will be discussed to provide you with an understanding of their appearance, cause or origin, and any possible ways to minimize or eliminate them. There are other artifacts not mentioned in this chapter. The discussion has been limited to those artifacts over which the MR operator has some reasonable control.

INHERENT PHYSIOLOGY

Motion Artifacts

In magnetic resonance imaging (MRI), whether as a result of gross body movement or a physiological process, motion is the most frequently encountered artifact. It has a multitude of appearances that can seriously degrade the image. The fundamental reason MRI is so sensitive to motion is the fact that MR images are based on a timing sequence. Motion can occur during RF pulses, between RF pulses, during sampling, and between phase encoding views[1].

Motion produces ghost images of the anatomy in the phase encoding direction. Motion can cause blurring and is proportional to the distance moved. This may result in fuzziness on the image or a lack of crispness or detail, as seen in Figure 14-1.

After exciting the spins in the imaging volume, the tissues respond releasing their energy over

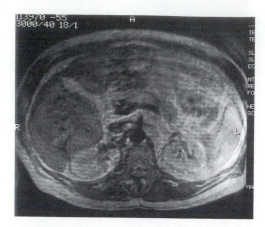

Figure 14-1. Motion caused by patient motion and breathing.

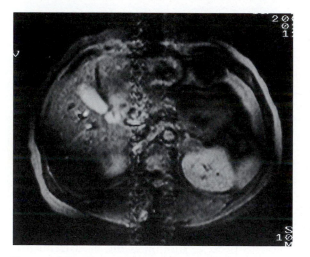

Figure 14-2. Aorta and vena cava motion.

time, producing a signal. Motion can be best divided into two types: gross body motion due to the patient moving and physiological motion, such as pulsations from the heart, fast arterial flow, slow venous flow [Figure 14-2], peristalsis in the bowel, cerebrospinal fluid pulsations, and respiration.

The motion of spins, combined with some temporal duration of data acquisition, means that the position of spins at the start of an experiment is different from that at the end[2]. Motion causes faint to prominent replications of the image to occur in the phase encoding direction. When the

data is collected, at the appropriate TE, the information gathered will have a phase, frequency, and amplitude. The phase and frequency is a result of the spins' location along the phase axis. However, the phase encoding process requires that the image data be acquired at distinct intervals over and over again to create the image.

Early investigators discovered that the appearance of an FID (free induction decay) was affected by diffusion or motion of the spins in a magnetic field gradient. Since data acquisition in MRI can be described as tailored data sampling of multiple unique FIDs, MRI will be similarly sensitive to movement of the spins[1]. Compensatory gradients, which create a balanced reversal of the effect of the original gradient, are used to eliminate the contribution to the phase shift from the frequency and slice select gradients. Gross patient motion, however, cannot be controlled by compensatory gradients. Since the information is gathered multiple times to create an image, if there is patient motion during the acquisition, the signal accumulates a phase shift and will be mismapped in the phase direction of the image.

Motion artifacts will be more apparent at higher field strengths. In higher magnetic fields there are more spins that will respond during the acquisition of the image. The more spins that are sensitive to the radio frequency pulse and that respond emitting a signal, the higher the amplitude of the resultant signal. Signal from tissues such as fat (on T1-weighted images) and cerebrospinal fluid (on T2-weighted images) will have higher amplitudes and can cause a more pronounced motion artifact. Since motion can have a number of causes there are also a number of solutions.

Sedation Sedation is an obvious solution to patient motion when the patient is not able to cooperate; a number of sedatives are available. It is important to monitor the patient's heart and breathing while they are sedated and to be prepared for any possible medical complications.

Sponges Often neglected sponges, pads, and nonallergenic tape can be used if you notice a patient is having difficulty remaining motionless during image acquisition. Patients frequently present unanticipated challenges. Sponges or pads not only support the patient's body, they also help to remind the patient which position to hold. If there is no support against the body there is no reference to guide the patient and assure that they have not moved.

Cardiac Gating Gating is a technique used to synchronize the collection of the MR data to the patient's physiological motion. Electrocardiograph (ECG) gating techniques trigger the imaging sequence during the same cardiac cycle consistently to collect the signal during the lowest velocity of arterial flow. Artifacts caused by cardiac pulsations can be decreased by synchronizing the imaging sequence to the R-to-R wave of the cardiac cycle. During this period the heart is at the end of diastole and is motionless for the greatest length of time. ECG gating is most effective when the heart beats in a normal and rhythmic pattern. Complications in synchronizing the imaging sequence to an irregular cardiac cycle occur with most imaging systems, especially those that do not have ample means of rejecting any "bad" data. While there is normally patient motion from and within the region of the heart, the artifact can be exacerbated if there is an irregular cardiac cycle, as seen in Figure 14-3.

Respiratory Gating Respiratory gating is available on imaging systems to minimize the motion artifact from patients who present with heavy breathing during the MR examination, as evident in Figure 14-4. Gating is performed by synchronizing the imaging sequence to the exhalation period of the patient's respiratory cycle, when the lungs and diaphragm are motionless for the greatest length of time. If images are acquired only during exhalation and with a normal respiratory cycle of 16–20 times a minute, respiratory gating can be a lengthy procedure. Since we do not normally breathe in a rhythmic and consistent manner the data is not acquired consistently and respiratory gating can in fact increase the motion artifact.

Breath Hold For cooperative patients, respiratory motion may also be controlled by obtaining breath hold scans acquired in only a few seconds. Generally these images have lower spatial resolution and signal-to-noise ratio than images acquired over a longer period of time; however, the technique can significantly decrease motion artifacts especially when imaging in the region of the abdomen.

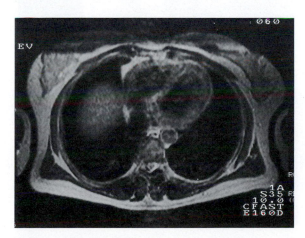

Figure 14-3. Cardiac motion.

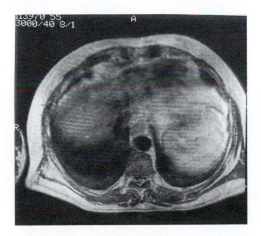

Figure 14-4. Breathing motion blurs image.

Swapping Phase and Frequency Encoding Direction Since motion artifacts are displayed in the phase encoding direction, swapping the phase and frequency encoding direction can minimize the display of motion on the image. This technique is frequently used when imaging the spine. Instead of artifacts from breathing, peristalsis, and cardiac motion that obliterate the spine and cord anteriorly to posteriorly, the phase encoding direction can be reoriented superior to inferior to limit the appearance of motion on the image, as seen in Figures 14-5 and 14-6. There is no time penalty for using this technique, however, caution is recommended when selecting the field of view and the imaging coil so that a wraparound artifact does not result.

Fast Imaging Fast imaging is a generic term used to describe rapid imaging techniques. The application is used to produce images in much shorter imaging times than would normally be accomplished. Shorter imaging times reduce

motion. Respiration and peristalsis become more manageable, increasing the success of abdominal imaging. CSF pulsatility and flow phenomena on T2 weighted spine images are not as apparent when fast scan pulse sequences are used.

Flow Artifacts

MRI excites protons simultaneously, then allows them to relax to equilibrium at their respective rate of relaxation. The process depends on the proton's availability both to absorb the radio frequency energy and to re-emit the absorbed energy. If protons are moving during the imaging process the same protons that absorbed the energy are not available to return a signal back into the original location and a flow phenomenon is created. This physiologic effect is capable of producing severe motion artifacts that are often difficult to eliminate.

Flow can be described in terms of its mechanism. The first type consists of effects that alter

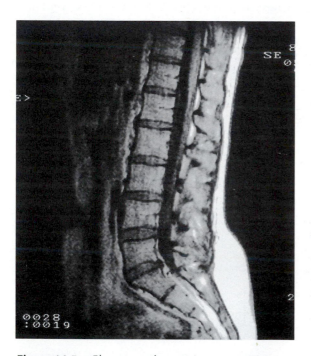

Figure 14-5. Phase encode anterior to posterior.

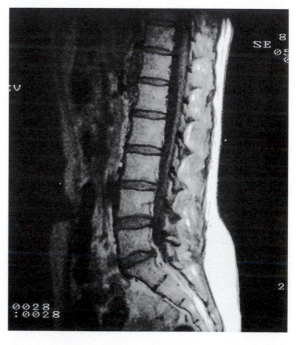

Figure 14-6. Phase encode superior to inferior.

T1 longitudinal magnetization. These are often called time-of-flight or velocity effects. They include entry flow, often called paradoxical or slow flow, and high flow void. They vary based on the pulse sequence and the series of events the spins have undergone during the imaging sequence.

The second type of flow mechanism is due to the effects of the spins as they experience different gradient magnetic fields. As these spins flow they move across a gradient and accumulate phase changes altering the transverse magnetization. Even echo rephasing, odd echo dephasing, and ghosting and harmonics are examples of this type of mechanism.

Flow-Related Enhancement This type of flow creates a high signal intensity and is also called entry phenomenon, slow flow enhancement, or paradoxical enhancement. The amplitude of the signal is determined by the type of spins that exists within the imaging volume. Stationary spins experience repeated excitation pulses and remain in their spatial location throughout the imaging data acquisition.

Outside the imaging volume, the spins are fully magnetized or unsaturated and have a large longitudinal magnetization. As long as these fully magnetized spins remain outside the imaging volume they do not affect the return signal. Unsaturated spins outside the imaging volume that move, such as slow laminar flow, will begin to move into the imaging volume. If they experience an RF excitation pulse, the now saturated spins will produce a large transverse magnetization and return a large amplitude of signal.

This high signal is called entry phenomenon and is capable of producing severe streaks across the image from the vessels within the image. The amount of the signal (entry phenomenon) is proportional to slice thickness and repetition time.

Even Echo Rephasing A second type of high signal intensity that can create artifacts due to flow is even echo rephasing. After excitation, spins that are exposed to a gradient will experience a phase dispersion. If they are stationary, these phase dispersions will refocus. However, if there

are spins that move through different gradient fields they will accumulate different phase dispersions depending on their velocity and vessel orientation.

During the imaging sequence, and after the initial 180-degree refocusing pulse, moving spins in laminar flow will not be back in phase and therefore will not return a large signal. If a second 180-degree refocusing pulse is applied to collect a second echo, the spins will come back in phase and will return a large (bright) signal. This will happen consistently as long as laminar flow is constant and the first and second echo times are symmetric. The first echo will exhibit a low signal intensity and the second echo will exhibit a large signal return due to rephasing. Often the second and fourth echoes exhibit vessel artifacts due to the high signal from the refocused spins.

High Flow Void The signal from flow can also cause a decrease in signal intensity, commonly described as a flow void. This occurs most often from rapidly flowing blood in spin echo pulse sequences that do not remain in the plane or field of view being exited by both the excitation and refocusing pulses so will not return a signal. As the velocity increases the signal intensity from the vessel decreases and the lumen gets darker and darker.

In gradient echo pulse sequences the signal from rapidly flowing blood returns because the protons are refocused by the gradient even after the protons have left the gradient field. Refocusing the gradients during gradient echo sequences, will affect the entire imaging area therefore spins that have moved in and out of the volume will often be refocused to some degree.

Turbulence Turbulence, which increases with velocity, dephases the spin's transverse coherence and produces a decay in transverse magnetization resulting in a loss of signal. Turbulence can create random fluctuations in the spins making it impossible to refocus or recover spin coherence. The regions of the vessel bifurcations and changes in direction and size of the vessel can accentuate turbulence and its effects.

Solutions

Solutions to flow artifacts are varied and will depend on the mechanism of flow. The most common compensatory adjustments will be described.

Presaturation   Presaturation pulses are used to eliminate the effect of entry phenomenon. These RF pulses, called presaturation bands or saturation bands, accomplish just what their name implies; they presaturate the flowing spins in the area adjacent to the imaging volume, as shown in Figure 14-7. As the imaging sequence begins and the saturated spins flow or move into the imaging volume, they are resaturated with subsequent applications of the RF pulse disproportionate to the saturation of stationary spins.

Presaturation bands can be placed in any plane necessary to limit the signal from nonstationary spins but careful placement of these bands is crucial to assure anatomy in the area of interest is not obliterated by the saturation of useful signal, as seen anteriorly and inferiorly in the image in Figure 14-8.

Because the sequence uses additional RF pulses at the start of the imaging sequence, RF power deposition to the patient increases. Since RF power is also a function of TR, number of slices, and scan type, the scan time may increase due to a compensatory increase in TR. The operator can perform other workarounds, such as decreasing the number of slice coverage, then reducing TR to maintain the original scan time.

Flow Compensation   Flow compensation is an application that uses a technique called gradient moment nulling to manipulate and refocus out-of-phase signals. During the period that gradients are on, flowing spins accumulate phase dispersions as they accelerate or slow down depending on the gradient polarity. This will cause flow artifacts as demonstrated in Figures 14-9 and 14-10, such as arterial and venous flow, cerebrospinal fluid (CSF) pulsations, respiratory motion, and peristalsis in the gastrointestinal track.

Flow compensation uses the technique of reversing the gradient magnetic field (gradient reversals) to refocus the spins that would

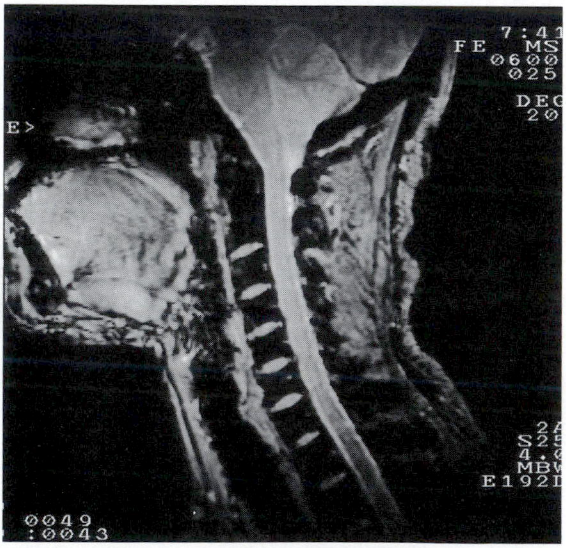

Figure 14-7.   Swallowing and CSF pulsations.

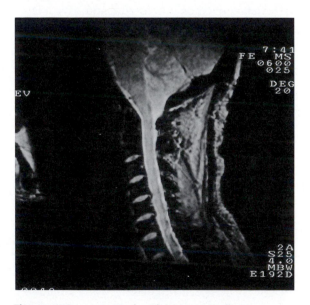

Figure 14-8.   Anterior bands correct swallowing motion. The inferior band may obliterate anatomy if too close.

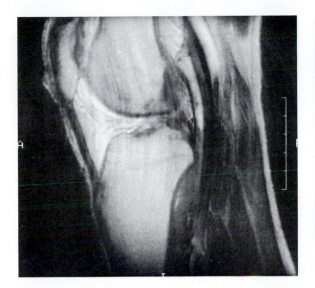

Figure 14-9. Popliteal artery motion.

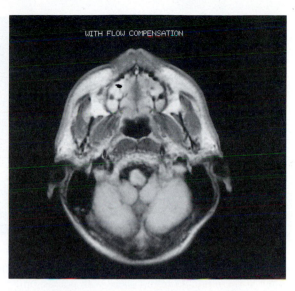

Figure 14-11. Flow compensation minimizes vascular and CSF flow.

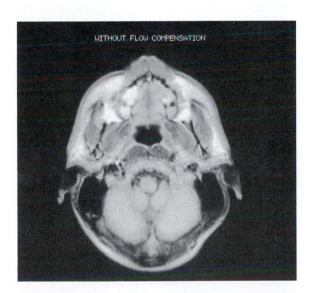

Figure 14-10. Vascular flow causes loss of detail in the posterior fossa region.

otherwise cause artifacts on the image. The technique is useful for decreasing the motion artifact in imaging sequences such as T2-weighted sequences, gradient echo sequences, and MR angiography, as seen in Figure 14-11.

ARTIFACTS CAUSED BY THE INHERENT PHYSICS OF MRI

Aliasing Artifacts

Aliasing or wraparound artifact occurs on MR images when the imaged object is undersampled (the object is larger than the field of view selected). This causes the undersampled area to become superimposed onto the opposite side of the imaged volume. The appearance is as though the image that was not properly sampled has been folded over onto the opposite side of the image, as seen in Figure 14-12A.

After applying the radio frequency pulse and during the spatial encoding process, a finite number of samples is assigned to the image. These samples have a phase and frequency value that will determine where in the matrix the signal belongs. Aliasing is due to the ambiguity in the assignment of frequencies to the MR signals. The data (signals) are collected at fixed time intervals and then are sent through a Fourier transform to be separated into their individual phase and frequency values. There is a finite number of

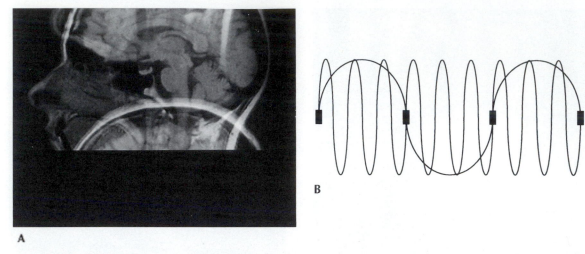

Figure 14-12. **A** An aliasing artifact. **B** Two different frequencies can have the same peaks, placing them in the same voxel (reprinted from Lufkin[4] with permission).

values available to create the data, based on the selected matrix size. Data from higher frequency signals can produce the same waveform as low frequency signals. Because the data is collected intermittently the Fourier transform is unable to differentiate the high-frequency signal from the low-frequency signal when their waveforms are similar.

As an example, consider the situation in which the applied magnetic field gradient has produced a linear gradation in precessional frequencies ranging from $+10\,kHz$ at one end of the imaged volume to $-10\,kHz$ at the other[2]. Signals received from the specified range of frequencies are given a specific location within the matrix. Because anatomy is still within range of the imaging coils but outside the field of view, the outside area is given an ambiguous level above or below $+10\,kHz$ and $-10\,kHz$. At least two frequencies will appear exactly the same for a given sampling rate, as shown in Figure 14-12B.

These higher frequencies may appear exactly the same as frequencies within the image. When the Fourier transform designates the levels and assigns their location within the matrix, both sets of frequencies and the corresponding anatomy are superimposed onto incorrect locations within the image volume. This misassignment of frequency creates an artifact in which the portion of the subject extending beyond the field of view appears within the imaged volume, but on the other opposite side of the actual anatomy, as shown in Figures 14-12A and 14-13.

Reorienting Phase and Frequency Axis

The aliasing artifact is generally seen in the phase encoding direction. Aliasing does occur in the frequency or readout direction of the image, however, in most MR imaging systems the frequency encoding direction has low pass filters to filter out frequencies outside the field of view that are above a certain frequency. There is also oversampling in the frequency direction by a factor of two which eliminates frequency wraparound. There is no filter in the phase direction therefore it is the phase component of the signal that generally causes the ambiguous signals to replicate within the matrix, as seen in Figure 14-14.

Reorienting the phase and frequency gradient direction when acquiring the data will change the direction of the filters and possibly eliminate the wraparound artifact. It is important to make wise choices when assigning phase and frequency gradient directions. The phase direction is usually

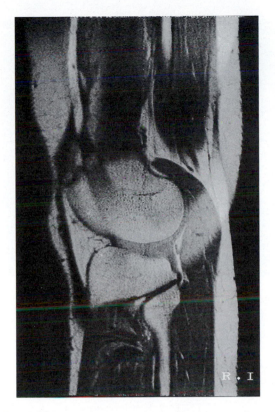

Figure 14-13. Wraparound from the opposite knee.

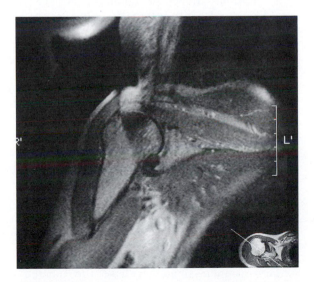

Figure 14-14. Superior to inferior wraparound on shoulder image.

placed in the short axis of the area of interest. If the long axis is used and the area in the long axis is larger than the field of view, reorienting can again cause an aliasing or wraparound artifact.

Field of View The field of view can be increased to ensure the scanned area falls within the imaging volume, minimizing the possibility of an aliasing artifact. By choosing a larger field of view there are more samples or frequencies to assign to the area of interest (compare the images in Figure 14-15). This will minimize the amount of ambiguity in the data collected since there are more frequency samples and therefore less ability for two frequencies to have the same phase or peak. This results in unique spatial locations and no aliasing.

No Wrap Technique An anti-aliasing technique known as a "no wrap" technique may be a useful tool to reduce or eliminate wraparound artifact. In this technique more frequencies are sampled in one or both encoding directions. Since aliasing rarely occurs in the frequency direction on most systems, due to the presence of low and/or high pass filters which remove unwanted frequencies, the use of no wrap in the frequency direction is not commonly used. However, no wrap in the phase direction is quite helpful. In this case, oversampling is performed in the phase direction but the data is not used in the reconstructed image. For instance, if a 256×256 matrix is acquired using phase no wrap, up to 512 phase levels can be acquired and reconstructed but only 256 will ultimately be used to create the displayed image. In this way, any frequencies that existed outside the field of view will not be used, thus eliminating the artifact. A caveat when using phase "no wrap" is the increase in scan time proportionate to the matrix size.

Surface Coils The use of surface coils is often helpful in minimizing this artifact. Because of the nature of the coil, surface coils have a sensitivity range beyond which the collected

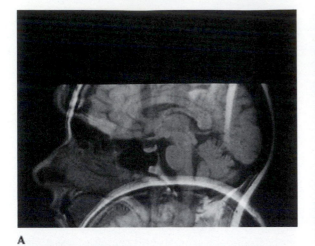

A

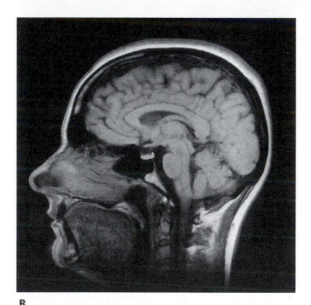

B

Figure 14-15. Field of view (FOV) comparison: **A** 13-cm FOV. **B** 26-cm FOV.

signal drops off, as seen in Figure 14-16. The coil is not sensitive enough to pick up perpendicular areas far beyond the radius of the coil. Frequencies outside this sensitivity range will not be received by the coil eliminating the aliasing artifact. Careful positioning of the patient to this coil is imperative to assure the signal picked up by the coils will

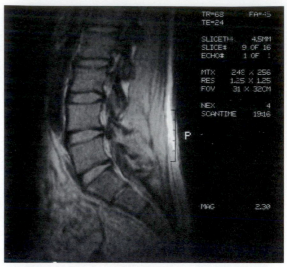

Figure 14-16. Surface coils minimize the wraparound artifacts.

include the area of interest and at the same time eliminate signal from outside the field of view.

Metal Artifacts

After motion, the most common artifact is probably metal artifacts, which manifests as a high intensity appearance where the signal has been misregistered and a void or loss of signal, in the area where the metal is located, as shown in Figures 14-17 and 14-18. Image quality is affected by metals due to the dependency on the homogeneity of the magnetic environment in the imaging system and around the patient. The better the field homogeneity the less overall image degradation will occur from metals.

Metals introduced into the magnet may distort the static magnetic field because of their own intrinsic magnetic properties. There are three main types of magnetic materials which may cause image artifacts: ferromagnetics, paramagnetics, and diamagnetics.

Ferromagnetic materials have the inherent ability to interact with the magnetic field by highly concentrating the magnetic lines of force

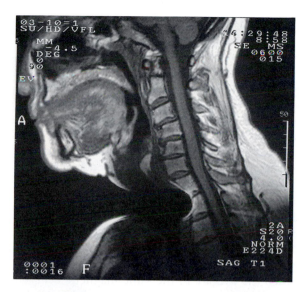

Figure 14-17. A metal artifact, probably on the patient's body.

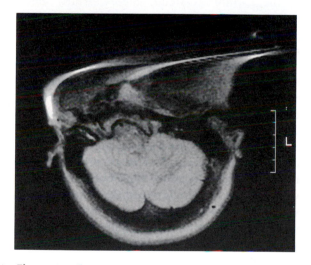

Figure 14-18. Ferromagnetic material in dental work.

and retaining the magnetism even after the magnetic influence has been removed [Figure 14-18]. Examples of ferromagnetics are cobalt, iron, and nickel.

Paramagnetic materials are able to concentrate lines of magnetic force to a lesser degree and therefore will only affect the magnetic field minimally. These materials will have an effect on the uniformity of the magnetic field, but unlike ferromagnetics, will not severely distort the main magnetic field. Paramagnetic materials include platinum, titanium, and iridium. Gadolinium and manganese are examples of ingestable paramagnetic substances used as contrast agents to affect the T1 and T2 relaxation times of the tissues.

Diamagnetic substances have the weakest magnetic properties and do not significantly alter the static or local magnetic field in areas where these materials are present. Mercury, copper, zinc, and gold are diamagnetic.

Nonmagnetic substances do not exhibit magnetic properties, however, they can distort the main magnetic field as electrical currents are induced into them by the gradients, creating a local magnetic field. The stronger the magnetic properties of the material, the more likely it is to cause mild to gross spatial mismapping of the anatomy in areas where these materials are located. This is secondary to the fact that the linear relationship between spatial location, phase angle, and frequency is no longer valid. MR images are created based on the deliberate and linear distortion of the static magnetic field to determine the spatial location of the information received from the patient in the imaging coil. The local magnetic field distortions that occur when metal is present can also cause rapid dephasing of the spins, which in turn causes a loss of signal and true T2 information.

Screening The best solution to eliminating metallic artifacts is first and foremost to screen the patient to remove or limit the amount of metal that enters the magnet scan room. Metal appliances, such as vena caval filter, joint prostheses, dental work, metal fragments, surgical clips, eye makeup, jewelry, hairpins, metal in clothing, and dentures, all can cause a warping of the main magnetic field at a specific location[3]. Patients should be changed into controlled garments, such as hospital clothing or sweats that have been tested to ensure that no magnetic material is present in them [Figure 14-19]. Patients should also be asked to remove eye makeup if their head

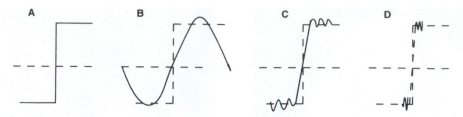

Figure 14-23. Truncation errors: **A** a tissue discontinuity encoded with Fourier series; **B** a single sine wave poorly approximates boundaries; **C** more terms improve approximation; **D** even more terms further improve approximation but the Fourier series is still truncated so the brightness oscillations persist. (Reprinted from Lufkin[4] with permission.)

There are several ways to minimize the truncation artifact on the image. With each of the methods there are trade-offs that must be considered individually to determine whether truncation on the image matters more than the potential consequence of the trade-off.

Matrix Size This is probably the most effective way to minimize the artifact. The larger the number of matrix steps the less ambiguous is the placement of the signal on the matrix by the Fourier transform. The distance between two interfaces decreases with increasing matrix size, therefore the intensity and the width of the truncation bands diminish. This can be a great asset in eliminating the artifact, demonstrated by Figure 14-24 which uses a 160×256 matrix. This technique will have no effect on the Gibbs phenomenon, which will persist regardless of the matrix size. The obvious consequence is the increase in scan time, if the phase steps are increased.

Pixel Size The smaller the pixel size the more accurate will be the edge detail. The interfaces between high- and low-intensity signals, if placed in different pixels, will be accurately represented and the Fourier transform will be able to distinguish the transition. This will minimize the fluctuations in the signal.

Filters Another method of minimizing truncation is to filter the raw data. Raw data is

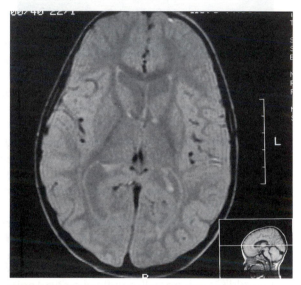

Figure 14-24. Brain image with 160×256 matrix demonstrates truncation artifacts on lateral portions of the brain.

stored in the time or frequency domain. Filters can be used to remove high frequency signals that cause the truncation artifact, however, it will not filter the first peak, which overshoots the interface and causes Gibbs phenomenon. As a matter of fact, the Gibbs artifact often is increased when these filters are used.

Overall, these artifacts are a result of the way in which MR images are acquired. An appropriate understanding is required in order to minimize and, more importantly, recognize artifacts and to ensure that they are not mistaken for pathology.

Radio Frequency Artifacts

Radio frequency artifacts are great nuisances to an MR image. They can appear unexpectedly on one image or several images within a set as a single line of artifact or multiple artifacts totally obliterating the area of interest.

Radio frequency artifacts can appear as discreet lines of noise or as "zipper" lines across the image in the phase direction, as shown in Figure 14-25. They appear as alternating bright and dark pixels along a single straight line across the image. Wideband noise containing multiple frequencies may diffusely degrade the entire image as seen in Figure 14-26.

The radio frequency artifact occurs perpendicular to the frequency encoding direction. The exact position of the artifact on the image depends on the frequency of interference relative to the central resonance frequency on the frequency encoded axis[6]. This artifact should be distinguished from the FID artifact, which only appears in the exact center of the image matrix and is parallel to the frequency encoding axis.

Most artifacts caused by radio frequency noise can be avoided using careful preparation by the MR operator and the service engineer. The most obvious cause of the artifact is RF penetration of the scanning environment. This can be the result of a leak in the Faraday cage responsible for keeping radio frequencies out of the scan room. The scan room is RF shielded using aluminum or copper which completely encloses the scan room. If there is a tear in the Faraday cage or in the door leading into the scan room, RF leaks can occur. This can be checked by taking a transistor radio into the scan room and securing the door. If you are able to pick up a radio signal anywhere in the scan room, there is a breech in the integrity of the RF cage and it should be checked. This is a crude method of checking for leaks and there are more precise methods available to the service engineer, however, it is available to the technologist and it does work.

Electronic devices often cause radio frequency artifacts on the image, as shown in Figure 14-26. Any electronic or motorized equipment should be either turned off, unplugged, and/or removed from the scan room unless it has been specifically shielded against RF leaks. This includes making sure the table electronics are turned off in the scan room and any meters, such

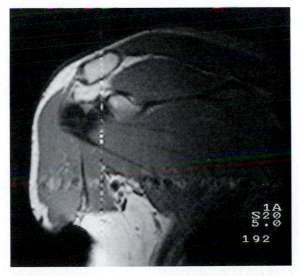

Figure 14-25. An RF discreet running superior to inferior with vascular motion running left to right.

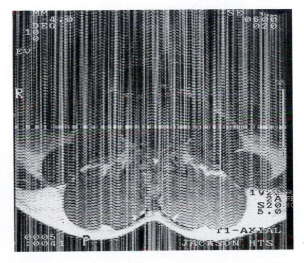

Figure 14-26. An RF discreet caused by motorized equipment.

as cryogenic meters, are turned off during the scanning process.

RF interference can also be the result of static electricity. Common sources of static electricity are wool blankets placed on the patient or kept in the scan room. The static from wool can significantly degrade the entire image set. It is wise not to allow your imaging facility to use wool blankets and to dissuade the patient from wearing wool inside the scanner. Indeed street clothes of any kind are suspect in causing artifacts on the MR image.

An often overlooked explanation for RF artifacts is interference caused by AC fluctuations such as light bulbs and alternating current in the room. Only direct current (DC) should be used in the imaging suite. If light bulbs are old they can begin to fluctuate and create RF interferences on the image. Additionally, careful attention to the shielding of electrical components within the scan room should be employed. The best solution to eliminating the potential for radio frequency artifacts is to have the service engineer perform frequent and thorough preventative system checks to identify and prevent these artifacts.

Free Induction Decay (FID) or Zipper Artifacts

In some MR systems, the MR signal is centered about the zero-line in the phase axis and is at a higher central reference frequency along the frequency encoding axis[7]. If there is system noise, a zero-line artifact or free induction decay (FID) artifact can occur. System noise causes a bright signal at the isocenter or central reference point with a linear dashed pattern along the frequency axis, as shown in Figures 14-27 and 14-28. This discreet artifact appears edge to edge on the matrix mimicking an RF discreet artifact. Depending on the signal processing, this artifact may appear as a star artifact. The star artifact manifests itself as a bright signal only in the direct center of the slice. It can be more apparent on half (HFI) and single acquisition studies. The artifact can often be verified by placing a grid on

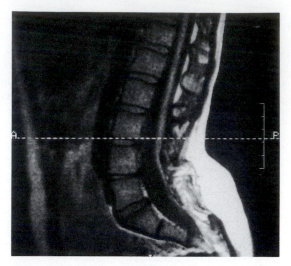

Figure 14-27.   FID artifact anterior to posterior in the sagittal lumbar spine looks like a "zipper."

the image and observing whether the artifact is in the center of the matrix. Since the star pattern can simulate pathology such as multiple sclerosis plaques, it is important to identify this artifact when it appears on the image.

The FID or zero-line artifact occurs because of the remnant FID that remains after the 180-degree pulse. The signal from each point in the image is represented by a sinc function that drops off rapidly about a given center point[7]. The normal sinc function has sidelobes that are minimal and are lost. Signals that fall within the normal amplitude range will be represented on the image as a single pixel with an appropriate shade of gray. Noise appears as a very high amplitude point with persistent sidelobes of the sine wave. The dashed pattern that is the usual display of this artifact is caused by the sidelobes parallel to the frequency encoded axis.

FID or zero-line artifacts are often inherent to the system and cannot be eliminated. Sometimes they can be minimized or periodically eliminated by adjusting the DC offset. This requires the assistance of the service engineer and after adjusting the artifact, it can drift back to its original appearance.

Acquisitions Increasing the number of acquisitions can minimize the effect of the FID artifact. When several encodes are averaged to produce the final image, the system recognizes it as noise and it is averaged out of the final image.

Shift in Central Reference Line Some manufacturers have eliminated the problems caused by the artifact by shifting the central reference line off to the edge when displaying the image. The artifact shows up at the edge of the matrix where there is no anatomy. This has become a more common practice and most imaging systems will no longer have the problem caused by the FID or zero-line artifact.

Herringbone Artifact

Herringbone artifacts challenge the technologist. This artifact appears as a faint to gross herringbone fabric pattern throughout the image. Others describe it as a screen door (compare Figures 14-29–14-31). It may be intermittent or constant, subtle or conspicuous but it is almost always accompanied by poor signal-to-noise ratio. It can appear in any direction and in many variations, however, it always occurs throughout the image on a single image or the entire image set. A simple indication that herringbone exists on the image is when the noise readings for the first and second echoes are different by more than 1.5–2 standard deviations.

RF Discreets Often herringbone artifacts are related to radio frequency discrepancies in the imaging system. These discrepancies are electromagnetic spikes picked up during data acquisition and stored in the time domain. Since these spikes occur during image acquisition, the time domain or raw data errors are translated onto the image, as shown in Figure 14-32.

Gradient Power Supply Another cause of herringbone is arcing (voltage surge) within the gradient power supply that results in very intense spikes while the data is being acquired.

A/D Converter Corrupt bits in the analog-to-digital (A/D) converter will cause spikes that can be recognized in the time domain as a fabric pattern artifact.

Fluctuating Currents Fluctuating currents caused by old light bulbs can cause degradation of the signal return and herringbone artifacts

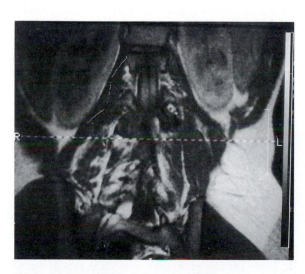

Figure 14-28. FID or "zipper" artifact.

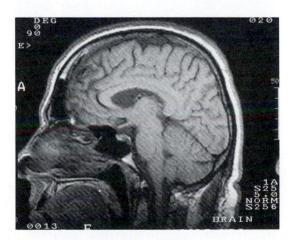

Figure 14-29. Herringbone. Figures 14-29–14-31 are for the same patient, same sequence, however the herringbone artifact appears different.

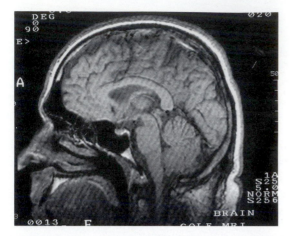

Figure 14-30.   Herringbone. This image has the typical fabric pattern appearance.

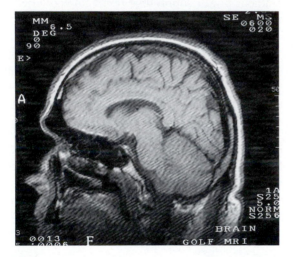

Figure 14-31.   Herringbone. Severe herringbone artifact ruins the diagnostic capability of the image.

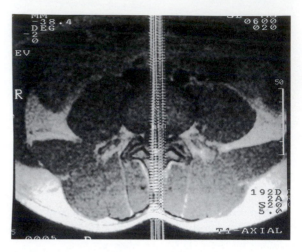

Figure 14-32.   RF discreets and herringbone.

on the image. These artifacts can be minimized using power conditioners to regulate the flow of current to the MR scanner. Light bulbs in the imaging suite should be changed regularly to eliminate the possibility of this occurrence.

The solution to this artifact is straightforward, contact your field service engineer to diagnose and repair the equipment. The solution could be replacing a gradient power supply, light bulbs, A/D converters, or a number of other imaging components that cause electromagnetic spikes.

Nonuniformity Artifacts

Intrepreting the results of a medical imaging procedure include analyzing the results of the exam by noticing the appearance of the structures on the image and whether or not there is uniformity within the tissues. It is sometimes necessary to acquire bilateral studies to make a diagnosis. Radiologists depend on their ability visually to determine and measure whether the image is normal or abnormal based on these comparisons. It is important as technologists to assist the radiologist by acquiring images in which the confidence level that any abnormality in the appearance of the image is due to the patient and not to the equipment.

Nonuniformity on an image can be subtle or very apparent. It is the challenge of the trained eye of the MR operator to identify this artifact and resolve the problem so that accurate images can be produced. Nonuniformity appears as a gray scale variation which is not representative of the patient. It may appear as an inhomogeneous brightness or darkness, as seen in Figure 14-33. It may appear in a corner of the image or in opposite corners. Keen eyes are a requirement.

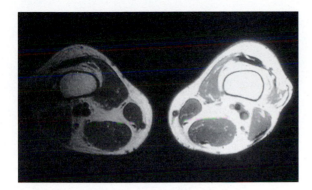

Figure 14-33. Bilateral knees with inhomogeneous brightness.

The cause of this artifact is often as subtle as its appearance.

Coil Positioning The imaging transmit and receive coils are designed to be placed in the direct center of the magnet and to approximate the size of the area to be imaged. The gradients, transmit and receive apparatus, and spatial encoding will function most accurately when the transmit and receive coils are placed in the center of the magnetic field. Each coil has a Q factor which dictates the patient load or size the coil can tolerate to accurately acquire the signal from the patient.

Make sure the patient's skin does not come in contact with the transmit coil. If a patient is large and is likely to come in contact with the coil, it is recommended that the technologist place a folded sheet or a sponge between the skin and the coil. If this is not done the image may show inhomogeneous brightness or a drop in the signal.

RF Energy Deposition The sequence selector determines how much RF power to transmit into the imaging coil and into the patient, and how much power will be received back from the patient and back into the receive coil. The amount of energy required to flip or tip the net magnetization out of the longitudinal plane is determined by the RF power level.

This procedure measures the signal coming from one or multiple slices, then determines how much wattage or RF current is necessary to perform the pulse sequence requested at the required frequencies.

Frequently metal coming from outside the image volume but still within the RF coil causes nonuniformity. The image will appear with either too much signal from the presence of metal or not enough signal to properly display the image. The images with signal that is too high will often clip. This means, that the amplitude of the return signal within the slice had to be limited by the Fourier transform so the computer could place a representative gray scale value in the pixel(s) to display the image.

With sharp eyes and meticulous scanning procedures, inhomogeneous artifacts can be minimized and often eliminated by the MR operator, allowing the clinician to have confidence in the accuracy of the image.

Partial Voluming Partial voluming occurs when the image displayed demonstrates overlapping anatomic structures within the same pixel. Instead of the image representing all the signals, the image is an average of the various signals within each pixel of the matrix representing the image. It can be minimized by acquiring thin slices and smaller pixel dimensions. This phenomenon can also occur because the patient was not positioned properly in the coil. Paging through the images adjacent to the image in question on the scanners display monitor is a good way to determine if inhomogeneous brightness is occurring as a result of partial voluming.

CONCLUSION

The objective of this chapter is to provide visual and written explanations for the numerous artifacts that are a part of MR imaging. As you have learned, there are many factors to consider when setting up the parameters for the imaging sequence. It is important to understand not only how to select these parameters to produce excellent image quality, but also to be able to recognize, understand, and manipulate the appearance of the image to avoid artifacts. If artifacts are unavoidable, it is your responsibility to ensure the radiologist or reader recognizes what is real on the image and what is artifactual.

REFERENCES

1. Haacke EM, Bellon EM. In: Potchen EJ, Haacke EM, Siebert JE, Gottschalk A, eds. *Magnetic Resonance Angiography Concepts and Applications*. Chicago: Mosby, 1992.

2. Heiken JP, Glazer HS, Lee JK, et al. *Imaging Artifacts. Manual of Clinical Magnetic Resonance Imaging*. New York: Raven Press, 1986.

3. Rothschild PA, Solomon M, Carlson. In: Cohen MD, Edwards MK, eds. *Magnetic Resonance Imaging of Children*. Philadelphia: Decker, 1990.

4. Lufkin RB. *The MRI Manual*. Chicago: Year Book Medical Publishers, 1990.

5. Czervionke LF, Czervionke JM, Daniels DL, et al. Characteristic features of MR truncation artifacts. *Am J Radiol* 151:1219–1228, 1988.

6. Young SW. *Clinical Applications of MRI Magnetic Resonance Imaging: Basic Principles*, 2nd ed. New York: Raven Press, 186, 1988.

7. Pusey E, Lufkin RB, Brown RKJ, et al. Magnetic resonance imaging artifacts: mechanical and clinical significance. *Radiographics* 6:891–911, 1986.

CHAPTER 15

Patient Issues: Making a Difference

Roger D. Freimarck

Historically, radiologic technologists have been required to provide their patients with the care necessary to ensure a successful, diagnostic examination as well as maintain a level of patient well-being. Ask five different technologists to define what patient care is and you may receive five very different responses.

Historically, managers of radiologic facilities have been required to provide their working staff with adequate training and equipment to ensure that patient care in their facilities is carried out with efficiency, professionalism, and a high degree of quality. Ask five different managers to define what patient care is and you may also receive five different responses.

Historically, both groups have been under-trained in the art of providing patient care and facilitating patient communication. To this day, patient care and communication in many typical radiology facilities is the result of on-the-job training and is a direct reflection of how much the management requires and expects.

Clinical magnetic resonance imaging is well into its second decade. In that period of time, there has been a virtual flood of information and recommendations regarding patient safety: the result of dealing with very powerful and potentially destructive magnetic fields. Additionally, there has been tremendous effort put forth to help all of us understand how best to use MRI in its varied technical and clinical applications. Yet there has been very little effort placed on helping us understand and appreciate how different MRI is in the area of patient care and communication, and how critical these areas are to a successful facility. All managers can appreciate one simple concept, an exam slot that goes unused as a result of these staff–patient issues is lost revenue and can be detrimental to future referrals. In fact, over the last several years, MR manufacturers have even developed an entire MR imaging system based on patient care and the patients' desire for "open" MR systems. These systems have been specifically designed with patient size and claustrophobia in mind, with much more physical room in the area of the system where images are generated. As a result, patients who are very large and/or claustrophobic are now referred to be imaged on one of these new patient-friendly systems. For this

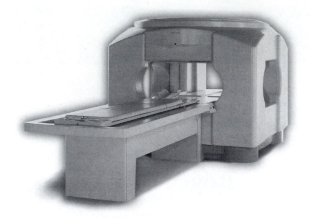

Figure 15-1. Toshiba's superconducting, open MRI system, 0.35 T. (Courtesy Toshiba America MRI, Inc.)

reason, many facilities are now installing an open system right next to their conventional standard systems in order to offer their patients and referring physicians both options [Figure 15-1].

This chapter is meant to give you information and advice on what your staff and facility should be providing your patients with in order to ensure image quality, exam tolerance, physical well-being, and emotional happiness. This information is applicable to all MR systems in clinical use today. However, it is most applicable to the more traditional "closed" type systems which utilize the familiar patient "bore" for imaging. Events which should occur before, during, and after an exam will be discussed. Specific patient magnetic safety issues, a topic which to date has been given a great deal of "press" and attention will not be discussed.

OVERVIEW

As a result of the critical focus on magnetic safety requirements, many facilities have equated patient care to compliance with these stringent requirements. In other words, the perspective goes something like this, "as long as we comply with all of our patient safety policies, we have met the bulk of our patient care requirements." What remains is that which takes place with all radiologic modalities, monitoring the patient's physical condition. However, a given number of MRI patients present themselves with symptoms atypical to other radiographic procedures: emotional anxiety and claustrophobia. Claustrophobia in particular can be very devastating to the patient, to the exam schedule, and to the facility bottom line. Dealing with these patient complaints has forced us to become better communicators and to show considerable concern for the patients' emotional well-being. The acquisition of these skills has not been a smooth process and managers and technologists have struggled with the reality of providing this aspect of patient care. The reality of the matter is simple: we must be just as concerned with the patient's emotional well-being as their physical state. To provide any less puts the success of any facility in extreme jeopardy.

For the purpose of this chapter, *patient care* is defined as any information about or interaction with the patient which has an impact on the quality of the exam images, the general "feeling" of the patient, and facility patient throughput. *Patient communication*, which is an aspect of patient care, is further defined as direct verbal contact with the patient by all MRI personnel.

BEFORE EXAM DAY

When does patient care begin? As strange as it may seem, patient care actually begins on the telephone, with the process of scheduling an exam. Whether you have a central scheduling area staffed by many, or a stand alone MRI department scheduling area staffed by one, the level of attention to details which will have an impact on exam quality and the patient's experience should be the same.

Along with the usual identification and safety information gathered, one must be certain that the exam requested is clinically correct for MRI. This is determined by matching the exam requested with the clinical symptoms justifying the request (note the assumption here that clinical information is available and therefore matchable). Given the aggressive national and local marketing MRI has received in the media over the years, many referring physicians often assume that MRI is the most clinically correct diagnostic exam for a whole host of clinical problems. They often do not consider that other exams, such as computed tomography or ultrasound, may be more appropriate due to either clinical symptoms or the patients inability to tolerate an MRI exam. For example, a request for a brain study on a patient with upper arm pain does not, on the surface, match up for MRI. A brain exam for a patient with arm weakness due to a possible stroke matches. A request for a brain study to rule out acute stroke on a comatose patient may best be done with perfusion or diffusion imaging, which may not be available at the site. In all cases, diagnostic specificity and potential exam quality should be addressed *before* the patient arrives in the MRI department. *Every* MRI facility should have definite guidelines for matching clinical information with a requested exam, as well as guidelines for when the red flag should be raised to examine other diagnostic possibilities. These guidelines should be determined as a result of radiologist, manager, and staff discussions. *Every* MRI scheduling person should have an idea of when to raise the red flag and seek further advice on appropriate scheduling.

Has the patient had a previous exam (in house, local, or outside) which should be compared with the exam currently requested? If so, the time to identify the "when and where" is now, not when the patient shows up and tells you they have had several previous exams in a neighboring state. Frequently the referring physician staff is aware of a patient having previous exams but does not automatically communicate this information to the MRI scheduling person. One of the most frustrating and embarrassing situations for a reading radiologist is to send a report to a referring physician that may have been different or could have been

more definitive had the exam been compared with previous exams. For example, a patient will frequently have a preop exam done in an outpatient MRI or CT facility and a postop exam done in the same facility where surgery was performed. Comparing the pre- and post-exams can be critical to the patient's prognosis, yet these patients may be scheduled with the clinical information of "rule out lesion" when in fact the information should have been "follow up to surgery, rule out reoccurring lesion." Simply put, the question of previous exams needs to be asked and answered initially during the scheduling process. Old exams, be they MRI, CT or appropriate plain films, should be on hand when the patient comes in. Anything less jeopardizes the quality and timeliness of the current study.

Does the patient's size or weight preclude the MRI from being attempted? As we all know, most MRI systems (with the exception of the new open systems) have a fixed bore size. The body part of interest must be able to be positioned in the middle of the magnet. Most systems also have a weight limit for the patient couch. Usually, as the patient approaches this weight limit, they also approach the size limit. The obvious exceptions are very short or very tall patients. Some exams, such as lumbar spine or lower extremity exams, can be performed with the patient's arms extended above their head. This can effectively temporarily reduce the body size but adds a dimension of patient discomfort, which can affect image quality. The scheduling process should identify the patient's weight. Knowing the patient's height is an added bonus. Knowing whether or not a patient will be a comfortable, a questionable, or a nonfit into the magnet will save everyone involved a great deal of hassle. It will also eliminate lost exam slots. For facilities which may have an open system in addition to the standard type system, there should be much thought given to how patient exams are assigned to the open system. For example, low field open systems may have difficulty offering exactly the same high resolution imaging produced by a higher field closed system in a reasonable scan time. It may not be proper to automatically assume that "any" exam can be done on the open magnet, particularly neurologic exams which require the greatest detail. However, when contrast differentiation is the predominate desire, low field imaging offers improvements over high field due to inherently better contrast curves. Thus the radiologist(s) responsible for reading the exams must set guidelines for when and how exams should be assigned to the low field open magnet.

Will the patient require sedation or medication to be able to tolerate the exam? Claustrophobia, pain, pediatric patients, and emotionally compromised patients can all be sources of lost exam slots if enough advanced planning does not take place, *even if the exam is to be done in an open magnet*. Identifying patients in the latter three categories is relatively easy. Identifying claustrophobia is not as straightforward. One school of thought is that asking *all* patients this question at the time of scheduling may in fact precipitate the symptom and cause unnecessary problems. The other school of thought is to ignore the issue unless the patient is said to be a known claustrophobe by virtue of a previous experience. My opinion is to compromise and choose selectively when to ask the question up front. Educating (and reminding) the referring office staff as to your scanner's size and weight limitations as well as typical scan times will allow them to identify potential claustrophobes without having to ask the dreaded question. A patient weighing 290 pounds will be a tight squeeze into any closed MRI system. Even slight claustrophobia could push this patient over the edge and a mild oral sedative may be appropriate. For patients who must travel a long distance for the MRI study, it may be wise to ask the question up front. This can eliminate confusion on the day of the exam and unnecessary rescheduling, particularly if they are traveling alone and on site sedation cannot safely be done. In general, I recommend that your staff ask the "C" question if the patient being scheduled is of questionable size or weight

and if they are traveling from a long distance. Proper arrangements for sedation and assistance can then be made up front for these "discovered" patients as well as for those who are known claustrophobes. Otherwise, I prefer to leave the issue of claustrophobia to the day of the exam. Pain medication and sedation for pediatric and emotionally compromised patients should be realistic and based on experience of success. It is beyond the scope of this chapter to suggest actual drugs and/or dosage or administration techniques for such patients. It should be noted, however, that sleep deprivation is one of the most often overlooked yet easiest tasks to perform with regard to preparation for successful pediatric exams. In general, identifying these four main groups of unique individuals at the time of exam scheduling gives a facility a much better chance of dealing successfully with the exam and pleasing the referring physician.

WHEN THE PATIENT ARRIVES

When the patient finally arrives for the exam, the process of on-going communication must continue. It goes without saying that all personnel coming in contact with the patient must be courteous and friendly. Many patients arrive in the MRI department extremely anxious, not knowing exactly what to expect, and perhaps full of horror stories told them by friends, relatives, or neighbors. A friendly face and kind words will get most patients off to a good start.

All MRI patients must participate in a safety interview, even for low field imaging. They must answer very specific and strange questions about their history, surgeries, metals, etc. Many interviewers simply forget to explain to the patient *why* the questions are being asked. One simple sentence can make all the difference to the patients acceptance of this process. "Because we use a very powerful magnet to make pictures of your body, I have several questions to ask you to help determine if the exam is safe to perform." They now know why the questions are being asked and how important it is to give accurate answers. *The interviewer must listen to the answers.* Frequently, the person doing the interview is not the technologist doing the exam. On more than one occasion in this country, a patient response indicating a possible safety hazard has not made its way to the scanning technologist. The result has been disastrous. Asking, listening, documenting, and passing on the information to the appropriate people is the key to a successful safety interview. Does your facility practice this information gathering process *all* the time?

Modern risk management guidelines dictate that your facility should have a written policy in place with regard to how you determine whether or not a patient with known metal inside their body is safe for imaging. Figure 15-2 is an example of such a policy. You may wish to use it as is or modify it for use in your facility.

For patients undergoing spinal exams, a valuable informational tool you may consider using in your facility is a form simply called the *spinal pain chart* [Figure 15-3]. This form, which contains anatomical drawings of the body, is filled out by the patient at the time of their exam. The patient simply draws appropriate letter symbols on the body figures, indicating exactly where and what type of symptoms they are experiencing *on the day of the exam*. Frequently, the clinical information obtained at the time of scheduling can be very vague at best and, may in fact change before the patient has the exam. A typical lumbar spine scan request will include "left leg pain" as the only clinical indication for the exam. Yet, when the radiologist knows precisely where the discomfort is and what it feels like today, proper attention can be focused on the part of the spine responsible for that area. The beauty of this simple form is that the information comes directly from the patient: it does not rely on third party interpretation. The form requires less than five minutes to complete and can obviously make the exam much more specific to the patient's needs.

Being dressed comfortably for an exam is an important aspect of patient care often overlooked. Most, if not all, male and female patients feel much more comfortable and relaxed if they are allowed to wear pants (pajama bottoms) and a standard gown. Most if not all facilities provide patient gowns. Fewer have pants available. I believe both are necessary and affordable. Robes should be optional. A robe may be somewhat confining which may actually increase claustrophobic feelings. Each patient should be provided with a lockable area for storing valuables during the exam. For liability issues, they should be strongly encouraged to use it.

If the scanning technologist has not spoken directly to the patient up to this point, communication must take place *before* the exam begins. In my opinion, there is absolutely no excuse for not taking the time to communicate with the patient before the exam (assuming the patient can communicate). In just a few minutes, the technologist can pass information on to the patient which helps them understand what to expect and how to participate in the exam and also allows the technologists to anticipate potential problem areas. The information should be realistic and inclusive of the entire exam. Each patient should be told why they are being enclosed in a shielded room, what they will hear and see, how long each portion of the exam will take, how many scans (pulse sequences) are the minimum for the exam, when they will be allowed to move or wriggle, how often they should expect to hear from you, and what they should do to get your attention. The choice of words used by the technologist during this preexam discussion can set the tone for the remainder of the exam. Saying "I am going to place you *into* the magnet" will frighten some patients before they even have a chance to be moved into scan position. Saying "I am going to place you *part way* into the magnet so that the area of interest is in the middle," is much less intimidating for most patients. Letting the patient know the magnet is always open on the ends is very helpful. For patients who are emotionally excited or borderline claustrophobic, one of the most powerful and calming statements they can hear from your technologist *before* the exam starts is, "if things become too

Date

Facility Name - MRI Department

Metallic Implant, Device and Foreign Body Safety Policy

Before a patient is placed in the strong magnetic field of the Magnetic Resonance Imaging scanner, it shall be determined by direct personal interview with the patient (or informed relative), whether or not the patient possesses any metal implants, devices and/or metallic foreign bodies which may be a contraindication for an MRI exam.

If the patient has a cardiac pacemaker in place and/or metallic clips in the brain (such as aneurysm clips), it is the policy of (facility name) that the patient should **NOT** be placed in the strong magnetic field. The referring physician or radiologist should then determine if an alternative exam (such as computed tomography) should be performed.

If the patient has other metal implants, devices and/or foreign bodies in their body, it is the policy of (facility name) to determine whether or not the implant, device or foreign body is safe to be placed in a strong magnetic field. This should be determined by obtaining pertinent clinical information from the referring physician. All implanted materials must be identified by name, model number and manufacturer. This information should be documented on the patient exam information form and then be compared to published lists of magnetic safety tested implants and devices. If the implant or device is approved for MRI, the exam can proceed. If the implant or device is not approved for MRI, the patient will **NOT** be imaged. The referring physician and attending radiologist will be informed and an alternative exam will be considered. If the implant or device is not exactly listed, the manufacturer should be contacted to determine magnetic compatibility. The radiologist should be informed of the outcome of this conversation and determine whether or not the patient can be safely imaged. All unidentified foreign bodies will be imaged at the discretion of the attending radiologist, and NOT the referring physician.

It is the strict policy of (facility name) to determine magnetic safety of all implants, devices and/or foreign bodies from approved sources such as the implant or device manufacturer, or from published lists of magnetic safety testing. There will be no exceptions.

Figure 15-2.   A foreign body safety policy.

uncomfortable, you may *stop* the exam." If the patient feels they have ultimate control over their destiny, they are much more likely to start the exam and endure being uncomfortable for the sake of completing the study. A patient who feels they are being forced to participate is much more likely to produce a suboptimal exam. The result may be rescheduling the exam with sedation or, if the patient had a particularly bad experience, they may not be willing to return at all. I would much rather have a patient call off the exam and be willing to come back.

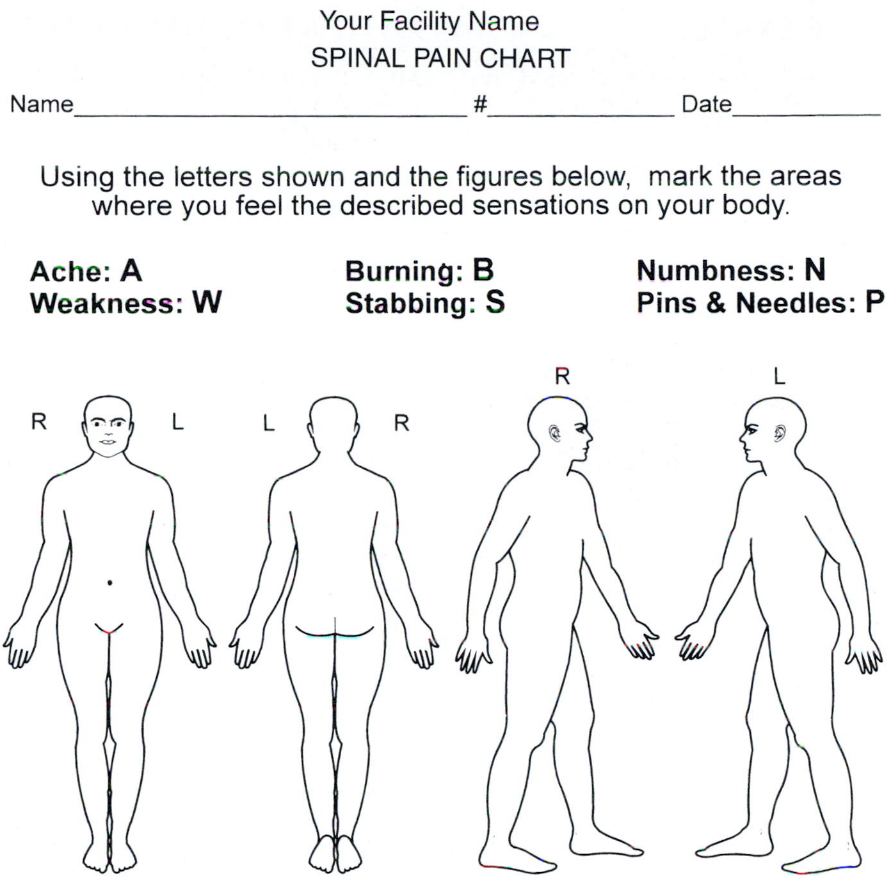

Your Facility Name
SPINAL PAIN CHART

Name_____ #_____ Date_____

Using the letters shown and the figures below, mark the areas
where you feel the described sensations on your body.

Ache: A   **Burning: B**   **Numbness: N**
Weakness: W   **Stabbing: S**   **Pins & Needles: P**

Figure 15-3. A spinal pain chart.

Magnetic field and radio frequency shielded exam rooms are not very conducive to making patients feel comfortable and cozy. The room must be completely sealed to ensure artifact free images and to comply with safety regulations regarding strong magnetic fields. To some patients, this room becomes the equivalent of a vault. They hear the door close and then silence. If the technologist has done a good job of patient preparation, most patients tolerate this enclosure quite well. After all, they know why the room must be sealed and how to reach the technologist, right?

Visitors should be encouraged to accompany the patient into the exam room, particularly when the patient is a child. Don't forget: visitors must also pass the magnetic safety interview to ensure they can safely be in the strong magnetic field next to the patient. *All* visitors must be cautioned about how they can and cannot interact with the patient during the study. Reading a magazine article out loud to the patient during a study can be very soothing. Many times, simply hearing another voice throughout the exam is all a patient needs to tolerate the exam. I would discourage having children in the exam room as visitors. They can become very disruptive and who knows what they can get into while your technologist is out of sight?

DURING THE EXAM

In my opinion, the most often violated responsibility of the scanning technologist is minimal or no conversation with the patient during the exam. It should be a commonsense rule for your technologists to talk with the patient frequently throughout the exam. Before each and every pulse sequence begins, the patient should be told what is about to occur, given any special instructions, and given some idea of how long it will last. After each pulse sequence is completed the patient should be asked how they are doing. They should also then be told how long before something else will happen and whether or not they may move a bit. Long periods of silence between pulse sequences can be very alarming and/or upsetting to most patients. There is no need for any patient to be uninformed about how the exam is progressing. If they are cooperating well and the exam is moving forward the patient should be complemented on how well they are doing. Words of congratulation can be very meaningful and conducive to enhanced cooperation. If the patient is not fulfilling their part of the exam, this should be communicated in a tactful way. Patients assume they are doing a good job unless told otherwise. Failure to communicate noncooperation can result in subsequent imaging sequences which are just as poor or worse. Words are cheap, powerful and above all, very effective. Appropriate words at the appropriate time can eliminate or at least lessen the devastating affects that patient claustrophobia can have on an active exam schedule. During the exam, the operating technologist *must* keep the patient intercom system adjusted to a level where they can hear the patient speaking, coughing, etc. *all* the time. Too many technologists turn the intercom volume down during the pulse sequence to avoid listening to the annoying machine sound. If they cannot hear the machine, they cannot hear the patient.

PATIENT COMFORT IDEAS

Most if not all equipment manufacturers have neglected patient comfort on the exam table. This should not excuse your technologists or your facility from doing the same. MRI-compatible table cushions and other padding devices can be very effective in the area of patient comfort. Simple sponge material purchased at a local foam shop can be easily cut into various shapes for custom padding around the various imaging coils used in scanning. A section of foam can be scanned along with the daily quality assurance phantom to determine artifact production. Most generic foam materials are artifact-free. The foam is cheap and can be discarded when soiled. Simple elbow pads with velcro closures are available and also very inexpensive. Padded elbows, especially for very thin patients can make a world of difference in the area of comfort. A simple bolster or several pillows placed under the knees will make most patients much more comfortable than lying flat. Most exam rooms are kept relatively cool. Blankets are a must for most patients and can be easily removed during the exam if the patient so desires. Patients with particularly sensitive hearing should be encouraged to use ear plugs. As a result of documented cases resulting in loss of hearing (patients who did not use ear plugs), all patients should be encouraged to use the plugs, particularly when using a high field system. One of the distinct advantages of low field imaging is the very low level of gradient noise produced by imaging, but do not take this for granted. Patients should be prepared for any noise, however little there may be. For higher field imaging, it may be wise to have a policy in place to inform those patients who decline the ear plugs of the potential problems. Unfortunately, to many patients, audible sounds of the exam may help to reduce claustrophobic feelings. Many MR systems incorporate mirror systems which allow the patient to see out one end of the magnet while in scan position. Most if not all patients find these devices comforting and very helpful. If your equipment does not offer this patient comfort device, I strongly recommend obtaining a pair of the mirrored glasses which perform very much the same function. They are relatively expensive but, as one who has used them, I can assure you the glasses will pay for themselves in very short order.

The use of sound and video systems as patient management tools has blossomed over the years. Due to marketing hype, many patients will show up on your doorstep expecting to listen to their favorite music or watch a full length feature film. Again, both are fairly expensive items to acquire but will pay for themselves eventually by salvaging exams otherwise unsalvageable. Be advised that these devices will not pay for themselves as quickly as the mirrored glasses. On a slightly negative note, sound and video systems may also add slightly to the length of an exam by virtue of set up and adjustment time. Additionally, raising the volume of a sound system using earplugs also raises the decibel level the patient experiences, a counterproductive measure.

PATIENT MONITORING

For those of you who have been involved with MRI during the early years, this scene will be familiar. A pediatric patient has been sedated with an oral dose of chloral hydrate. After much waiting, the child has finally fallen asleep and is placed on the exam table. The enormously expensive machine is prepared for this "high tech" exam. At the last minute, a five cent styrofoam cup is placed upside down on the child's abdomen. This cup is meant to provide the technologist visual assurance that the child is breathing by moving up and down throughout the respiratory cycle (it is entirely possible for chest movement to occur without air moving in and out of the lungs). Believe it or not, there are many MRI facilities who still employ this archaic

method of physiologic monitoring. Your facility should employ the services of either a pulse oximeter and/or an apnea monitor to provide definitive clinical information on the status of a sedated or physically compromised patient.

Every MRI facility should have clear policies in place which define when a patient should be placed on a physiologic monitor. Common sense should tell your technologists when this is necessary but it should still be in writing.

Often, there is a fine line between providing standard imaging department patient care and providing the patient with nursing services. Each MRI facility must make a decision as to whether or not a registered nurse should be part of the working staff. Having a nurse on staff has obvious advantages. Nurses have received a vast amount of formal training in all aspects of patient care. As such, in my opinion, administering sedation and medications, introducing intravenous lines for contrast media injections, injecting contrast media, providing proper patient monitoring, and dealing with life-threatening emergencies are best handled by a registered nurse. Also, in my opinion, technologists are very capable of learning to perform all of the above but require proper training. *However, they should learn by means other than on-the-job training.* Unfortunately, many MRI facilities who have their technologists performing these tasks have resorted to this traditional approach. There is tremendous medical legal risk for these facilities. It is not inconceivable that, by having a nurse on staff, a typical facility can image one or two more patients in a given week due to more efficient magnet time. This more than pays for the expenses associated with the nurse and provides this valuable service for many patients.

AFTER THE EXAM

Patient care should not end with the last knock of the last imaging sequence. Part of the overall

MRI experience for patients is how they are ushered out once the exam is complete. Upon exam completion, the technologist should not encourage the patient to review their images. However, for those patients asking to do so, the technologist should not refuse to show some example images. Images which do not show obvious pathology should be used to give the patient some idea of how "fantastic and clear" the images are. Remember, this patient is someone's friend, relative, or neighbor. All you have done up to this point to promote a positive experience could backfire if the patient senses you are no longer interested. When requested, have your technologist take a few minutes, show a few images, and answer appropriate questions. Obviously the technologists cannot give the patient diagnostic information regarding the exam, but they can be upbeat and commend the patient for "pretty pictures." Most patients are content knowing that only the radiologist is allowed to release clinical information. As the patient departs, your technologist or front desk personnel should give the patient a realistic idea of when the results will be sent to their doctor's office. Frequently, this is when you will discover the patient has an afternoon appointment and the doctor expects the results of the exam. Otherwise, the patient will not be bothering their doctor earlier than necessary. Your referring physicians will appreciate this bit of patient communication.

SUMMARY

MRI facilities are complex in many varied ways. The modality is highly technically oriented and very, very expensive. Clinical expectations of the modality are great – especially of the newer open MR systems. Often, in our rush to have our facilities become technically superior by offering our referring physicians the latest clinical diagnostic developments, we overlook our responsibilities to our patients. The above information is meant to be used as a guideline for providing your patients with the basic care and attention necessary to make your facility equally superior in the "people" sense. Rules and policies can never be formulated to cover all possibilities. Intelligent people know when rules must be followed, when to deviate, and when to develop new ones. Patient care in MRI is unique in many ways. Managers of MRI facilities must realize that this technology can lend itself to lengthy periods of boredom for the operator. As such, one of the duties most frequently dropped or glossed over is patient care and communication as I have defined it. The technical aspect of magnetic resonance can, and usually does, overpower the patient aspect. We must do our best to see that our staff technologists pay close attention to both.

CHAPTER 16

MRI Safety Concerns

Gregory L. Wheeler

GENERAL CONSIDERATIONS

Magnetic fields are measured in gauss (G), tesla (T), or kilogauss (kG), with 1 T equal to 10 000 G. According to the most current recommendations and guidelines provided by the United States Food and Drug Administration (FDA), clinical MR systems are permitted to function on a routine clinical basis at static magnetic field strengths of up to 2.0 T[1].

There are significant safety issues concerning the static, time-varying, and RF oscillating magnetic fields. We will discuss the safety issues of each of these magnetic fields and recommend safe practices to minimize the risk of injury to a patient, volunteer, family member, and/or the medical staff.

The International Non-Ionizing Radiation Committee of the International Radiation Protection Association (IRPA/INIRC), in cooperation with the Environmental Health Division of the World Heath Organization (WHO), has developed health criteria documents on magnetic fields (UNEP/WHO/IRPA 1987) and radiofrequency fields (UNEP/WHO/IRPA in press)[2]. The committee emphasizes that in the application of MR, the following issues deserve special attention.

1. Magnetic resonance (MR) in vivo examinations should be performed only when there is a potential clinical advantage to the patient.
2. An assessment of risks and benefits of the MR examination should be made, and the decision to proceed must be based on the relationship between the patient and the physician.
3. Consideration should be given to the clinical advantages and disadvantages of MR compared to other diagnostic techniques.
4. Where MR examinations form parts of a research project, the project should be guided by rules of human ethics: informed consent of the patient should be obtained.
5. MR equipment users must be adequately trained in the principles and operation of the equipment, indications and contraindications for use, record keeping requirements, safety aspects, and precautions.

295

6. Manufacturers should supply complete documentation about patient exposure levels for their equipment, and these safety guidelines should be considered in the design of equipment and facility layout so that exposures to magnetic and radio-frequency fields are within the levels recommended for patients[2].

BIOEFFECTS OF STATIC MAGNETIC FIELD

There are two main concerns regarding the issue of safety and the static magnetic field. The first deals with the bioeffects associated with exposure to the static magnetic fields. The second deals with the effects of the forces exerted by the magnetic fields of the MR systems on certain metallic objects[2].

Mechanism of Interaction

The mechanism of interaction for static magnetic fields is the polarization effect imposed by the static magnetic field. Static magnetic fields cause the alignment of magnetic substances based on the substance's degree of magnetic susceptibility.

MRI energy field	Mechanism of interaction
Time-varying	Induced current
RF oscillating	Thermal heating
Static	Polarization

Regardless of the type of MRI energy field considered, there is a level of intensity, the threshold intensity (I_T), below which no response is elicited. Below I_T, MRI is entirely safe. Above I_T the response to MRI exposure first increases slowly and then more rapidly until 100 percent response is observed[3].

There have been a number of articles regarding the potential bioeffects of static magnetic fields. Most of the studies have concluded that static magnetic fields of up to 2 T produce no substantial harmful bioeffects. There have been no alterations in cell growth and morphology, DNA structure and gene expression, pre- and postnatal reproduction and development, visual functions, nerve bioelectric activity, animal behavior, visual response to photic stimulation, cardiovascular dynamics, hematologic indices, physiological regulation and circadian rhythms, or immune responsiveness[2].

No adverse health effects are expected from exposure of the head and/or trunk to magnetic flux densities up to 2 T, or from exposure of the limbs to magnetic flux densities up to 5 tesla[2]. There has been speculation concerning the bio-effects of intense magnetic fields on growth rate, mutation, fertility, and blood cell count in mammals. Experiments on the developing embryos of pregnant mice who were exposed at various times during gestation, did not show any statistical alterations in the offspring when compared with nonexposed control mice[4]. From the review of the biological effects of magnetic fields, it can be concluded that no adverse health effects are to be expected from short-term (hours) exposure to static magnetic fields up to 2 T.

Cell and Nerve Function

An adequate investigational study on the absolute safety of electromagnetic fields used in MRI has not been established to date and therefore leaves the issue to controversy. Researchers have shown that deoxygenated sickled red blood cells in vitro will align against or perpendicular to a static magnetic field[5]. This phenomenon is attributed to paramagnetic anisotropy retained by the heme of the hemoglobin S that is polymerized by deoxygenation[6].

There have been several studies performed to assess neuropsychiatric and cognitive function alterations related to exposure to MR procedures. These investigations did not identify any effects associated with exposure to static magnetic fields of the MR systems, either with respect to cognition, acute or chronic behavior changes, or memory alterations[2].

Normal subjects exposed to static magnetic fields of a 4.0 T MR system reported unusual sensations including nausea, vertigo, and a metallic taste associated with alteration in nerve function as a result of interaction with direct exposure to or movement through the high-intensity static magnetic field (e.g., stimulation of the vestibulolabyrinthine complex may explain the vertigo)[7]. It is suggested, based on the information reported, that exposure to static magnetic fields of MR systems of up to 2.0 T does not appear substantially to influence nerve function in human subjects[2].

Cardiovascular Function

There have been findings in respect to the cardio-vascular effects of exposure to static magnetic fields. As blood, a conductive fluid, flows through a static magnetic field it induces a biopotential. This induced biopotential is typically exhibited by an augmentation of T-wave amplitude as well as other nonspecific waveform changes that are apparent on the electrocardiogram[2]. The increase in T-wave amplitude is directly proportional to the intensity of the static magnetic field such that, at low static magnetic field strengths, the effects are not as predominant compared with the higher ones[8]. Elevated T-waves are associated with ischemia and myocardial infarction, so it is important to evaluate the patient before and after the examination to assure that the elevated T-waves are the result of the exposure to the static magnetic field.

Temperature

Static magnetic fields do not cause an alteration in the skin and body temperature of humans or laboratory animals. There have been conflicting reports about the effects of the static magnetic field on temperature, suggesting that static fields can increase and/or decrease skin and body temperatures. Further research suggests that the temperature increases observed may be the result

of instrumentation that may have been perturbed by the static magnetic field. Investigations conducted in laboratory animals and human subjects indicated that exposure to intense static magnetic fields and/or gradient magnetic fields does not alter skin and body temperatures[9].

Magnetophosphenes

Although their precise etiology is still unclear, magnetophosphenes are believed to result from direct excitation of the optic nerve and/or retina by currents that are induced by rapid gradient magnetic fields or alternatively, eye or head movements within a static magnetic field[10]. Clinical MR systems are currently limited to static magnetic fields up to 2.0 T. Within this field strength limit there have been no reports of magnetophosphenes, however there have been reports of the presence of magnetophosphenes in field strengths as high as 4.0 T.

BIOEFFECTS OF TIME-VARYING (GRADIENT) MAGNETIC FIELDS

Time-varying or gradient magnetic fields have a number of important applications in MR imaging. These applications range from superimposing spatial magnetic field variations on top of a homogeneous static magnetic field for spatial localization, to rephasing, dephasing, and refocusing magnetic moments at different amplitudes and for various durations.

There are at least two possible bioeffects related to gradient magnetic fields during the MR procedure. One is associated with induced currents and voltages that may result in power deposition and subsequent tissue heating while the patient is exposed to the gradient magnetic fields during the MR procedure[18]. Sufficient evidence exists to support the finding that the thermal effects that result from the gradient's time-variations during the MR imaging procedure are essentially negligible, and therefore, are considered clinically insignificant.

The second bioeffect is the possibility that neuromuscular stimulation may occur. This is a direct result of the direct stimulation or induced voltages that exceed the threshold for achieving neural action potential discharge[2].

The factors responsible for inducing a physiologic response to an induced voltage are as follows.

1. The strength of the static magnetic field.
2. The orientation of the gradient magnetic field.
3. The orientation of the gradient magnetic fields being switched relative to the patient's tissues.
4. The size of the greatest diameter of the patient's body.
5. The frequency of the stimulus.
6. The duration of the induced voltage.
7. The shape of the waveform, the width of the pulse.
8. The sensitivity of the tissue.
9. Other factors that can all affect the threshold at which a response or measurable effect is observed[2].

Therefore the effects of time-varying (gradient) magnetic fields on the human body is significant enough to warrant investigation and possible limits on the magnitude of the induced currents from MR imaging procedures. There is reasonable cause to investigate whether the magnitude of induced currents from clinically applied MR procedures might be sufficient to induce seizures, magnetophosphenes, alterations of nerve conduction velocity, peripheral nerve stimulation, skeletal muscular contractions, or even cardiac arrhythmias[2].

The effect induced currents or voltages have on the tissues during the MR imaging procedure requires the knowledge of the amplitude of the induced current and the induced current densities. To calculate the induced current densities it is important to know the electrical conductivity or resistivity of the induced current loop. This is determined by the tissues through which the induced voltage will attempt to induce a current flow[2].

Mechanism of Interaction

Time-varying magnetic fields are able to induce electric currents in human tissues. According to Faraday's Law of Induction, exposure of any conductor to time-varying magnetic fields will induce a voltage in a conductor that is oriented perpendicular to the time rate of change of the magnetic field[2]. When a body is placed into the MR system and the time-varying magnetic field coils are activated, two results are simultaneously achieved. Not only is there the creation of a gradient magnetic field, but there is also the potential of inducing voltages within the tissues of (and/or other electrical conductors on or in) the patient in the bore of the MR system and its three orthogonally oriented sets of gradient coils[2].

Time-varying magnetic fields (gradients) for a typical MR imaging procedure have peak gradient amplitudes approximately 0.5 to 1.0 G/cm and are achieved in a rise time of 500 μs or more. There is a greater magnetic field over time, or dB/dt, as one proceeds farther away from the center and toward the ends of the gradient coils, where the time rate of change of the gradient magnetic fields (dB/dt) is the greatest[2].

It is difficult to correlate the induced body currents with the magnetic flux change of the different magnetic field gradients occurring in pulse sequences from MR equipment. Pulse sequences generate RF waves with wave shapes that deviate from sinusoidal, making it difficult to predict the biological effects during stimulation.

The United States Food and Drug Administration (FDA) has issued safety guidelines and suggested operating limitations for MR imaging devices regarding the gradient magnetic fields associated with MR imaging procedures. The specific wording of the guidelines issued in 1988 is as follows:

> Rate of change of magnetic field: Limit patient exposure to time-varying magnetic fields with strengths significantly less than those required to produce peripheral nerve stimulation...[11]

Cell and Nerve Function

Recommendations on limiting the exposure to time-varying magnetic fields are based primarily on effects of induced currents on excitable cell membranes in the nervous system and muscles, and to a certain extent on more subtle effects on other cells[12].

Theoretically, transient magnetic fields can either stimulate or impair electrical impulses along neuronal pathways in tissues[3]. The rate of change over time of the magnetic field, expressed as dB/dt, is measured in T/s. Because some cells and tissues are electric conductors, the transient magnetic field gradients may induce electric current, the normal function of nerve cells and muscle fibers may be affected[2]. The threshold current density of time-varying magnetic fields is determined by the tissue conductivity and the duration of time the time-varying field has been energized.

Clinical experience indicates that no adverse health effects are to be expected when the rate of change of magnetic flux density does not exceed 6 T/s.[2] It is important to consider each individual situation based on the patient's electrocardiogram (ECG) and abnormalities present.

With regard to nerve function in the time-varying magnetic fields, peripheral nerve stimulation occurs before effects on the function of the heart are induced and can be used as a primary criterion for the assessment of MR safety. A draft of the MRI Guidance Update for dB/dt was issued by the Office of Device Evaluation, Center for Devices and Radiological Health, on October 11, 1995. This draft is a revision of the previous document published April 21, 1995, and outlines several modifications to the prior levels of concern. For example, it was decided that painful peripheral nerve stimulation be the target threshold to avoid (as opposed to simple twitching or simple biologic detectability of this low level of stimulation) and that an exam be terminated if the patient complains of severe discomfort or pain[2].

There is also a "Warning" section in the document stating that special patient populations should be studied only in controlled clinical settings and under the supervision of the Institutional Review Board. This special patient population group included children, pregnant women, epileptics, patients with metallic implants, cardiac arrhythmia, peripheral neuropathy, comatose patients, or patients who are unable to communicate[13]. The *Guidance for the Content and Review of a Magnetic Resonance Diagnostic Device 510(k) Application* document, issued on April 21, 1995 and revised on October 11, 1995 further states:

> Operators of the MR systems are to be warned by the MR system manufacturers regarding the types of imaging techniques available on the specific MR system that may produce peripheral nerve stimulation. They also need to be provided with a description of the types of sensations of peripheral nerve stimulation that are capable of being produced. Whenever these techniques are used, operators are to be instructed to inform the patient that peripheral nerve stimulation may occur, describing the nature of such sensations to the patient.

> The MR operator is to maintain constant contact with the patient during the procedures in which peripheral nerve stimulation may be induced. The patient is to be instructed not to clasp their hands (to avoid creating a conductive loop), if they experience severe discomfort or pain. In these instances, the MR procedure must be terminated and a report regarding the incident should be completed and immediately submitted to the manufacturer of the MR system, as well as the FDA[13].

Cardiac Muscle and Cardiovascular System

Cardiac muscle stimulation is important to evaluate during the application of the time-varying magnetic fields (gradients). The best approximation of the current density that will be experienced as a consequence of using gradients during the MR procedure is $1\,\mu A/cm^2$ for a dB/dt of $1.0\,T/s$. MR imaging systems routinely produce current densities of approximately $3\,\mu A/cm^2$ for a dB/dt of $3.0\,T/s$. This is below the level where biologic effects are expected. By comparison, roughly $15-100\,\mu A/cm^2$ are needed to produce tetanic contractions of the skeletal muscles involved in breathing, whereas $0.2-1.0\,\mu A/cm^2$ appears to be the threshold current density required to produce ventricular fibrillation in the human heart (at frequency ranges of 20–200 Hz for sinusoidal voltages)[14]. Seizure induction thresholds seem to be even higher.

While the calculations suggest that the threshold currents required to induce ventricular fibrillation in a healthy heart are significantly greater than those achieved during the MR imaging procedure routinely, it is important to recognize that higher amplitude gradients with faster rise times and faster pulse sequences will increase the current densities proportionally.

Magnetophosphenes

Magnetophosphenes result from direct excitation of the optic nerve and/or retina by currents that are induced by rapid gradient magnetic fields, or alternatively, by rapid eye motion within a static magnetic field[15]. Persons experiencing this visual sensation report seeing "flashes of light" in the eyes.

Although there have been no cases of magnetophosphenes reported for fields of up to and including 1.9 T, magnetophosphenes, metallic taste, headache, and symptoms of vertigo seem also to be relatively reproducible symptoms associated with rapid motion within the static magnetic field of 4 T MR systems[7]. It is apparent that magnetophosphenes result from the gradient magnetic field effects of induced voltages and currents that are produced from motion in the environment of the static magnetic fields (i.e., changing magnetic fields inducing electrical

voltages)[2]. While these magnetophosphenes are biologically detectable, they are not necessarily harmful.

Neural Stimulation

It is important to discuss the possible and likely neural stimulation effects due to the increasingly rapid pulse sequences. As the gradient coil technology advances gradient amplitudes and rise times are increasing. Whereas years ago many MR systems would have had 1 G/cm maximum gradient amplitudes with 600–700 µs rise times, today it is not uncommon to find clinical MR systems with 15 G/cm maximum gradient or more magnetic field strengths and 300–500 µs rise times[2].

Echo planar imaging, the fastest pulse sequences design currently being introduced to the MR imaging community, uses ultrafast gradient coil applications of about 2.5 G/cm maximum amplitudes and < 300 µs rise times. Uncontrolled, involuntary skeletal muscular contraction and/or twitching has already been reported and investigated in human subjects. This is believed to represent direct peripheral muscle stimulation induced by echo planar imaging sequences[16]. Patients have experienced feelings similar to electric shocks or tingling along the spine and the nose.

It is important that the patient's body does not complete a loop, thereby increasing the potential for these effects. The patient's body establishes a loop whenever the hands are clasped, the legs and/or arms are crossed or the knees and/or feet touching. The threshold for these gradient magnetic field-induced bioeffects has been observed at and beyond 60 T/s[17].

BIOEFFECTS OF OSCILLATING (RF) MAGNETIC FIELDS

The range of radiofrequencies (RF) used to excite the spins within the body is between 1 and 100 MHz. This is a small portion of the frequencies in the nonionizing electromagnetic radiation range of 0–3000 GHz. This must be distinguished from the ionizing electromagnetic radiation range that is associated with X-rays and gamma rays.

Mechanism of Interaction

The RF field is an electromagnetic energy field that consists of an oscillating electric field and a similar orthogonal magnetic field. These energy fields interact simultaneously with matter and according to the nature of the matter. The electric field component can induce heating in matter and induce high-frequency electric currents, while the magnetic field component acts as a rapidly transient magnetic field, relevant due to the potential for heating both superficial and deep tissues[3].

Depending on the pulse sequence design, radiofrequency power levels can range up to 16,000 W. As the radiofrequency pulses are applied they are transmitted from the transmit/receive rack through the bulkhead of the scan room into the transmit coil where there are losses in energy transmitted due to transmit cable losses. There are losses due to coupling and reflection of the RF back into the RF amplifier, and losses when the RF is received due to coil inefficiencies, and even RF signal loss.

RF Absorption

With the application of the oscillating (RF) magnetic field the tissue will absorb the RF energy based on the patient's size and body habitus, the tissue's sensitivity, and the duration and the type of RF pulses the patient is subjected to. Shellock and Kanal[2], to authors of *Bioeffects of RF Electromagnetic Fields*, state the following.

> The physical dimensions and configuration of the tissue in relation to the incident wavelength are important factors that determine the relative amount and pattern of energy that is absorbed during exposure to RF radiation. If the tissue size is large in relation to the incident wavelength, energy is predominantly absorbed on the surface. If it is small relative to the wavelength, there is little absorption of the RF power. The most efficient absorption of RF energy occurs when the tissue is approximately 50% the size of the incident wavelength; this frequency of maximum absorption is known as the "resonant frequency."

The resonant frequency, achieved when the applied radiofrequency matches the frequency of oscillating of he precessing spins within a magnetic field, causes the spins to absorb the RF energy with an increased ability to penetrate superficial tissues and directly heat internal sites within the body. A rise in body temperature is most often reported with exposure to oscillating (RF) fields.

The rise in tissue temperature from oscillating (RF) magnetic fields is caused primarily from magnetic field induction instead of the electric fields, therefore the heating effect to the patient will occur most common to the superficial areas of the body and periphery with least heating in the center.

Specific Absorption Rate (SAR)

The physiologic measure of intensity of RF energy is the specific absorption rate (SAR) with units of W/kg. During MR procedures, most of the RF power transmitted for imaging or spectroscopy is transformed into heat within the patient's tissue as a result of resistive losses. It is for this reason that the primary bioeffects associated with the RF radiation used for MR procedures are directly related to the thermogenic qualities of this electromagnetic field.

The pattern of RF absorption or coupling of radiation of biologic tissues depends primarily on the organism's size, anatomic features, the pulse duty cycle, the duration of exposure, the density and conductivity of the involved tissues, and other variables.

The thermoregulatory system regulates heat loss by means of convection, conduction, evaporation and radiation. If the thermoregulatory effectors are not capable of totally dissipating the heat load, then an accumulation of storage occurs, along with an elevation in local and/or overall tissue temperatures[18].

Biologic effects of RF are associated with the SAR. The SAR, in turn, is related to the RF power density as it varies in time (temporal) and space (spatial). Maximum permissible exposure limits are expressed as power density. They are set approximately 100 times lower than levels known to cause a response. The thermal reactions to a given SAR can vary considerably based on the patient's thermoregulatory system and the presence of conditions that may affect the system's efficiency.

Recommended Safe Levels of Exposure

The US Food and Drug Administration provides recommendations for two alternative safe levels of exposure to RF radiation during MR procedures, primarily in an effort to control the risk of systemic thermal overload and thermal injury. Either the specific SAR levels or temperature criteria that follow may be used by MR imaging personnel when performing MR imaging procedures.

1. The exposure to RF energy below the level of concern is a SAR of 0.4 W/kg or less averaged over the body, and 8.0 W/kg or less spatial peak in any 1 g of tissue, and 3.2 W/kg or less over the head.

2. The exposure of RF energy that is insufficient to produce a core temperature increase of 1 °C and localized heating to no greater than 38 °C in the head, 39°C in the trunk, and 40 °C in the extremities, except for patients with impaired systemic blood flow and/or perspiration (i.e., patient with compromised thermoregulatory systems)[1].

Rapid Pulse Sequences

Currently there is a trend to design faster and faster pulse sequences with which to gain diagnostic information using MR in shorter times. This trend has given rise to a number of rapid or fast pulse sequences that are depositing RF into the tissues of the body at an incredibly rapid rate. For example the fast spin echo, fast gradient echo, and magnetization transfer may use SARs that easily exceed whole body averaged SARs of 4.0–8.0 W/kg. The main reason for the increased RF deposition is the increase in 180-degree RF pulses used in the pulse sequence at incredibly rapid rates. Not to exclude echo planar imaging pulse sequence that deposits RF at a rapid rate in a short time. Larger field of views that require RF transmission using the body coil increase the RF deposited increasing the potential problem in MR imaging examinations.

PATIENT SAFETY CONSIDERATIONS

The FDA issued the tentative findings of the Radiologic Devices Panel on May 9, 1988 concurrently with its recommendation that magnetic resonance diagnostic device be reclassified from class III (pre-market approval) into class II (performance standards). In Part V, The Panel's View of Device Related Risks and Benefits, Section A: "Risks to Health" states the following.

Risks to health identified in the petitions included:

1. Adverse effects of whole or partial body exposure to the static magnetic field.
2. Adverse effects of exposure to time-varying magnetic fields.
3. Adverse effects of absorption of energy from radiofrequency magnetic fields.
4. Hazards from high acoustic noise levels.
5. Hazards from laser beams.
6. Electrical and mechanical hazards.
7. Insufficient image or spectral quality resulting in reduced clinical utility.
8. Other potential hazards addressed by labeling[1].

It is because of these identified risks that we discuss individual safety issues when considering subjecting a person to a magnetic resonance imaging procedure.

Screening for Safety Considerations

All individuals, including patients, volunteers, staff, custodial workers, emergency team, and visitors must be screened before exposing them to magnetic fields and the MR system. It is crucial to conduct a careful screening procedure to ensure the safety of anyone who enters the magnet environment. Included in this screening should be a questionnaire designed specifically to determine if there is reason to believe that a person undergoing the magnetic resonance imaging procedure would experience an adverse reaction to the exposure to electromagnetic radiation. The questionnaire should be clear and unambiguous to determine the following.

1. What surgery the patient has had in the past.
2. If there are any implanted materials or devices that are magnetically, mechanically, or electrically activated.
3. Whether the patient may be pregnant or has any unresolved metallic foreign bodies in their body.

A diagram of the human body should be provided on the questionnaire so that the patient can indicate the area of interest and more importantly the position of any object that may interfere with the safety of the patient or the interpretation of the MR images. Even with a completed questionnaire by the patient or individuals that will be exposed to the electromagnetic field, it is important to conduct an oral interview prior to exposing the individual, to further ensure the individual's safety.

In 1994, the Safety Committee of the Society for Magnetic Resonance published screening recommendations and a questionnaire that encompassed all the important safety issues[19].

These recommendations were developed to be a consensus of standard care for all MR centers.

Safety Considerations for Biomedical Implants

Over the past 15 years there have been numerous studies and investigations on the safety of performing MR imaging procedures on patients who have biomedical implants or devices. Shellock and Kanal make the following recommendation.

> With respect to the ferromagnetic qualities of metallic implants, materials, and devices, investigations have generally demonstrated that an MR procedure may be performed safely in a patient with a metallic object if it is nonferromagnetic or if it is attracted only minimally by the static magnetic field in relation to the in vivo application of the object (i.e., the associated deflection force or attraction to the magnetic field is insufficient to move or dislodge the metallic object in situ)[2].

Therefore, patients with any of the following or similar devices that could be adversely affected by the electromagnetic fields used in MR imaging should not be examined with this modality[20].

- Internal or external cardiac pacemakers.
- Implantable cardioverter defibrillators.
- Cochlear implants.
- Neurostimulators.
- Bone-growth stimulators.
- Implantable drug-infusion pumps.

Cardiac pacemakers have associated risks with MRI related to the possible movement of the device, damage to the reed switch, changes to the mode of operation, electromagnetic interference, and induction of current in lead wires. Of particular concern is the possibility that the pacemaker wire(s) or other similar intracardiac wire configuration could act as an antenna in which the gradient and/or radio-frequency electromagnetic fields may induce sufficient current to cause fibrillation, thermal injury, or other potentially dangerous event[2]. It is for these reasons and risks that patients with residual external pacing wires, temporary pacing wires, thermodilution Swan–Ganz catheters, and/or any other type of internally or externally positioned conductive wire or similar device are excluded[2].

MR facilities are recommended to rely on peer-reviewed literature regarding the safety of performing MR procedures in patients with potentially hazardous magnetically, mechanically, and electrically activated objects. MR users are recommended to contact manufacturers of the devices to determine their composition and to determine if they are safe when exposed to the magnetic fields used in the clinical setting.

Any electrically conductive material that can be removed should be removed from the patient prior to a MR imaging procedures. Care should be exercised to ensure that any wires that are not removed from the electromagnetic field do not create a loop that can run the risk of acting like an antenna inducing current into the wires and potentially harming the patient.

Cochlear implants use a high-field strength cobalt–samarium magnet in conjunction with an external magnet to align and retain a radio-frequency transmitter coil on the patient's head, while other types of cochlear implants are electronically activated[21]. Subjecting patients with cochlear implants to an MR imaging procedure is strictly contraindicated due to the probability of injuring the patient or the operation of the cochlear implant device.

Other materials such as magnetic sphincters, magnetic stoma plugs, magnetic ocular implants, dental implants, tissue expanders with magnetic ports, and other devices that are magnetic can move or torque in the presence of an electromagnetic field and therefore should be removed.

The presence of an electrically, magnetically, or mechanically activated device is usually considered to be a contraindication for an MR procedure[2]. Anyone who has the above device types should be excluded from the MR imaging procedure unless the device has been shown previously to be unaffected by the electromagnetic field or has an acceptably low risk of injuring the patient.

Safety Considerations for the Pregnant Patient

Safety is an important, controversial, and individual issue when performing MR imaging procedures on pregnant patients. The guidelines issued indicate that the safety of MR when used to image the fetus has not been established or provided[2]. It is important to identify individuals who suspect that they may be pregnant before exposing them to electromagnetic fields. It is also important to inform them that there are no known deleterious effects to the use of MR procedures during pregnancy and to determine the risk versus the benefit to the clinical finding.

According to the recommendations provided by the Policies, Guidelines, and Recommendations for MR Imaging Safety and Patient Management issued by the Safety Committee of the Society for Magnetic Resonance Imaging in 1991, MR procedures may be used in pregnant patients if other nonionizing forms of diagnostic imaging are inadequate or if the examination provides important information that would otherwise require exposure to a diagnostic procedure that requires ionizing radiation[1]. The policy has also been adopted by the American College of Radiology and is considered to be the "standard of care" with respect to the use of MR procedures in pregnant patients[22].

There are a lot of indications for the use of MR imaging procedures in pregnant patients, despite the wide body of data regarding the potential bioeffects. Therefore, in cases where the referring physician and radiologist can affirm that the outcome of the MR examination requested during pregnancy has the potential to change or alter the care or therapy of the mother or fetus, an MR procedure (i.e., MR imaging, angiography, or spectroscopy) may be performed with informed consent, regardless of the stage of trimester[23].

Shellock and Kanal state the following.

The predominant issues related to MR procedures are:

1. The possible effects of the static magnetic field of the MR system.
2. The risks associated with exposure to the gradient magnetic fields.
3. The potential adverse effects of the radio-frequency (RF) electromagnetic fields.
4. Possible adverse effects related to the combination of the three different electromagnetic fields.
5. Possible adverse effects related to the use of MR imaging contrast agents[2].

Safety Considerations for Pregnant Health Care Personnel

Safety considerations for the pregnant health care worker are also individual and somewhat controversial. Since there are no indications that the use of clinical MR imaging during pregnancy has produced deleterious effects, similar considerations should be applied to health care workers.

A survey of reproductive, healthy, female MR operators was conducted in 1991. A questionnaire addressing their menstrual and reproductive experiences was sent to female MR technologists and nurses at most clinical MR facilities in the United States[24]. The data indicated that there were no statistically significant alterations in the five areas studied for MR workers relative to the same group studied when they were employed outside of the MR environment[24].

More specifically, it is recommended that pregnant health care workers be permitted to perform MR procedures, as well as to enter and attend the patient in the MR scan room, regardless of the trimester. Health care workers should not be in the MR scan room during the imaging procedures and especially while the time-varying magnetic field and oscillating (RF) pulse is being administered.

These recommendations are based not on indications of adverse effects, but rather from a conservative point of view and the feeling that there is insufficient data pertaining to the effects of the other electromagnetic fields of the MR system to support or allow unnecessary exposures[2].

Safety Considerations for Use of Contrast Agents on Pregnant Patients

The administration of an MR imaging contrast agent to a pregnant patient should occur only if the benefit justifies the potential risk to the fetus and the patient signs a written informed consent acknowledging that any associated risks are currently unknown[25].

MR contrast agent product literature does not currently support the use of gadolinium-based contrast agents on pregnant patients because of the lack of studies on safety. It is known that the contrast agent crosses the placenta and is excreted by the fetal bladder. From there the contrast agent is then swallowed by the fetus, where it is once again filtered and excreted into the urine. This process continues many times. The rate of clearance for the contrast agents from the fetal circulation system and the amniotic fluid is unknown.

It is therefore recommended that the risks versus the benefits of using the contrast agent during pregnancy be carefully evaluated in each case and should be used only if the benefits outweigh the potential and associated risks.

Safety Considerations for Auditory Effects

Acoustic noise is produced when the electromagnetic forces created by the gradient coils cause motion or vibrations against their mountings. This noise, often heard as a "knocking," "chirping," or "tapping" noise, occurs during the rapid alterations in the current within the gradient coils. This noise is a safety consideration when performing a MR imaging procedure on patients.

Gradient
ated and me
Hurwitz et
sound levels
A-weighted s
The report
field-induced
within recog

The US
indicates tha
with the ope
to be belov
by pertinent

There is
to reduce th
noise of the
encouraged
10–20 dB.

A signifi
noise cause
accomplishe
active noise
que with
reduction
reported w

A signif
use earphc
acoustic nc
certainly a
patients. I
intercom t
can talk t
presence c

**Safety C
Contras**

The use a
agents in
the rise.
MR ima
mechanis
gadoliniu
nontoxic.

Gado
electrons

use of MR contrast agents. These reactions include sneezing, dyspnea, throat irritation, laryngismus, rhinorrhea/rhinitis, and coughing. Dermatologic reactions include rash, flushing, hives, erythema, skin discoloration, swelling, and tingling in the digits, among others. Many of these patients have previous histories of allergic reactions and respiratory difficulty, such as asthma.

Reactions have been reported with the use of each of the approved MR contrast agents. Anaphylactoid reactions involve respiratory, cardiovascular, cutaneous, and possibly gastrointestinal and/or genitourinary manifestations[30].

Special Patient Population Considerations

There are special patient populations that should be closely evaluated prior to the administration of MR contrast agents. This group includes patients with renal insufficiency, renal failure, Wilson's disease, sickle cell-anemia, and pregnancy.

There is the potential for increased levels of gadolinium ions to accumulate in patients that have renal failure. There are studies that indicate that administering contrast agents to patients with impaired renal function has not been established as safe. There have been several studies that have reported that these agents should be well tolerated[31].

Patients who have elevated levels of copper (such as with Wilson's disease) or zinc have not been fully evaluated. The toxicity levels in these patients will depend on such factors as the glomerular filtration and renal clearance rates, as well as their blood copper levels[32].

The FDA has indicated concern in the package insert information regarding the use of gadolinium-based MR imaging contrast agents in patients with sickle-cell anemia. According to the package insert for these agents, the enhancement of magnetic moments may potentiate sickle erythrocyte alignment[33]. There have been in vivo studies that have shown that the deoxygenated sickle erythrocytes will align perpendicular to the externally applied magnetic field.

The concern is for the theoretical possibility of inducing vaso-occlusive complications. However, there has not been any evidence to show that any of the contrast agents actually precipitated a sickle-cell crisis.

Contrast agents are administered directly into the blood stream. In a pregnant patient the contrast agents will cross the placental barrier and are then filtered into the fetal bladder. From the fetal bladder, the agents are excreted into the amniotic fluid. The contrast agent, within the amniotic fluid, is then swallowed by the fetus subsequently and then is either passed through the gastrointestinal tract of the fetus or is filtered and excreted in the fetal urine. The process repeats again.

There is no data available to show the clearance rate of MR imaging contrast agents in the fetus. Therefore, a conservative approach is recommended against the administration of any of the gadolinium-based contrast agents to pregnant patients unless there is a compelling clinical reason for their use.

Breast feeding mothers who are to have contrast agents during MR imaging procedures are recommended to express their breasts and not breast feed for 36–48 h to ensure that the nursing child does not receive an appreciable quantity of the contrast.

Metallic Foreign Bodies

Patients with a history of metallic foreign body injury involving bullets, shrapnel, metallic fragment or foreign bodies to the eye should be thoroughly evaluated before being exposed to the magnet field. Magnetic fields can cause serious injury to patients who have metallic objects in their body as a result of the magnetic field moving the foreign body.

The risk of injury depends on the ferromagnetic properties of the foreign body, the geometry and dimension of the object, and the strength of the static magnetic field of the MR system[2]. There is a significant risk when the foreign body is in or near a particularly sensitive site such as a vital neural, vascular, or soft tissue structure.

Patients with unresolved intraocular ferrous foreign bodies are at risk of significant eye injury. The single reported case of a patient who experienced a vitreous hemorrhage resulting in blindness occurred during an MR imaging procedure performed on a 0.35 T magnetic field system. The patient had a 2.0×3.5 mm intraocular metal fragment that became dislodged while the MR system was being excited[34].

Plain film radiography has been shown to be an acceptable tool for ruling out residual or existing metal fragments within the body. Research has shown that small intraocular metallic fragments as small as $0.1 \times 0.1 \times 0.1$ mm can be detected using plain film radiography[35]. Therefore, it is recommended that patients or individuals with a suspected intraocular foreign body undergo a plain film radiograph to rule out residual metallic fragments.

Claustrophobia and Anxiety

Patients who will undergo a MR imaging procedure may be at risk in experiencing psychological disturbances before, during, or after the procedure. These disturbances differ in severity and can delay or prohibit the imaging procedure. Claustrophobia and anxiety are considered to be conditions and not contraindications to MR imaging.

The sensations of apprehension, tension, worry, claustrophobia, anxiety, fear, and panic attacks have been suggested to originate from one or more factors involved in the MR procedure, including the following.

1. The confining dimensions of the interior of the MR system (e.g., the patient's face may be 80–250 mm from the inner portion of the MR system).
2. The prolonged duration of the examination.
3. The gradient-magnetic-field induced acoustic noise.
4. The temperature and humidity within the MR system.
5. The distress related to the restriction of movement.
6. The possible stress related to the administration of an MR imaging contrast agent[36].

It has been reported that dysphoric psychological reactions can affect as many as 65 percent of the MR imaging population. As many as 10–20 percent of that population will be unable to complete the examination because of their reactions, which include fear of dying, paresthesia, heart palpitations, nausea, dyspnea, faintness, and often vertigo.

The overall environment of the MR system can be changed to optimize the management of this population of patients. Open-air architecture designs are now available and have reduced the sense of apprehension for patients who would otherwise present with claustrophobia and anxiety. Manufacturers now design MR imaging systems that have air flowing through the bore or gantry of the system, lights have been installed to reduce the closed-in feeling, and MR imaging suites have built in windows and skylights to bring as much light into the room as possible.

Some authors suggest that it would be advisable to identify patients ahead of time who are at risk for presenting with claustrophobia and anxiety. Others feel that the suggestion of claustrophobia to the individual can incite an anxious response that might not otherwise occur. This author does not recommend asking a patient if they are claustrophobic during the screening procedure.

Patient anxiety can also be reduced by allowing properly screened relatives or friends to accompany the patient into the examination room. This familiarity can reduce patient anxiety.

Technologists are strongly advised to communicate frequently with the patient, especially those that present with anxiety, during the examination. The level of contact the technologist maintains with the patient can be a large factor in the patient's feeling of safety within the magnet.

Imaging centers have begun to use aromatherapy to reduce the feelings of claustrophobia and anxiety. Aromatherapy oils can be placed directly on the patient or on a tissue close to the patient's head and nose. Some imaging centers place the oils directly onto the coils, allowing the patient to smell the oils and be relaxed during the procedure. It has been suggested that the aromatherapy oils that work best to reduce anxiety are cucumber, green apples, lavender, and vanilla.

It may be necessary to sedate patients with severe anxiety, claustrophobia, or other psychological problems such as a panic attack. Special precautions should be taken before, during, and after the administration of sedatives to ensure that the patient continues to breathe during the imaging procedures. Physiological monitoring of the patient during sedation is strongly recommended. A study conduced by Avrahami in patients with panic attacks who were unable to undergo MR imaging, reported that treatment with intravenous diazepam caused the symptoms to disappear rapidly and permitted completion of the examination in every case[37].

Shellock and Kanal recommend the following techniques for managing patients with psychological problems.

1. Prepare and educate the patient concerning specific aspects of the MR examination (e.g., MR system dimensions, gradient noise, intercom system, etc.).

2. Allow an appropriately-screened relative or friend to remain with the patient during the MR procedure.

3. Maintain physical or verbal contact with the patient during the MR procedure.

4. Use MR-compatible headphones to provide music to the patient and to minimize gradient-magnetic field induced noise.

5. Use an MR-compatible television monitor to provide a visual distraction.

6. Place the patient in a prone position inside the MR system.

7. Place the patient feet first instead of head first into the MR system.

8. Use special mirrors or prism glasses.

9. Use a blindfold so that the patient is not aware of the close surroundings.

10. Use bright lights inside and at either end of the MR system.

11. Use a fan inside the MR system to provide adequate air movement.

12. Use relaxation techniques such as controlled breathing or mental imagery.

13. Use systematic desensitization.

14. Use medical hypnosis.

15. Use a sedative or other similar medication[2].

PHYSIOLOGIC MONITORING DURING THE MR PROCEDURE

Due to the widespread use of MR imaging contrast agents and sedatives, and the potential for adverse effects related to these drugs, it is advisable and recommended that MR-compatible monitoring devices be readily available in all MR imaging facilities. Physiological monitoring devices should be used if there is a possibility that the patient's physiological condition may change during the course of the examination.

Every MR facility should address with all staff and support staff, including custodial service, the procedures for responding to an emergency in the MR facility. This will avoid delays and confusion in the event that a patient is in respiratory or cardiac distress during the examination, or at risk of losing their life.

Fatalities and severe injuries have occurred in association with MR procedures, which may have been prevented with the proper use of monitoring equipment and devices[38]. Therefore, MR users must carefully consider the ethical and medicolegal ramifications of providing adequate patient care, which includes identifying those patient who require monitoring in the MR setting and a proper protocol to ensure their safety using appropriate devices[38].

In 1992, the Safety Committee of the Society for Magnetic Resonance Imaging published guidelines and recommendations regarding physiologic monitoring of patients during MR imaging procedures. This information indicates that all patients undergoing MR procedures should at the very least be visually and/or verbally monitored, and that patients who are sedated, anesthetized, or are unable to communicate should be physiologically monitored and supported by the appropriate means[21]. Recent guidelines issued by the Joint Commission on Accreditation of Healthcare Organizations indicate that all patients who receive sedatives or anesthetics require monitoring during the administration and recovery from these medications[39].

Potential Hazards with Physiologic Monitors

There are potential hazards with the use of physiologic monitoring devices. Monitoring devices must be checked for the possibility of ferromagnetic components and unshielded RF components. Ferromagnetic materials in the static magnetic field can be attracted and pulled towards the magnetic field. These devices, depending on their design, amount of ferromagnetic material, and length of time the devices are in the magnetic field, can act as "missiles" seriously injuring anyone who may be in their path.

Devices that have ferromagnetic components should be kept as far away from the static magnetic field as possible and should be fixed in position. The physiologic monitoring devices that use radiofrequencies must be RF shielded and RF filtered before using them in the MR scan room. Extraneous radiofrequencies can distort MR images when they are picked up by the transmit and/or receive coils.

Physiologic monitoring devices used to monitor MR patients include electrocardiographs, respiratory rate monitors, and pulse oximeters. A noninvasive heart rate and blood pressure monitor may also be used to obtain intermittent recordings of the patient's heart during the MR imaging procedure.

Commercially available, specially modified, pulse oximeters using hard wire cables have been used, with moderate success, to monitor sedated and anesthetized patients during the MR procedure. These devices work intermittently during the operation of the MR system because of interference from the time-varying (gradient) and oscillating (RF) magnetic fields. Of greater concern is the fact that many patients have been burned using pulse oximeters with hard wire cables during MR procedures, presumably as a result of excessive current being induced in inappropriately looped conductive cables attached to the patient probes in the pulse oximeter[40].

SAFETY CONSIDERATIONS FOR PATIENTS WITH BIOMEDICAL IMPLANTS, MATERIALS, AND DEVICES

Patients with biomedical implants, materials, and devices should be screened carefully prior to MR imaging to determine and rule out potential risks. The presence of biomedical implants in a patient exposed to an electromagnetic field risks injuring the patient, inducing electric currents in conductive materials, moving or dislodging the device if it is ferromagnetic, and causing image artifacts impairing the diagnostic usefulness of the images.

Most of the research gathered and assembled for the MR imaging community has been provided by Frank G. Shellock and Emanuel Kanal. The authors published a first and second edition of *Magnetic Resonance Bioeffects, Safety, and Patient Management*, that I have often referred to in this chapter. Shellock and Kanal had previously published papers as far back as 1991 on the policies, guidelines, and safety recommendations for MR imaging. Their numerous publications provide appendixes that list the implants, materials, and devices that have been tested for attraction and deflection forces during exposure to static magnetic fields[2]. They also provide words of advice and caution when using these lists. Manufacturers may change the composition of an implant or device without being required to report and seek approval from the FDA. Therefore, it is further suggested that MR facilities consider contacting the company that manufactured the device to determine if there are any alterations in the component.

I defer, respectfully, to their wisdom, efforts, time, and comprehensiveness in gathering and presenting the data for the benefit of the medical community. My compilation here is only a small reflection of the work previously compiled and published by Shellock and Kanal.

Temperature

The studies on temperature elevations on patients with metallic biomedical implants have been encouraging. Reports show that only minor changes in temperature have been measured during MR imaging. Therefore, heating is not considered a significant risk to a patient with biomedical implants or devices. There has never been a report of a patient being seriously injured as a result of excessive heat developing in a biomedical implant or device (with the exception of burns that have occurred as a result of induced current in electrically conductive devices)[2].

Studies have evaluated deflection forces, attraction forces, or other aspects of interaction between static and/or gradient magnetic fields and biomedical implants, materials, and devices with ferromagnetic properties. The investigations have demonstrated that MR procedures may be performed safely in patients if the metallic object is nonferrous or is only minimally attracted by the magnetic field[41].

Each implant, material, device, and object (particularly those made of unknown materials) should be evaluated using ex vivo techniques before performing an MR procedure in a patient[41]. This will provide immediate data on the potential adverse risks based on the amount of deflection or attraction and the degree of ferrous material present prior to exposing the patient to the magnetic field.

Aneurysm Clips

Test results have shown that the majority of aneurysm clips have ferromagnetic properties. They are considered to be a contraindication in a patient who is to undergo an MR procedure[42]. Because of the safety implications related to performing an MR procedure in a patient with an aneurysm clip, each aneurysm clip should be tested in vivo, either before implanting the device in a patient who may undergo MRI or before exposing a patient who has this implanted device to an MRI procedure. If, when tested, there is no movement or torque, the lot number, name brand, and mode of operation should be noted and recorded for future reference.

If an aneurysm clip is found to be ferromagnetic, it should not be used for surgery. It must not be implanted into a patient who may undergo MRI in the future. Gordon C. Johnson of the Center for Devices and Radiological Health, Food and Drug Administration, in response to the need for caution during MRI imaging of patients with aneurysm clips, has suggested the following:

> To minimize the possibility of inadvertently imaging a patient with a magnetically active metallic implant, implanting physicians should provide patients with information about the type and identity of their particular implants and suggest, where appropriate, that patients carry an alert card or wear a medical alert bracelet or necklace identifying them as having such an implant. In addition, physicians who order MR procedures should carefully screen patients and inform the MR imaging facility of any metallic implants the patient may have. MR imaging facilities should review their procedures to be sure that all patients are adequately screened for the presence of metallic implants before MR imaging[43].

Hemostatic Vascular Clips

None of the various hemostatic vascular clips that have been evaluated were attracted by static magnetic fields up to 1.5 T[41]. Most hemostatic vascular clips are made from nonferrous forms of stainless steel and tantalum. It is still recommended that these clips be tested ex vivo prior to the MR examination, although none evaluated have showed deflection.

Carotid Artery Vascular Clamps

Carotid artery vascular clamps were tested and showed deflection when exposed to a 1.5 T magnetic field. In general, vascular clamps are considered safe for patients undergoing MR procedures because they are only "slightly" ferromagnetic. However the Poppen–Blaylock carotid artery vascular clamp is considered a contraindication to MR procedures as it demonstrated substantial attractive force. With the exception of the Poppen–Blaylock clamp, patients with metallic carotid artery vascular clamps have been imaged by MR systems with static magnetic fields ranging up to 1.5 T without experiencing any discomfort or neurologic sequelae[44].

Vascular Access Ports

Vascular access ports and catheters are used to provide long-term administration of chemotherapeutic agents, antibodies, and analgesics. They are implanted in a subcutaneous pocket over the upper chest wall with the catheters leading to the jugular, subclavian, or cephalic vein.

Three of the implantable vascular access ports showed measurable attraction to the magnetic fields. However, it is felt that these forces are relatively minor, and these implants are considered safe to scan.

Some manufacturers are developing nonmetallic devices said to be "MRI compatible" and state that they will not cause image distortion, which is also a concern. Another concern that manufacturers are investigating is the degradation of the vascular port in long-term use. It has been shown that vascular access ports with metallic reservoirs may be more acceptable for long-term use than those with plastic reservoirs.

Surgical Clips

Most surgical clips become anchored by fibrous tissue and they are generally considered to be safe. It is recommended that the type of clip be evaluated ex vivo to determine ferrous content prior to scanning. Surgical clips can produce artifacts on the image.

Ocular Prostheses

According to *MR Procedures and Biomedical Objects*, by Shellock and Kanal, of the different ocular implants and devices tested, the Fatio eyelid spring, the retinal tack made from martensitic (i.e., ferromagnetic) stainless steel (Western European), the Troutman magnetic ocular implant, and the Unitech round wire eyelid spring were attracted by a 1.5 T static magnetic field[45].

A patient with the Fatio eyelid spring may experience some discomfort due to interaction with the static magnetic field, however it is not likely to injure the patient severely. Retinal tacks made from martensitic stainless steel and the Troutman magnetic ocular implant may injure a patient undergoing an MR procedure.

Heart Valves

The heart valves tested generally showed deflection in a 2.0 T static magnetic field. However, the amount of deflection is considered to be less than the normal displacement from the force exerted by the beating heart. Therefore, although patients with most valvular implants are considered safe for MR, because there are valves whose integrity are compromised, careful screening for valve type is advised[2].

Otologic Implants and Devices

Patients who have cochlear implants should not be exposed to strong magnetic fields. Cochlear implants made by 3 M/House, 3 M/Vienna, and Nucleus Mini 20-Channel showed definite deflection at 1.5 T. They are a definite contraindication to MR imaging.

Cochlear implants are made of ferromagnetic materials and are also activated by electronic and/or magnetic mechanisms. Some manufacturers of the implants issue warning cards for patients to carry.

Of the other otologic implants, only one, a McGee piston stapes prosthesis, showed deflection in the presence of the magnetic field. The manufacturer has recalled this type of otologic implant and patients who received these devices have been issued warnings to avoid MR procedures[46].

Penile Implants

It has been reported that two penile implants, OmniPhase and Duraphase, showed deflection when exposed to the magnetic field. Patients with any of these types of implants are advised not to undergo the MR imaging procedure to avoid potential discomfort. None of the others listed and tested are contraindicated.

Biopsy Needles and Devices

Commercially available biopsy needles and devices (i.e., guide wires, stylets, marking wires, biopsy guns, etc.) have been evaluated with respect to compatibility with MR procedures, not only to determine ferromagnetic qualities but to also characterize imaging artifacts[47]. The results of the study indicate that most of these were not useful for MR-guided biopsy procedures because of their ferromagnetic and artifactual qualities.

Recently biopsy needles and devices have been constructed of nonferrous materials for use with MR-guided biopsy procedures. Appendix I, in *MR Procedures and Biomedical Objects*, by Shellock and Kanal, provides an extensive list of recently developed and available nonferrous needles and devices.

Intravascular Coils, Filters, and Stents

The compatibility of the various types of intravascular coils, filters and stents has been tested. Several of them exhibited ferromagnetic properties. However, these devices typically become embedded in the vessel wall because of tissue in-growth within approximately 6 weeks from their implantation[48].

The displacement or dislodging of intravascular coils, filters and stents is therefore unlikely. Patients with these devices have undergone MR imaging procedures using magnetic fields that included 1.5 T without incident. It is further recommended that the MR imaging procedure should not be performed if there is suspicion that the device is not secured properly or is inappropriately aligned.

Orthopedic Implants and Devices

Orthopedic implants, in general, are non-ferrous and are safe for patients undergoing MR imaging procedures. Orthopedic implants can cause artifacts and image distortion, however, they are not likely to become dislodged during exposure to magnetic fields.

Only the Perfix screw was attracted to the magnetic field and in its application is firmly embedded in bone. It can cause a significant amount of image distortion if present during the MR imaging procedure.

Halo Vests and Devices

MR procedures should be performed only on patients with specially designed halo vests or cervical fixation devices made from nonferromagnetic and nonconductive materials that have little or no interaction with the electromagnetic fields generated by MR systems[49]. Halo vests can be constructed from either ferromagnetic or non-ferromagnetic materials, or a combination of both. There are commercially available devices that are composed of nonferromagnetic materials, however, they still run the theoretical risk of inducing an electric current in the ring portion of the halo device. Additionally, there is a potential for the patient's tissue to be involved in part of this current loop, so that there would be the concern of a possible burn or electrical injury to the patient[50].

There have been no reports of injury associated with imaging patients with halo vests during an MR imaging procedure, however there has been a report of an incident of "electrical arching" without injury.

It may be inadvisable to permit patients with certain cervical fixation devices to undergo MR procedures using a magnetization transfer contrast (MTC) pulse sequence because of the subtle motion or vibration of the halo rings that create the sensation of heating. Other comparable pulse sequences should also be avoided when performing MR imaging procedures on patients with halo vests.

Breast Implants and Breast Tissue Expanders

Breast tissue expanders and mammary implants are used for breast reconstruction following mastectomy, for the correction of breast and chest-wall deformities and underdevelopment, for tissue defect procedures, and for cosmetic augmentation[2]. These expanders have either an injection site or a remote injection dome that is used for needle placement for saline injections.

Two of the prostheses, the Becker and the Siltex have a choice of a standard injection dome or a microinjection dome. These ports contain 316 L stainless steel to guard against piercing the port with a needle. Several of the breast tissue expanders are constructed with magnetic ports to allow for a more accurate detection. Hence they are attracted to a magnetic field and can cause injury to the patient in an MR exam.

Image distortion is a concern with some of these devices. The amount of image distortion caused by the metallic ports should not interfere with the diagnostic quality of the image unless the device is in the scanned region of interest. It is recommended that patients with breast tissue expanders that have metallic components be identified so that the individual interpreting the MRI images is aware of the potential for artifacts.

Dental Implants and Materials

Most dental implants showed deflection when exposed to magnetic fields used by MR imaging procedures. The amount of deflection can be an annoyance due to magnetic susceptibility, especially with gradient echo pulse sequence.

Only dental implants that have a magnetically activated component present a potential problem for patients who may undergo an MR imaging procedure. Other dental implants and materials are held in place and are not at risk of becoming dislodged or moving during an MR imaging procedure.

CONCLUSION

Safety in MR imaging procedures is an important and still controversial issue. The MR community continues to provide data on the safety of exposing patients in various conditions to magnetic fields. A special thanks to Frank G. Shellock, Emanuel Kanal, and others for their research, time, and effort in gathering and bringing this data to the community.

There are other biomedical objects that have been tested and reported by Shellock and Kanal. They provide a well-organized and thorough report on the safety of these objects and I defer to their findings.

With education, careful planning, and thorough histories from patients the MR imaging environment can be a relatively safe environment for MRI staff, patients, and their families.

REFERENCES

1. Food and Drug Administration. Magnetic resonance diagnostic device: panel recommendation and report on petitions for MR reclassification. *Fed Reg* 53:7575–7579, 1988.
2. Shellock FG, Kanal E. *Magnetic Resonance Bioeffects, Safety, and Patient Management*, 2nd ed. Philadelphia: Lippincott-Raven Publishers, 1996.
3. Bushong SC. *Magnetic Resonance Imaging, Physical and Biological Principles*, 2nd ed. St. Louis: Mosby, 1996.
4. Weiss M, Herrick R, Tabor K, Contant C, Plishker G. Bioeffects of high magnetic fields: a study using a simple animal model. *Magn Reson Imaging* 10:689–694, 1992.
5. Brody A, Sorete M, Gooding C, et al. Induced alignment of flowing sickle erythrocytes in a magnetic field: a preliminary report. *Invest Radiol* 20:560–566, 1985.

6. Murayama M. Orientation of sickled erythrocytes in a magnetic field. *Nature* 206:420–422, 1965.
7. Redington R, Dumoulin C, Schenck J, et al. MR imaging and bioeffects on a whole body 4.0 Tesla imaging system. In: *Book of Abstracts, Society of Magnetic Resonance in Medicine.* Berkeley, CA: Society of Magnetic Resonance in Medicine, Vol. 1, p. 4, 1988.
8. Dimick RN, Hedlund LW, Herfkens RJ, Fram EK, Utz J. Optimizing electrocardiographic electrode placement for cardiac-gated magnetic resonance imaging. *Invest Radiol* 22:17–22, 1987.
9. Shellock F, Schaefer D, Crues J. Exposure to 1.5 T static magnetic fields does not alter body and skin temperatures in man. *Magn Reson Med* 11:371–375, 1989.
10. Barlow H, Kohn H, Walsh E. Visual sensations aroused by magnetic fields. *Am J Physiol* 148:372–375, 1947.
11. Food and Drug Administration. Guidance for content and review of a magnetic resonance diagnostic device 510(k) application. *Fed Reg*, 1988.
12. Tenforde T, Budinger T. Biological effects and physical safety aspects of NMR imaging and in vivo spectroscopy. In: Thomas S, Dixon R, eds. *NMR in Medicine: Instrumentation and Clinical Applications.* Medical Monograph No. 14. New York: American Association of Physicists in Medicine, 493–548, 1986.
13. Guidance update for d*B*/d*t* for the "guidance for content and review of a magnetic resonance diagnostic device 510(k) application" document. Office of Device Evaluation/Center for Devices and Radiological Health. Robert A. Phillips, Computed Imaging Devices Branch. Rockville, MD, 11 October 1995.
14. Budinger T. Nuclear magnetic resonance (NMR) in vivo studies: known thresholds for health effects. *J Comput Assist Tomogr* 5:800–811, 1981.
15. Lovsund P, Nillson S, Reuter T, Oberg P. Magnetophosphenes: a quantitative analysis of thresholds. *Med Biol Eng Comput* 18:326–334, 1980.
16. Budinger T, Fisher H, et al. Physiologic effects of fast oscillating magnetic field gradients. *J Comput Assist Tomogr* 15:909–914, 1991.
17. Erhardt J, Lin CS, Magnotta V, Fisher D, Yuh W. Neural stimulation in a whole body echo-planar imaging system. In: *Book of Abstracts, Society of Magnetic Resonance in Medicine.* Berkeley, CA: Society of Magnetic Resonance in Medicine, vol. 3, 1372, 1993.
18. Gordon CJ. Thermal physiology. In: *Biological Effects of Radiofrequency Radiation* EPA-600/8-83-026A, 4-1 to 4-28, 1984.
19. Shellock FG, Kanal E. SMRI Report. Policies, guidelines and recommendations for MR imaging safety and patient management. Questionnaire for screening patients befor MR procedures. *J Magn Reson Imaging* 4:749–751, 1994.
20. Perrson BRR, Stahlberg F. *Health and Safety of Clinical NMR Examinations.* Boca Raton, FL: CRC, 1989.
21. Kanal E, Shellock FG. Policies, guidelines and recommendations for MR imaging safety and patient management. *J Magn Reson Imaging* 2:247–248, 1992.
22. Shellock, FG, Kanal E. SMRI Report. Policies, guidelines and recommendations for MR imaging safety and patient management. *J Magn Reson Imaging* 1:97–101, 1991.
23. Smith F. The potential use of nuclear magnetic resonance imaging in pregnancy. *J Perinat Med* 13:265–276, 1985.
24. Kanal E, Gillen J, Evans J, Savitz D, Shellock FG. Survey of reproductive health among female MR workers. *Radiology* 187:395–399, 1993.
25. Kanal E, Shellock FG. *Safety Manual on Magnetic Resonance Imaging Contrast Agents.* New York: Lippincott-Raven Healthcare, 21–22, 1996.
26. Hurwitz R, Lane SR, Bell RA, Brant-Zawadzki MN. Acoustic analysis of gradient-coil noise in MR imaging. *Radiology* 173:545–548, 1989.
27. Goldman AM, Gossman WE, Friedlander PC. Reduction of sound levels with antinoise in MRI imaging. *Radiology* 173:549–550, 1989.
28. Oksendal A, Hals P. Biodistribution and toxicity of MR imaging contrast media. *J Magn Reson Imaging* 3:157–165, 1993.
29. Kanal E, Applegate G, Gillen C. Review of adverse reactions, including anaphylaxis, in 5260 cases receiving gadolinium-DPTA by bolus injection. *Radiology* 177(P):159, 1990.
30. American College of Radiology. *Manual on Iodinated Contrast Media.* American College of Radiology, 1991.
31. Niendorf H, Dinger J, Haustien J, Cornelius I, Alhassan A, Clauss W. Tolerance data of GD-DTPA: a review. *Eur J Radiol* 13:15–20, 1991.
32. Cacheris W, Quay S, Rocklage S. The relationship between thermodynamics and the toxicity of gadolinium complexes. *Magn Reson Imaging* 8:467–481, 1990.
33. Brody A, Sorette M, Gooding C, et al. Induced alignment of flowing sickle erythrocytes in a magnetic field. *Invest Radiol* 20:560–566, 1985.
34. Kelly WM, Pagle PG, Pearson A, San Diego AG, Soloman MA. Ferromagnetism of intraocular foreign body causes unilateral blindness after MR study. *Am J Neuroradiol* 7:243–245, 1986.
35. Mani RL. In search of an effective screening system for intraocular metallic foreign bodies prior to MR – an important issue of patient safety. *Am J Neuroradiol* 9:1032, 1988.
36. Melendez C, McCrank E. Anxiety-related reactions associated with magnetic resonance imaging examinations. *JAMA* 270:745–747, 1993.
37. Avrahami E. Panic attacks during MR imaging: treatment with IV diazepam. *Am J Neuroradiol* 11:833–835, 1990.

38. Kanal E, Shellock FG. Patient monitoring during clinical MR imaging. *Radiology* 185:623–629, 1992.

39. Joint Commission of Accreditation of Healthcare Organizations. *Accreditation Manual for Hospitals.* 1993.

40. Kanal E, Shellock FG. Burns associated with clinical MR examinations. *Radiology* 175:585, 1990.

41. Shellock FG, Crues JV. High-field strength MR imaging and metallic bioimplants an in vitro evaluation of deflection forces and temperature changes induced in large prostheses. *Radiology* 165(P):150, 1987.

42. Becker RL, Norfray JF, Teitelbaum GP, et al. MR imaging in patients with intracranial aneurysm clips. *Am J Roentgenol* 9:885–889, 1988.

43. Johnson GC. Need for caution during MR imaging of patients with aneurysm clips. *Radiology* 188:287, 1993.

44. Teitelbaum GP. Metallic ballistic fragments: MR imaging safety and artifacts. *Radiology* 175:855–859, 1990.

45. Shellock FG, Morisoli S, Kanal E. MR procedures and biomedical implants, materials, and devices: 1993 update. *Radiology* 189:587–599, 1993.

46. Applebaum EL, Valvassoori GE. Effects of magnetic resonance imaging fields on stapedectomy prosthesis. *Arch Orolaryngol* 11:820–821, 1985.

47. Shellock FG, Shellock VJ. Additional information pertaining to the MR-compatibility of biopsy needles and devices. *J Magn Reson Imaging* 6:441, 1996.

48. Teitelbaum GP, Bradley WG, Klein BD. MR imaging artifacts, ferromagnetism, and magnetic torque of intravascular filters, stents, and coils. *Radiology* 166:657–664, 1988.

49. Shellock FG, Swengros-Curtis J. MR imaging and biomedical implants, materials, and devices: an updated review. *Radiology* 180:541–550, 1991.

50. Shellcok FG, Slimp G. Halo vest for cervical spine fixation during MR imaging. *Am J Roentgenol* 154:631–632, 1990.

CHAPTER 17

MR Facility Organization and Management

Edie E. Cox

INTRODUCTION

This chapter is written primarily for the technologist who aspires to manage, direct, or own an imaging facility. For those who are uncertain as to what role if any, they intend to play in management, there is still much practical information herein. As a technologist, even if you are not managing your facility's staff, you are always managing patients, and the same principles apply. Take pride in and enjoy any role you play in your facility's successful operation.

INTELLIGENT STAFFING PATTERNS

Your imaging facility is not successful (or unsuccessful) by itself. It is only the people who work there and the combination of their talents/ efforts which make your facility successful. Choosing the right individual for a specific position is difficult enough, but assembling a team whose talents complement each other is no less than an art form. The crux of choosing such a team is developing the appropriate game plan or pattern within which each staff member will peform his/ her function. The objective of this game plan is to use combinations of staff members whose individual talents can be used to the company's best advantage. It is from this perspective that intelligent staffing patterns are formulated.

With this goal in mind, imagine your imaging center at its best – operating smoothly, providing reliable and timely results to its referring physicians, offering a high level of care and professionalism to its patients, and being a source of pride and professional gratification to its staff members. Let's analyze the scene. Who would be working at your imaging center? A receptionist, a technologist, a transcriptionist, a radiologist, and possibly a manager or an accountant. How many of each? Are there other positions to fill?

Task Identification

Start your analysis by identifying all the tasks which need to be performed on a daily basis for your center to operate at its best. Here is a sample list of tasks.

- Patient scheduling.
- Patient reception.
- Scanning patients.
- Film interpretation.
- Transcription.
- Notifying physicians.
- Insurance confirmation.
- Billing and collections.
- Accounting.
- Patient transportation.
- Marketing.
- Management.
- Filing.
- Prescan confirmation of patients.
- Cleaning.
- Patient interview and history taking.

The various tasks are virtually endless and are somewhat site-specific in nature. Be as detailed as possible when assembling your list. After having assembled such a list, combine tasks that are compatible. Insurance confirmation, prescan confirmation of patients, and patient reception are compatible tasks. For example, it makes sense that after a physician refers a patient, one person may ascertain insurance coverage, contact the patient, confirm the appointment time, rule out any contraindications, and determine transportation needs. When speaking to the patient, he/she can also discuss what portion of the charges the insurance company will pay and whether the patient is willing and able to pay the balance and on what terms. When the patient does arrive for the appointment, reception is much more time-efficient because both parties know in advance the patient's particular situation.

Continue combining tasks until you feel you have arrived at the most logical combinations, with regard to your facility's needs. You are actually constructing skeleton job descriptions with which you can now more easily recognize job skills individuals must possess to fill specific positions. Before beginning the actual interview process, consider a few more issues.

What imaging modalities does your facility offer? During what hours does your market require access to each of these modalities? Remember, the idea is to construct staffing patterns and operating policies to allow your center to function at its best and its fullest potential. Compare your skeleton job descriptions with your optimal hours of operation. What portion of hours of operation should a particular position fill? Examine each position and choose work schedules that facilitate completing tasks assigned to each position within a given time. For instance, it's impractical for the person who confirms insurance to work evening hours, during which insurance companies don't operate. However, for the person who performs collections, evening hours may be the most practical, in that he can reach patients at home in the evenings. In this manner, evaluate each of the skeleton job descriptions you've formulated. Once this is accomplished, you'll know who you want, what skills they must possess, and what shift they must be available to work. This is the first half of the equation in formulating intelligent staffing patterns.

Computing Packages

The second half of the staffing equation has more to do with what your facility has to offer its employees than what they have to offer the facility. Pay, benefits, bonus programs, and continuing education opportunities are all aspects of a plan which will attract and keep quality people. Here is a list of suggestions to consider when formulating your compensation packages.

Pay Pay good employees more than they can get elsewhere, and they won't go elsewhere. Turnover is much more costly than it would first appear.

Raises Give raises on the basis of performance, not according to a calendar. Reward the behavior you desire as soon as possible. Delayed rewards don't have the impact of timely ones.

Bonuses Create a bonus system based on your company's financial performance. Understand that a company's performance is the result of income minus expenses. Employees are only one of a company's expenses, but collectively they represent a very large portion. Bonuses should encourage employees to contribute to their company's performance by being as productive as possible, minimizing the need for more employees. If the bonus plan is structured such that the bonus "pot" is divided up among employees, the fewer employees there are, the greater their individual portions of the pot. Likewise, it is fairer to make the bonus plan contingent upon the number of hours an employee works. Full-time employees have a greater influence on company performance and should be rewarded commensurately.

Vacation Time Offer the option to take money instead of time.

Sick Time Offer little or no *paid* sick time. Pay only for performance.

Opportunity for Promotion Within the Company Hire from within when possible.

Continuing Education Evaluate conventions, seminars, and other opportunities to provide continuing education. Attempt to enhance staff members' knowledge by hand-picking the most beneficial seminars and paying staff to attend.

Company Meetings Pay staff members to attend; pay overtime, if necessary. Don't expect them to "donate" their valuable time for the company's benefit.

Make company meetings a forum for interaction and participation. Because staff members deal with the center's challenges on a daily basis, they have the best understanding of them. Reward productive ideas.

Turnover Successful companies are successful only because they are made up of good people. Good people will not stay for long in a place where they are undervalued. Turnover is costly. Each staff member develops a rapport with staff members from referring physicians' offices. They accumulate small experiences and tidbits of information over time that are virtually unteachable to their successors, no matter how good a training program your facility provides. In addition, during the time a new staff member is being trained, competency and efficiency are reduced by more than just the one staff member missing. Because the staff member is occupied with training, his/her usual duties are put on hold, or at least slowed down a great deal. Turnover is expensive. Costs include not only time and money, but opportunity costs due to lost rapport and intimacy with referring physicians and their staff. Devise your compensation packages to reward performance and you will attract, and most importantly, keep good people.

Okay, you've thoroughly pondered compensation packages. It's time to give some thought to a few suggestions about interviewing, hiring, and firing.

Your Ad Don't bait your hook with squid if you intend to catch mullet. Run an ad to appeal to the person you want to hire. State the hours, the rate of pay, benefits, general geographic location of your facility, a brief synopsis of the job itself, and an address to mail resumes. An ad like this will be expensive, but so is your time. You don't need to waste any of it interviewing people who can't work the evening shift, if it's the one you're trying to fill. Something *not* to state in your ad, your facility's name and address. No kidding. Your favorite referring physician's key employee will respond to your ad, knowing he/she will be recognized for the outstanding employee he/she is. If you do hire this person, you can bet that your facility will no longer be that referring physician's favorite imaging center. If you don't hire this person, this person is going to wonder why he/she isn't good enough to work at your facility.

** SAMPLE FORM **

CONTRAINDICATIONS CHECKLIST:	YES	NO
1. IMPLANTED ELECTRONIC DEVICES?	_____	_____
2. INTRACRANIAL SURGICAL CLIPS?	_____	_____
3. INTRACRANIAL METALLIC OBJECTS?	_____	_____
4. INTRAORBITAL METALLIC OBJECTS?	_____	_____
5. SHRAPNEL?	_____	_____
6. COCHLEAR IMPLANT?	_____	_____
7. PACEMAKER?	_____	_____
8. DORSAL COLUMN STIMULATOR?	_____	_____
9. PREGNANT?	_____	_____
10. EPICARDIAL PACER WIRES?	_____	_____
11. INFERIOR VENA CAVA UMBRELLA?	_____	_____
12. OTHER POSSIBLE CONTRAINDICATION?	_____	_____

Figure 17-2.   Contraindications checklist.

prefers, it's a nice idea to follow up by sending flowers or some other small gift for having inconvenienced him/her.

Unfortunately, the size of your facility, and the patient volume may dictate just how far you can reasonably go with regard to service. For many hospital facilities, a simple act, such as sending flowers, may be impossible to administrate. Just the same, it is wise to be as service-oriented as your situation allows. At the very least, acknowledge the patient has been inconvenienced and offer a sincere apology. Try to accommodate patient needs as much as possible and as often as possible.

Patient impressions of your facility are all important. Therefore, it is paramount that any areas which patients will occupy are clean and neat. Check there are no dirty gowns in the rest rooms and changing areas; and make sure the tech areas and scan room appear clean and organized.

Practice consideration for the patient's privacy by minimizing the number of people who interact with the patient once he/she is undressed and gowned for the exam. If at all possible, it is most courteous to perform any necessary introductions while the patient is still clothed, and thus on an equal footing.

** SAMPLE FORM **

PATIENT INFORMATION

Name: _____ Date of Birth: _____

Home Address:_____

 City/State:_____ Zip:_____

Employer: _____

Employer's Address: _____

Spouse's Name: _____ Spouse's Work Phone: _____

Closest Relative Not Living With You:

_____ Phone: _____

Are you covered under any secondary insurance benefits? ____ yes ____ no
(i.e. Medicare, supplemental, etc.)

 If "yes," please list company and policy number, if known:

_____

Whom May We Thank For Referring You? _____

Figure 17-3.   Patient information form.

During the exam, be attentive to the patient's needs, fears, and concerns. Explain the procedure, how long it will take, and what the patient will hear, see, and feel. Discuss when and from whom the patient will receive the results of his/her exam. Offer to answer any questions the patient may ask that are within your scope of expertise, but *never, never* diagnose. No matter how good we become at recognizing pathology, it is beyond our role as technologists to offer a patient anything that remotely resembles a diagnosis. To do so is to interfere with the patient–doctor relationship already established.

** SAMPLE FORM **

CONSENT FORM

In consideration of services rendered by ___XYZ IMAGING CENTER___ , I agree to pay all charges incurred on the account of the patient specified below and accept full responsibility for payment of services performed by XYZ IMAGING CENTER. I also understand that ___XYZ IMAGING CENTER___ will file my insurance claim as a courtesy to me, and that any amounts not covered by my insurance will be paid by me.

If this is a Workmen's Compensation claim, I understand that the above paragraph does not apply to me, unless it is determined that my injury is not work-related.

I authorize payment of medical benefits in the amount of $_____ to _XYZ IMAGING CENTER__ .

I authorize ___XYZ IMAGING CENTER__ to release any and all information requested by any insurance company billed, in order to complete my insurance claim. I authorize and direct the insurance company to pay _XYZ IMAGING CENTER__ directly, any and all benefits up to the amount of my bill.

I authorize any other medical providers/facilities to release my medical records to _XYZ IMAGING CENTER__ .

I authorize _XYZ IMAGING CENTER_ , to sign my name to any cheque written in both our names, where such cheque is in payment for its services.

I understand that there may or may not be a financial relationship between _XYZ IMAGING CENTER__ and the health care provider who referred me. Further, I understand that I have the right to go to the imaging center of my choice and that upon request, ___XYZ IMAGING CENTER___ will provide me a list of alternative centers.

I CERTIFY THAT I HAVE READ AND UNDERSTAND EACH PARAGRAPH OF THE ABOVE CONSENT FORM.

_____
Patient

_____
Parent or Guarantor

_____
Date

Figure 17-4.   Consent form.

Once the exam has been completed, escort the patient back to the rest room/changing area. Once he/she has changed, have someone escort the patient out of your facility. Offer once again to answer any questions the patient may have and by all means, thank him/her for coming to your facility.

A tool you can employ to gauge how well your facility is answering patient needs is a patient comment card [Figure 17-5]. Patient comment cards are also great marketing tools when sent to referring physicians, as patient endorsements.

Postexam Strategies

A few patient management issues come into play after the exam. They are the timely delivery of results and/or films to the patient's referring physician, the return of any outside films to the appropriate destination, and billing and collections.

It is good medical practice to deliver results as quickly as possible. Therefore, if possible at your facility, arrange for reports to be faxed or phoned to the offices of referring physicians as soon as they are available. In the best of circumstances, you might actually train the radiologist to phone referring physicians with results. It is a great way for the radiologist and the referring physician to build a rapport.

Develop a method by which outside films are sent to a destination designated by the patient or referring physician. Don't underestimate the tendency for outside films to disappear into the ether! I suggest that receipt of outside films should be documented on the patient's film jacket or on a ledger of some sort. If feasible, record the number of films received, the date of receipt, what kind of films they are (X-ray, CT, previous MRI), where they're from, and where they should be sent. From this point on, the outside films should stay with the patient's jacket until they have been used for comparison and results have been delivered to the referring physician. When the patient's study has been completed and is ready to be stored, the outside films should be removed from the patient's jacket and sent via mail or delivery service to the previously designated destination. This also should be documented on the patient's jacket or ledger book, that is, which outside films went to which destinations, by what methods, and on what dates.

It is good practice not to loan out original films. You will save your facility much time and aggravation involved in hunting down originals for your top referring physician after someone else has checked them out. Offer copies or, better still, offer duplicate originals. Many facilities are equipped with a laser imager or similar technology capable of duplicating multiple sets of originals. Duplicate originals are exactly the same quality as originals and are therefore preferred over copies. Of course, there is a catch to producing duplicate originals. Producing duplicate originals necessitates knowing in advance when duplicates are needed, and how many will be needed.

Duplicates made from a copy machine are *always* poorer in image quality than the originals. In addition, a nonradiologist physician who received copies may not realize they are copies and make incorrect assumptions about the quality of the study.

The last postexam interaction you or someone from your facility will have with the patient is billing/collections. Typically, the patient will be left with some portion of the fee to pay out of pocket. Optimally, this amount is collected at the time of service. Unfortunately, the out of pocket amount can be quite large and because of this, only a portion of it may be collected at time of service. Terms of payment for the balance should be arranged with the patient during the initial prescan phone conversation or at some time *prior* to the patient receiving service. Accommodating the patient's financial needs increases the likelihood of getting paid. Therefore, if possible, make it easy for the patient by providing him/her with a payment schedule and a supply of self-addressed, stamped envelopes, or by billing

** SAMPLE PATIENT COMMENT CARD **

YOUR COMMENTS COUNT

Thank you for choosing _____ Imaging Center for your exam! We work very hard to make your experience with us as enjoyable as possible. Your feelings are important to us, so we offer this comment card as an opportunity to gain your input.

1. How was our front office staff?
   □ Friendly □ Professional □ Unfriendly □ Rude

2. Were we   □ on time for your exam?
              □ late for your exam?

3. If we were late, did you feel that the amount of time you waited was excessive? □ Yes □ No

4. How was our technical staff?
   □ Friendly □ Professional □ Unfriendly □ Rude

5. Was the exam explained to your satisfaction? □ Yes □ No

6. Were you made as comfortable as possible during your exam?
   □ Yes □ No - What could have improved your comfort?

   _____

7. Is our atmosphere as comfortable and as private as you would like it to be? □ Yes □ No - What didn't you like?

   _____

8. If you used our courtesy van was our driver friendly and professional? □ Yes □ No

9. How would you rate your overall visit with us?
   □ Excellent □ Good □ Fair □ Poor

10. Would you recommend us to others? □ Yes □ No

11. Who is the physician that referred you to us?

12. Comments: _____

   _____
   _____
   _____
   _____
   _____

_____
Your Name (*Optional*)   Date of Exam

Figure 17-5. Patient comment card.

the patient monthly and enclosing the same. Unfortunately, your facility will experience a certain number of patients who agree to terms of payment and don't follow through. This is common in any business, but is a particularly sensitive issue in medicine. Many people feel that medical care is a right and that they are entitled to it, whether they are able to pay for it or not. Because of the sensitivity of this issue, the task of collections requires a fair amount of tact and diplomacy. You must always bear in mind that patients can and will speak with their referring physicians about their experiences with your facility, particularly if the experience was very very good or very very bad. You must decide on a case-by-case basis how hard you are willing to push a patient to pay, bearing in mind the effect it will have on the referring physician or others he/she might tell. What portion of your receivables are you willing to walk away from to preserve goodwill?

The goals to be accomplished by practicing effective patient management are twofold. First, strive to practice a high degree of care and professionalism. Your patients deserve no less, and your facility will achieve a reputation for treating patients with compassion, diplomacy, and professionalism. Second, strive to practice in an efficient manner. The more efficiently you can work, the more favorably affected is the bottom line, and thus your facility's financial success.

STAFF CONTINUING EDUCATION

Budgeting for continuing education is vital to any sound management game plan. Professional personnel, such as technologists, radiologists, and nurses, are required to obtain continuing education to maintain their license. Requirements vary from state to state for each license, therefore it is prudent to ascertain your state's requirements.

Continuing education should be a part of your facility's budget, not only for professionally licensed personnel, but for *everyone*. No matter how well your facility's staff performs, there will always be room for improvement. Continuing education is a source of new ideas and concepts, without which any improvement is impossible. Conventions, seminars, trade shows, and manufacturers' courses generally offer classes approved by your state's licensure department for continuing education credit. Though not always approved for continuing education credit, journal subscriptions are great sources of new ideas and techniques for technologists and radiologists.

Additionally, there are several in-house practices your facility can adopt to continually educate technologists. If possible, when technologists find themselves with spare time, they should observe and ask questions while the radiologist interprets films. Another educationally productive use of technologists' spare time is to experiment with new scanning sequences. Keep a list of untried sequences to run. Restrict your experimental efforts to sequences which improve the diagnostic value of a scan or sequences which save time (without compromising diagnosticity), so as to improve throughput. Technologists may also engage in a case review program. After cases have been interpreted, technologists should review both the films and the report, and follow up by questioning the radiologist any time there is something present that the technologist doesn't understand. This serves two purposes. Not only is this a good method for technologists to become proficient at recognizing pathology, it also serves to double-check the accuracy of the interpretation. No matter how good, radiologists are only human. The number of misreads that occur is inversely proportional to the number of eyeballs that look at a film. The radiologist will appreciate you for *diplomatically* pointing out a possible error in interpretation or dictation.

Another educationally productive in-house tool is technologist/radiologist meetings. These meetings are a great forum in which to do the following.

Discuss interesting cases
Discuss changes or improvements in technique

Review normal anatomy versus abnormal anatomy or variants

Discuss equipment capabilities and limitations

These meetings will also enhance technologist/radiologist rapport and communication.

The entire staff of your facility will also benefit greatly by attending customer service seminars at least once per year. Many times we adopt methods or procedures that are convenient for us, but are not terribly service-oriented and sometimes downright obstructive, from our customer's (patients and referring physicians) point of view. Customer service seminars are excellent sources of ideas with which to fine tune our operating policies and phone interactions with patients, referring physicians, and insurance adjusters.

A wise manager will budget for continuing education. When staff members are asked to pay for continuing education themselves, management then loses control of the quality and quantity of the continuing education staff members receive. Well-chosen continuing education is not an expense, it is an investment in performance.

TECHNOLOGIST INDEPENDENCE

Technologist independence is a goal every facility should strive to achieve. It is particularly important for those facilities which operate in the absence of a radiologist. Technologist independence is the product of two factors, education and advance planning.

Education

Although we've explored the topic of education in the previous section, education is such an important issue, it merits a few more thoughts. An educated technologist easily recognizes pathology and is able to make more intuitive judgments about how to proceed upon discovering the pathology. An educated technologist possesses the skills required to work with and defuse anxious or angry patients. An educated technologist is able to troubleshoot equipment problems *prior* to calling an engineer; this saves both money and time. An educated technologist is a valuable asset to any imaging facility and is able to command top dollar for his/her skills.

Advance Planning

Advance planning is the second factor contributing to technologist independence. Much time, money, and anxiety can be saved by anticipating events. Start by identifying events which occur with some frequency and which require alternative actions. Your list should include the following, plus any situations that are particular to your facility.

The technologist discovers pathology; this is either anticipated or unanticipated.

The patient requires sedation; this is either anticipated or unanticipated.

The patient requires contrast; this is either anticipated or unanticipated.

The patient is difficult or uncooperative; the patient either completes the exam or doesn't complete the exam.

A medical emergency occurs.

Let's continue by evaluating each event separately and exploring various options. Assume that at your facility the radiologist is available, at best, infrequently for consultation.

The Technologist Discovers Pathology

As a technologist, when you find pathology it is your responsibility and your obligation to take the appropriate course of action. A plan can be devised, in advance, with an appropriate course of action, that is in accordance with a patient's best interest. Many times you will discover pathology that was anticipated via the referring physician's clinical exam and resultant prescan diagnosis. If you have a protocol manual, this situation is best handled cookbook style, according to protocol. Details to address in such a manual might include standard and alternative scan sequences, positioning tips, reconstruction parameters, and filming parameters. Seek the radiologist's help in devising a protocol manual. It is the most practical advance planning tool you'll ever have.

Not quite as frequently you'll discover pathology which was not anticipated via your referring physician's diagnosis. If the radiologist is available for consultation, then do so. This is your best option. If the radiologist is not on site for immediate consultation, evaluate to the best of your ability, how serious the situation is. If the situation appears to be life-threatening, now or any time before the patient is to return to his/her referring physician, continue scanning and attempt to reach the radiologist. If the radiologist is unavailable, attempt to reach the patient's referring physician. Explain your concerns and ask how to proceed. Be as delicate and as diplomatic as possible with the patient. Do not diagnose, but express to the patient the urgency of the situation and explain how he/she should proceed, according to the orders received from the radiologist or the patient's referring physician.

If the situation does not appear to be life-threatening, evaluate to the best of your ability whether to take extra images. If the pathology is best evaluated by another modality and is well visualized on more than two sequences of your standard protocol, there is no need to waste the patient's time or your time acquiring additional views. If this is not the case, determine what extra views would be the most advantageous. Depending on the location and extent of the pathology, you may elect to perform one or two extra sequences in a different plane or with a different pulse sequence. If you feel that you need more than two supplementary views to adequately evaluate the pathology, it may be prudent to seek the radiologist's opinion before continuing. The patient might be better served

by having a second MRI study to specifically evaluate this newly discovered pathology. This is a call only the radiologist and the patient's referring physician are qualified to make. Complete the originally requested exam (you may still find the originally anticipated pathology) and discharge the patient, as usual.

If, indeed, you do elect to perform extra views, assess the amount of time you'll need to do so. If you have enough time to complete them and the patient is willing and able, perform the extra views, in addition to standard protocol. If there is no time available or the patient is unwilling or unable to complete extra views then and there, schedule the patient at his/her earliest convenience to return. Make certain to inform the referring physician's office of these events and how soon they can expect results. When you have the opportunity, find out the radiologist's choice of sequences for extra views.

The Patient Requires Sedation

The next event to plan for in advance is patient sedation. If it is known in advance that the patient is anxious, claustrophobic, or in pain, arrange for the referring physician to prescribe an appropriate medication. Ask the patient to bring it with him/her to the appointment, and schedule the patient's appointment so there is time for the medication to take effect once administered. It is prudent to arrange transportation for patients who will be arriving or leaving under the influence of medication. If it is not possible to arrange transportation, encourage the patient to bring a companion who can drive, once the patient is medicated. If no companion is available, make arrangements for the patient to stay at your facility until he/she can safely drive home. Additionally, if a physician or other appropriately licensed medical personnel will not be available to administer the medication, you should make certain it is prescribed in a form the patient can self-administer, according to his/her physician's instructions.

Unfortunately, many patients don't anticipate being as fearful, claustrophobic, or uncomfortable as they sometimes become before completing (or sometimes before even beginning) their MRI exam. It is not conservative practice, and in most cases, not legal for technologists to administer any medications, other than radionuclides or contrast agents for imaging purposes. Therefore, it is optimal and advisable to have available (or available on short notice) a medical professional who is appropriately licensed to prescribe, dispense, and administer medications. In most states, registered nurses are licensed to dispense and/or administer medications, although they cannot generally prescribe them. For many facilities, having a registered nurse available to dispense and administer sedation is a sufficient remedy for the sedation dilemma. In most cases, the necessary prescription can be obtained by phone from the referring physician or the radiologist. This is significantly less expensive than having a physician on staff full-time. However, dispensing and administering sedation in the absence of a physician may expose your facility to significant liability. Personnel in charge of risk management should be consulted before any such policy is adopted as protocol.

The Patient Requires Contrast

Fortunately, most times you will have the luxury of knowing in advance that a patient requires contrast. Realistically, you cannot expect referring physicians to understand when contrast is and isn't indicated. Indications for contrast should be conspicuously listed for personnel who schedule patients. Scheduling personnel should be instructed to consult the radiologist or a technologist upon receipt of any unfamiliar diagnoses or upon any unusual requests for contrast.

If you discover unanticipated pathology which requires contrast, you should attempt to consult the radiologist. If the radiologist is not present, you should determine, to the best of your ability, how serious the situation is. As with noncontrast extra views, if the situation warrants, you should contact the radiologist or referring physician and ask for his direction. Again, be as diplomatic as possible with the patient; don't diagnose but explain the situation is urgent and requires prompt action.

If the pathology is not life-threatening, evaluate to the best of your ability, what contrast views are needed and how much time it will take to complete contrast views. If there is time available and the patient is willing and able to complete contrast views, contact the radiologist. Optimally, the radiologist is available and can be present during contrast administration and for a prudent length of time postadministration. If a radiologist is not available, it is wise to arrange for other medical personnel with licensure in advanced life support procedures to be present during and after contrast administration. This, too, might pose a higher risk of liability were a patient to experience a reaction to the contrast material. Risk management personnel may elect not to allow administration of contrast in the absence of a radiologist, if it is determined that the risk is too great or liability too costly. Even though the rate of reaction to gadolinium MRI contrast materials is low in both the number of occurrences and degree of severity, today's society is litigious and consequently liability is a very serious issue.

If a radiologist or other appropriate medical personnel is available, you should continue scanning, but wait until he/she is physically present to administer contrast and continue with contrast views. If a radiologist/other qualified medical personnel is not available, complete the requested exam and schedule the patient for postcontrast views. Notify the referring physician's office and let them know how soon they can expect results. Again, when you have the opportunity, confirm with the radiologist that the postcontrast sequences you've chosen are satisfactory.

The Patient is Difficult or Uncooperative

Fear and anxiety can manifest themselves in behaviors ranging from hysterical crying to belligerence. Each individual copes with stress differently. Technologists need to learn that what may seem like a personal attack is really only an expression of fear and anxiety. It is much more advantageous (and professional) to learn how to defuse this behavior, rather than to return it with hostility, which only adds fuel to the fire. Here are some techniques and suggestions for defusing difficult or uncooperative behavior.

- *Never argue* or assume a confrontational position with a patient. Instead, hear the patient out. Let the patient relieve some pressure.
- *Sympathize with the patient.* Let the patient know that if you were in his/her position, you might very well feel the same way.
- If the patient's concerns are legitimate, not just an emotional response to a stressful situation, *solve* the patient's problem quickly or find someone who can take appropriate action to solve the patient's problem.
- If the patient's concerns are *only* emotional in nature, attempt to *reorient* the patient's perception of his/her present situation. Emphasize the positives and give as little attention as possible to the negatives. Review for the patient the benefits which will result from having endured a temporarily uncomfortable or unpleasant situation.
- *Reassure* the patient that he/she is taking the optimal course of action, given his/her present options.

Many times this process of listening, sympathizing, addressing concerns, and reassuring the patient will convince him/her that you are not an opponent. This method facilitates trust and a cooperative spirit between patient and technologist, ultimately benefiting both.

Infrequently, and fortunately so, you will encounter patients whose trust and cooperation you cannot gain. Don't fault yourself for these negative interactions – resolve to learn anything you can from them and try harder the next time.

Again, in this situation, there is no advantage in returning the patient's undesirable behavior with hostility. If you become convinced over the course of an interaction that you are not going to appease the patient, be as agreeable as possible and bring the interaction to a close quickly. Allow little time and opportunity for the situation to escalate. Once it is over, contact the patient's referring physician and explain what occurred. Apologize for any inconvenience and ask the physician how your facility may resolve the situation. If possible, follow the physician's suggestion and do it promptly. Otherwise, avoid flatly telling the physician no and offer similar solutions that you can manage.

It is optimal to complete each exam having met or exceeded both the patient's and referring physician's expectations. It is very important to satisfy the patient, but remember that physicians are a source of many referrals and their satisfaction is paramount.

A Medical Emergency Occurs

This is the single most important event to plan for. Fortunately, it doesn't occur often, which is all the more reason to plan ahead. Procedures infrequently followed are all too easily forgotten.

If your facility is hospital-based, an emergency plan is almost certainly in place. Generally, there is a code team which can be summoned very quickly in such an event. If your facility is an outpatient center, but is physically attached to a hospital, you may have access to the hospital code team or emergency room staff. Make sure to determine *before* you have any emergency that the hospital can, indeed, respond to an emergency within your facility. Many times, insurance or liability problems exist and, even though physically connected, a hospital may not be prepared to respond to an emergency in your facility.

If your facility does not have ready access to a code team, then it is prudent to devise your own emergency plan. Consult your risk management personnel and/or insurance carrier upon completing your plan, and ascertain that your plan does not expose your facility to any unnecessary liability. Here are some suggestions for devising a plan.

- Have each staff member licensed in basic cardiopulmonary resuscitation (CPR).
- Have a crash cart available.
- Assign personnel specific and alternate duties.
- If it is not possible to have present at all times someone who is licensed to use the crash cart, be ready to administer basic CPR, to dial 911 or the emergency phone number in your area, and to quickly prepare for the arrival of emergency personnel.
- Have someone cue other staff members that an emergency has occurred, so that they know to perform their assigned emergency duties.
- Have a staff member outside your building to meet emergency personnel, and to escort them quickly to the site of the emergency.
- If an emergency occurs outside the scan room, ask anyone not involved in treating the emergency to exit. Have someone clear the area of any obstructions before emergency personnel arrive.
- If the emergency occurs within the scan room, it is imperative to remove the patient from the scan room before emergency personnel arrive. Clear the area of people and obstructions. It is a good idea to close the door to the scan room after the patient has been removed, to preclude the entry of personnel not familiar with the effects of strong magnetic fields.
- If other persons, who are not staff members within your facility, can see or hear emergency activity, have a staff member inform them that a medical emergency is ongoing. Ask them to remain calm and to be patient. Reassure them that normal operation will resume as soon as possible. Inform them just as soon as the situation is over.
- Resume normal operation as soon as possible. It is prudent practice not to converse about the emergency with subsequent patients or any other nonstaff members.
- Practice your plan two or three times per year and whenever there is staff changeover.

Sometimes advance planning means nothing more than thinking through a situation before it occurs. Other times, as in medical emergencies, advance planning means a carefully thought out, written, and practiced agenda. Use your judgment in deciding how much attention a given situation requires and remember that any planning is better than none at all.

WORKING WITH AND FOR THE RADIOLOGIST

It is a radiologist's responsibility to interpret to his/her best ability, the imaging studies that a technologist performs. In this sense, technologists and radiologists are teammates and as such are directly dependent on each other. An interpretation can only be as accurate and as thorough as the images and clinical information it is drawn from. As the saying goes, "garbage in, garbage out." Therefore, it is a technologist's responsibility to provide the radiologist with as much information as possible.

Clinical Information

MR is an exquisitely sensitive imaging modality, but is unfortunately not terribly specific. In other words, MRI is capable of detecting even subtle pathologies, but many of these pathologies have very similar MRI appearances. It is because of this that the patient's clinical presentation and medical history play such an important role in correctly diagnosing MR findings. With that in mind, let's continue by exploring the clinical information needed to accurately interpret MR findings.

Diagnosis A suspected diagnosis should be obtained from the referring physician at the time the patient is scheduled.

Referring Physician   The referring physician's name, specialty, and phone number should be made available to the radiologist, who may need them to consult the physician during film interpretation.

Symptoms   The patient's symptoms should be explained in as much detail as possible. Include the length of time the patient has been experiencing them, as well as their onset. Was onset following an incident of trauma, or was it gradual over months or years? If onset was posttraumatic, describe the mechanism of injury. If onset was gradual, question the patient about his/her past medical history. Has he/she had cancer or any other systemic disease which might explain or contribute to his/her present condition?

Treatments   Some therapeutic treatments can affect MR image appearance. Radiation therapy, for instance, will alter bone marrow signal in treated areas. Postsurgical changes can also be confusing. Be sure to get treatment descriptions and dates.

Current Medications   The patient's current medications may create MR signal alterations or may contraindicate sedation for the exam. For example, a patient taking steroids may have decreased uptake of MRI contrast material, thereby affecting contrast appearance. For a patient who is already taking a muscle relaxant or pain medication, sedation may be contraindicated altogether.

Physical Appearance   A patient's physical appearance can help to confirm the information he/she has given. It can also lead you to wonder about its accuracy. Many substance abusers are understandably uncomfortable explaining to each medical professional they encounter the exact nature of their illnesses. Before diagnosis, it is entirely possible the patient is unaware of the nature of his/her illness, as is the case with many patients who have cancer, AIDS, or multiple sclerosis.

Results of Other Imaging Studies   It is always beneficial to the interpreting radiologist to have access to the results of previous related imaging studies. It is particularly helpful to have the actual films handy for comparison. Many times this can narrow a differential diagnosis from four or five likely possibilities to one or two.

Presenting Your Findings

Most of the diagnostic information needed by a radiologist is contained in the films and images themselves. Obviously, it is essential that technologists are able to recognize pathology. It is not essential that technologists are able to correctly identify it, although this can be helpful. The ability to recognize pathology comes through experience. It is of great educational value to review cases postinterpretation and to ask questions when you encounter diagnoses you don't understand or recognize.

Ask the radiologist what you might have done to make a particular scan easier to interpret. Discuss alternative parameters such as different planes, TR times, filming techniques and so on. Inquire as to anything you might do in the way of an improvement the next time you encounter a similar case. This type of interaction will yield a wealth of practical information and will help educate the radiologist as to your equipment's capabilities and limitations. Try to spend as much time as possible interacting with the radiologist in this way.

Here are some ideas you may wish to employ in an effort to improve the readability of any studies you turn in to the radiologist for interpretation.

Point out or notate anything of interest or concern on the films.

Help the radiologist by providing reference images, measuring grids, and page numbers on the films.

Notate significant changes in technique or any other factors that affect scan quality or image appearance.

Organize previous studies so it is clear to the radiologist which study is current and is to be interpreted, and which studies have been read.

Organize any films for comparison so the radiologist knows they are available.

Realize that working *with* the radiologists is much more beneficial to you, your center, and your patients than simply working *for* them. You and the radiologist are teammates, not adversaries. Work to achieve two-way communication, flexibility, and a good understanding of each other's needs and limitations, then you will become a valuable asset to your facility and a valuable teammate in the eyes of the radiologist.

DEALING WITH REFERRING PHYSICIANS

Every interaction anyone from your facility has with a referring physician or his/her staff should be looked at as a moment of truth. Each moment of truth is an opportunity to leave either a negative, neutral, or a positive impression about your facility. Negative, or even neutral impressions do not gain further referrals. The retail industry has conducted numerous studies to evaluate why customers quit doing business with one company, in favor of a competitor. There are many reasons, but the single most common reason is an attitude of indifference on the part of an employee of that company towards its customers. Remember, to the person on the other end of that phone line, *you* are the company. An attitude of indifference on your part will be interpreted as the attitude of the entire company. This indifference is no reward for someone who has just awarded your company their business.

Let's identify and examine what there is to gain from your interactions with referring physicians and their staff. Also, let's identify and examine what referring physicians and their staff members hope to gain from these interactions with you, and the mutual good that comes from each of you getting what you want.

Let's start by identifying things to be gained by interacting with a physician or one of his/her staff members. Most important is the opportunity to win and keep his/her *referral business*. To facilitate winning and keeping his/her referral business, you should obtain *adequate information* to properly perform the tasks he/she has requested. And since neither party has all day to accomplish a given task, you should effect a *time-efficient interaction*. Let's examine these things separately.

Referral Business

Winning and keeping a physician's referral business is crucial to the very survival of your facility, let alone its success. Radiology is a capital-intensive business and particularly so are MRI centers. In most places, competition has become fierce, as more and more centers chase fewer and fewer reimbursement dollars. In a highly competitive market, referring physicians have many options and a variety of motivations for going elsewhere. Don't give them reason to go elsewhere, via poor service or that fatal attitude of indifference. Reward them for referring patients to your facility by providing them with prompt, reliable service in a friendly helpful fashion.

Information

The second thing you set out to gain from these interactions is adequate information. Information, such as patient diagnosis and history, contraindications, and current insurance information, is crucial to your ability to get the job done right first time. Obtaining adequate information is purely a mechanical matter. Identify the information most frequently needed and devise forms and checklists to help guide you through time-efficient interactions. The key to thoroughness lies in being prepared. The forms at the end of this section are examples of preparation devices – a fax form for patient referrals [Figure 17-6] and a scheduling form for over-the-phone referrals [Figure 17-7]. The

EXPLANATION OF THE SCHEDULING

FAX SHEET

This form is intended to be distributed to referring physicians offices, along with patient information brochures and prescription pads. It should be given out in the form of a "master copy," from which the office staff can make as many copies as needed.

This form can be used in two ways. If a referring physician's office calls to refer a patient who is present at the time, the patient may merely arrange an appointment time that is convenient over the phone, and then be on his or her way. The referring physician's office can then fill out this form and fax it to your facility at their convenience.

If a referring physician's office wishes to schedule a patient who is not present, they may fill out this form and fax it to your facility. You may then phone the patient, arrange an appointment time, and call the referring physician's office to notify them that the appointment has indeed been made.

Figure 17-6.   Scheduling fax sheet and explanation.

scheduling form is multiple pages, one of which is the bill. These forms, once written, will also help control the amount of time it takes to interact, which is of course, goal number three.

It is important to both parties that these interactions be time-efficient. It's smart for you, and in addition it shows courtesy and concern for their time. There are helpful habits you can develop to enable you to direct conversations and to hasten information collection. For example, when someone calls, greet them with a smile on your face and identify your facility. Offer your name, as well. Ask them what you can do for them and allow them plenty of time to explain. Then help them, if possible. If you can't, connect them with someone who can. When someone calls to refer a patient, make sure to take the minimum amount of information necessary to schedule the patient. Request a fax of any other information or obtain it from the patient. This will make your facility the path of least resistance for referring patients. If you must transfer your caller to someone else, explain what your caller wants, so he/she doesn't have to explain

SCHEDULING FAX SHEET

TO: _____   (FAX: _____)

FROM: DR. _____   (PHONE: _____)

PATIENT NAME   _____

PATIENT PHONE   _____

TYPE OF SCAN / AREA _____

DIAGNOSIS _____

TYPE OF CLAIM (CIRCLE ONE):

    AUTO   -   DATE OF ACCIDENT _____

    HEALTH

    WORK COMP. -   DATE OF INJURY   _____

            -   AUTHORIZED   Y   N

            -   SOCIAL SEC. #   _____

INSURANCE CO. _____

INSURANCE PHONE (   ) _____

POLICY HOLDER _____

POLICY / CLAIM # _____

PLEASE CHECK ONE:

    PATIENT HAS BEEN SCHEDULED _____

    CALL PATIENT TO SCHEDULE   _____, THEN CALL OUR OFFICE WITH

    APPOINTMENT TIME.

Figure 17-6 (*continued*).

twice. It's gauche and just poor service to ask your caller to call back. He/she can't possibly know when the person they need to speak with will be available, and you'll have to handle the call twice.

What does your caller hope to gain by interacting with you, or why do people buy quarter-inch drill bits? Because they want quarter-inch holes. Likewise, what your caller wants is solutions to problems. In addition, your caller wants good feelings and wants to put forth the minimum amount of effort to get these solutions to problems and good feelings. Let's examine separately solutions to problems, good feelings, and minimized efforts.

Solutions to Problems

When a referring physician orders a scan of a patient's lumbar spine, he/she is really after a diagnosis upon which to base a treatment plan. When a staff member calls to schedule a patient for an MRI, what he/she really wants is to encounter the path of least resistance. Just like you, he/she has at least a dozen other tasks to accomplish in an inadequate period of time. Meet his/her needs by being efficient and friendly. Get patients scheduled as quickly as possible. Call the referring physician's office to say when the patient is scheduled and when to expect results. Keep a list of patients who are available on short notice. Upon the all too common occasion that someone cancels on short notice, call one of your short notice patients and surprise his/her referring physician with quicker results than expected.

Giving your caller what he wants means more than just being nice on the phone. It means actually setting up your procedures to accommodate his/her needs. Examine your workflow patterns and company policies. Are they inefficient? Are they downright obstructive? Can physicians expect to speak to the radiologist whenever they need to, or just every other rainy Tuesday on a full moon? Do your hours accommodate patients who work during weekdays? Hire specifically for the evening shift and/or the weekend shift, depending on the hours your market favors. When you make copies of films, do you include a copy of the report, too? Do you charge for copies? All these things go together to paint a perceptual picture of your facility in the minds of the people who do business with you. If you're consistently flexible and willing to accommodate, you will achieve preferred status over your competitors.

EXPLANATION OF THE

SCHEDULING/STANDARD INSURANCE FORM

The following page is a form designed to be attached to a (triplicate) standard insurance form - currently the HCFA-1500. This form is to be carbon-coated on the backside (as are pages one and two of the attached HCFA-1500). Information written on the front page will be transferred to the three pages of the HCFA-1500. The front page is used for scheduling only. The shaded areas are to be filled in when the patient is being scheduled, and the balance of information is to be obtained upon patient confirmation. The three pages of the HCFA-1500 are your bill - one copy for the patient's insurance company, one copy for the patient, and one for your receivables file.

Figure 17-7. Scheduling/standard insurance form and explanation.

desirable than being the only game in town. However, if you're the only MRI center in town, then chances are, there are no established referral patterns and you will have to educate local physicians as to when and why to refer for MRI. This is tougher than you may think. Physicians can be very old dogs when it comes to learning new tricks. Evaluate your location with regard to proximity to referral sources, that is physicians and hospitals.

Accessibility is another primary consideration in site selection. Remember, the vast majority of your patients will be traveling to your center for the first time. If your location is on a major thoroughfare, nearby well-known local landmarks, and has easy access in and out of the parking lot, you will suffer far fewer late patients and no-shows. Not only do they wreak havoc with your schedule, they cost your company a lot of money.

Here is a quick reference, in outline form, of the information to be gathered and evaluated before site selection. There is no perfect site, but knowledge of both strong and weak areas is essential before you can establish a successful postinstallation marketing program.

Research before selecting site

I. Location
  A. Proximity to competitors
    1. Are they successful?
    2. Why are they successful? Physician investors, competition, location, hospital alliances?
  B. Proximity to referral sources
    1. Are they the right specialties?
II. Accessibility
  A. Major thoroughfare
  B. Near well-known local landmarks
  C. Traffic light or left-hand turn lane
  D. Well lit and highly visible
    1. Safety
    2. Conspicuity

III. Referral patterns
  A. If well established
    1. Who are local physicians using now?
    2. Why are they using these facilities?
    3. How often? Reduce by 50 percent.
    4. Can you outservice your competitors?
  B. If not well established
    1. Is there a sufficient patient population?
    2. Are the right specialists nearby? Chiropractors, orthopedic surgeons, neurologists, neurosurgeons?
    3. Are they old dogs?
    4. How long will it take to teach them? Double it.
    5. Do you have enough operating capital to get you through the education curve?
IV. There is no perfect site
  A. Identify and evaluate assets.
  B. Identify and evaluate deficit areas.
  C. How do they compare? Do the assets outweigh the deficits, or do you have a better option?

Postinstallation Marketing Postinstallation marketing is a process of information distribution best accomplished by asking yourself a few what and how questions. What information do I distribute, in what format, and how do I distribute it? There are a multitude of options. Choose them carefully according to what will be useful to and well accepted by your market. For example, radio advertising in a conservative market may do you more harm than good. Here are some methods and materials to consider.

Brochures directed toward referring physicians. Make sure to include information on the radiologists, your equipment, your hours of operation, indications and contraindications, and so on.

Brochures directed toward referring physicians' office staff. Include information on patient scheduling, hours of operation, which managed care organizations and insurance companies you work with, payment plans, transport, if offered, and so on.

Brochures directed toward the patient. Include information explaining why the doctor has ordered an MRI, what the experience will be like, what it will show, how long it will take, contraindications, and a map.

Educational scan conferences and lectures/luncheons.

Ads in newspapers, medical journals, and magazines.

Specialty items such as pens, posters, coffee cups, calendars, clipboards, flashlights, and so on.

Some physicians prefer prescription pads over patient information brochures. Be sure to print a map on them.

Videotape is a different media for informational brochures.

Any marketing materials you choose to develop may be distributed by mail or in person. If a referring physician's location is some distance from your center, the best option may be the mail. However, if the referring physician is nearby your center, a hand delivery is most effective. A hand delivery affords your center the opportunity to make eyeball-to-eyeball contact with someone from that referring physician's office. It is an opportunity to establish a relationship and if you're very fortunate, it will grow into an ongoing relationship requiring management.

Relationship Management   There is simple human nature at the crux of any ongoing business relationship. People want to do business with people they like and trust. Every imaging center should have one individual whose sole responsibility is to establish and maintain relationships with referring physicians and their office staff. Give them that person to like and trust. Optimally, your center has a full-time marketing person or physician consultant, for the purpose of developing and managing relationships with your entire base of referring physicians. This person should continually attempt to expand this referral base by seeking out and meeting new physicians and their staff members.

Depending on your market, this base can become quite large. For this reason, successful marketing requires a lot of time and is difficult for a technologist, office manager, or radiologist to do well, in addition to his/her primary responsibilities. That's not to say it's impossible when done part-time, but expectations of success should be realistic. The more time and effort expended, the quicker and more voluminous are the fruits of your labors.

The relationship management aspect of marketing involves the entire staff of your center. Each staff member needs to understand how delicate these relationships are and treat them accordingly. Every interaction between someone from your facility and a referring physician or one of his/her staff is an opportunity to make a favorable impression or to reinforce an existing relationship. Therefore, we are *all* involved in the marketing effort to a considerable degree.

CHAPTER **18**

Evaluation of Magnetic Resonance Imaging Equipment

Bartram J. Pierce

During this time of explosive medical technology, the technologist can play a very important role in the evaluation and selection of magnetic resonance imaging systems. No one in the radiology department has more hands-on imaging experience than the technologist. The technologist spends more time operating the system, dealing with the patient, and looking at images than does the radiologist. The technologist knows how to get the most from his/her equipment; the shortcuts, the idiosyncracies, and the strategies to obtain the best diagnostic scan. The majority of radiologists seldom have time for the logistics of image production. Their only concern is to receive a diagnostic study. No one knows better than the technologist what it takes to turn an appointment book into a stack of diagnostic images. The technologist is the most logical choice to contribute valuable input in the evaluation of equipment, whether upgrading the current system or purchasing a new one.

Depending on your rapport with your radiologists you may or may not figure prominently in the evaluation and decision-making process. You may be given the job of gathering the necessary information for their decision. Whatever the situation in your facility, as a technologist, you

can give the radiologist valuable insight into what it takes to operate the system on a daily basis, therefore playing an important and vital role in their decision-making process. A plethora of upgrades, new systems [Figure 18-1], and third-party equipment is available in today's market; to illustrate the process of evaluation, this chapter considers the purchase of new magnetic

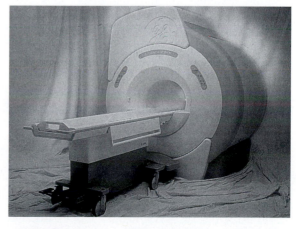

Figure 18-1. General Electric Medical Systems latest magnetic resonance imaging system, the Signa Horizon LX MR/i. (Courtesy GE Medical Systems.)

351

resonance systems. The methods discussed can be applied to many other situations.

CHOOSING FIELD STRENGTH

The selection of field strength is determined by many factors, most of which are out of the hands of the technologist. Your group of radiologists and/or administrators will make this decision based on the following information.

Referring physician's needs and expectations.

Exam mix (neuro, orthopedic, etc.).

Competing systems in the area.

Patient load and reimbursement figures.

Radiologist preference.

State Certificate of Need procedures.

Various field strength attitudes in your referring area.

Cost or financial considerations.

Once your radiologists and/or administrators have made the decision on which field strength they wish to purchase, it then becomes a matter of gathering the proper information on the MR systems that fit their criteria. It is essential to collect and organize all the information available in a format which allows comparison of the magnet systems on an equal basis. This contributes to making a correct and informed decision which will benefit the facility, the practice, and most of all the patients. The value of the technologist in this process is one of information gatherer and hands-on reviewer.

USE OF A TIME LINE

After making the decision to purchase a new system and before gathering information, it is advisable to develop a time line to keep the process on track and moving forward. A time line is simply a list of decisions and crossroads that will be encountered during the long process of evaluating and choosing a new system, accompanied by a deadline for each stage. There is an immense amount of information to sift through and it is quite easy to get bogged down and frustrated without a plan. It is also very helpful to define what major decisions need to be made and when they need to occur in order to meet the installation deadline. The time line can be as detailed or as general as you wish to make it, but at the very least it should list all the major decisions and tasks up to the installation deadline [Table 18-1] and first patient scanning. Take some time and thought when putting together the time line. It should have reasonable, realistic time goals. Dates for the completion of tasks should be adhered to if at all possible. The selection, construction, and installation of a new magnet system can be a long and involved process fraught with set backs. Sticking to the time line may give you a feeling of accomplishment as you complete each step. If used correctly it will also eliminate frustration and prevent frantically rushing to meet a deadline. Table 18-2 is a simple time line.

Table 18-1

Time Line Items*

Contact all vendors
Information matrix complete
Radiologist evaluation
Magnet system finalists
Site visits
Final recommendation
Finalize bid
Joint venture presentation
Place order
Detailed site plans
Delivery date
Construction begins
Facility ready for magnet
Applications
First patient scanning

*A sample list of items that might be included in a time line for installation. Add and delete any items to the time line that you feel are necessary to keep the process moving and on track.

Table 18-2

Time Line*

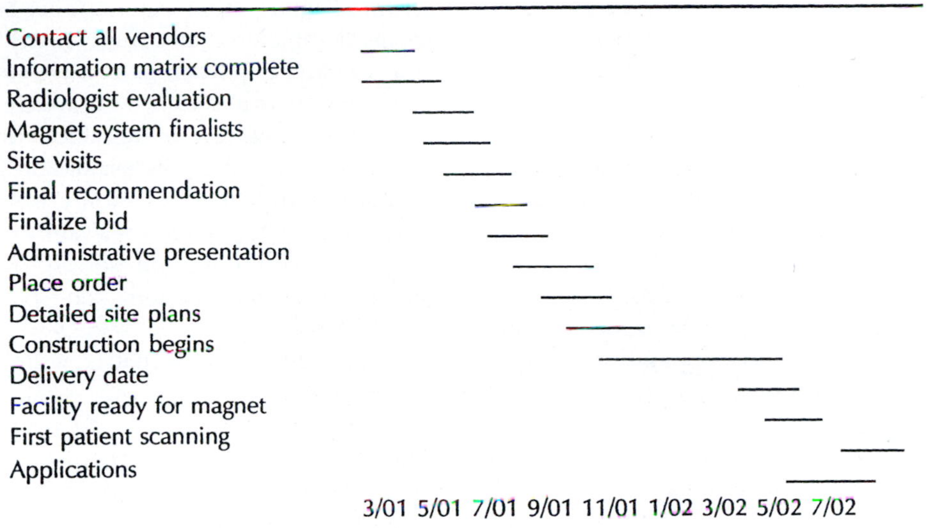

Contact all vendors	
Information matrix complete	
Radiologist evaluation	
Magnet system finalists	
Site visits	
Final recommendation	
Finalize bid	
Administrative presentation	
Place order	
Detailed site plans	
Construction begins	
Delivery date	
Facility ready for magnet	
First patient scanning	
Applications	

3/01 5/01 7/01 9/01 11/01 1/02 3/02 5/02 7/02

*Set a time line like the one above. Make every attempt to adhere to the dates outlined on the time line in order to keep the project on track.

INFORMATIONAL MATRIX

An informational matrix arranges all the information you have gathered in a form that makes comparison easy and straightforward. It is simply a listing of everything you think is essential to be able to compare multiple systems. This is necessary because of the large number of systems to choose from, the complexity of these systems, and the manufacturers use of different terminology to describe the same thing. In this scenario it sometimes becomes extremely difficult to compare apples to apples and oranges to oranges. For example, General Electric talks about its fast spin echo (FSE) sequences while Siemens talks about its turbo spin echo. These are essentially the same pulse sequence but with different names. To make things even more difficult every MR system comes as a standard system with different accessories or optional items, such as coils, pulse sequence packages, and different camera/VCR interfaces. Comparing the different options can

be confusing without some way of keeping all the information straight.

Once you have established a time line, the process of gathering and organizing all the necessary information begins. Prepare a folder or binder for each system and/or vendor you will be considering. Each folder should contain the following.

1. Promotional material for each system
2. Product data or specification sheets
3. Correspondence with the vendor
4. Documentation of all pertinent conversations

By keeping detailed records of each vendor's participation you lessen the chance that problems or discrepancies will crop up. This is especially true for phone conversations and meetings, where what you hear and what the vendor means may not be the same, or problems when the vendor promises you one thing and, at a later date, offers another.

The informational matrix can be set up as elaborately or as simply as you wish. Sit down with your radiologists and/or your administrators and develop a shopping list of options and features that you wish to be included in your system. This will give you a place to start and give the vendor an idea of how your system is to be configured. For instance, if you know you won't be performing MR angiography (MRA) or cardiac studies, it is not necessary to spend valuable time comparing these features. Once you have developed your shopping list it is time to contact the vendors or manufacturers you wish to deal with.

Contact all the manufacturers that make systems similar to the one your group has decided to pursue. Try not to ignore any vendor just because you may not get along with the representative or because you may have heard something bad about the company. With this approach, everybody starts on an equal footing. If a company is not interested or does not have the product you desire you will find out soon enough. Once you have contacted the vendors you will soon start to receive volumes of information about every conceivable system, containing every conceivable feature and option.

Not all people involved in the decision-making process may be technically oriented. You may need to have two or three matrices, containing different information each for a different audience. You may need one matrix for the radiologists, one for the referring physicians, one for the banker or finance company, and one for the state. If available, setting up a matrix on a computer spreadsheet will make it easier to make changes and pull out just the information you need for a particular audience. Whatever you decide, start your matrix off with as much information as available. Don't be afraid to make the matrix extremely detailed, you can always trim it down later. A suggestion is to set up two matrices in the beginning, one with mostly technical information and one with

mostly nontechnical information. Table 18-3 is a list of items you may wish to include in your technical information matrix. This list is by no means complete or all-inclusive. Add any items you may find important and delete any items not applicable to your site. The nontechnical matrix can also be used to catalog factors or items that are very important to the evaluation process and decision, and factors you don't wish to forget. Add anything you think is relevant to installation, service, applications, and so on. Examples of nontechnical information can be found in Table 18-4.

When setting up the matrix, write the features or options on the left-hand side. Prepare two columns for each system being considered. The first column is to denote whether the feature or option is available from that vendor and maybe to identify the vendor's acronym for it. The second column is to indicate whether said feature is part of the basic package or an optional item. If known, include the cost of the optional feature in this column. An example of information included in the second column is listed below.

1. Inc/basic: included in the basic system configuration and the quoted price

2. Inc/optional: included in the system configuration and quoted price but could be removed to decrease expenditure.

3. Optional: not included in the system configuration or the quoted price but can be purchased at an additional cost.

4. WIP: feature is currently work in progress and unavailable to most sites

Pay especially close attention to any item listed as work in progress or investigational, especially if it is a feature your site is very interested in. Vendors have a tendency to promote their work in progress as available features. How long before this feature will be available in the field? Is the work in progress (WIP) still in the research and development (R&D) stage or is it in beta testing (clinical trials)? If it is in clinical testing, ask for a

TABLE 18-3

Items to Include in a Technical Information Matrix*

Pulse sequences

Volume Imaging

Fast spin echo

MR angiography

Coils
   linear
   quad
   phased array

Presaturation

Fat saturation

Offset FOV

Multiangle obliques

Spectroscopy

Echo planar imaging

Perfusion/Diffusion

Functional imaging

Gating
   cardiac
   peripheral
   respiratory

Cardiac sequences

Cardiac evaluation software

Camera interface

Camera upgrade

VCR interface

Online storage: # images

Archive system
   Magnetic optical discs
   DAT type
   Storage capacity

Music system

CCTV system

Additional console

Workstation

Magnet subsystem

Cryogens
   type
   boiloff rate
   refill interval

Shimming type
   (active or passive)

5 Gauss fringe field
   radial
   axial

Gradient subsystem
   strength
   rise time
   % duty cycle
   cooling

RF subsystem
   RF power amplifier output
   transmitter type (digital)
   receiver type (linear/phased array)
   # of channels (1/4)
   body coil
   type (high pass)
   dimensions

Head coil
   type
   dimensions

Computer subsystem
   magnetic disk capacity
   amount of image store (256 vs 512)
   optical disk capacity
   amount of image store (256 vs 512)
   image store
   recon time (ms) 256×256
   recon time (ms) 512×512
   processor bits (32/64)
   processor speed (MHz)

DICOM compatible

Upgradability

Patient transport
   vertical height
   horizontal travel
   horizontal speed
   accuracy
   patient weight
   motor driven
   detachable table
   creature comforts (pads, armrests, etc.)

Operator console
   # of monitors
   type of monitor (color)
   size of monitor
   image display (# pixels)
   interface (keyboard/mouse)
   operating system interface
   DICOM compatible

*Add or delete items yourself. This list is not all encompassing.

list of the beta sites so you may call and talk to the test engineers. If there are any features or options that are WIP during your evaluation, be sure to get the vendor to put the anticipated release date in writing. Table 18-5 shows an example of how to set up the informational matrix between two systems profiling some common technical factors.

Table 18-4

A Sample Listing of Items for Inclusion in a Nontechnical Information Matrix*

Applications	cryogens
length	refill interval
# techs	Service dispatch
location	Parts dispatch
hot line	Response time
publications	phone
Line conditioner	on site
UPS system	Uptime guarantee
Upgrades	RF shielding costs
operational	Additional room costs
software	Shipping
hardware	Rigging
Service contract	Mobile service
amount	supply/arrange
hours of service	cost
hours of service, PM's	Payment terms
hours of service, cryo	

*Anything necessary for the comparison of the two systems should be included in the list.

If you have difficulty compiling all the information needed and/or seeing the various manufacturers' systems, you might consider attending the annual meeting of the Radiological Society of North America (RSNA). It often helps tremendously to see the equipment or systems you are interested in. This annual meeting showcases the latest technological advances and all of the major manufacturers, as well as the smaller players, have a presence there. Displays contain images of actual scans, discussion of all features including works in progress, and technical information of each system. Some manufacturers even set up actual MRI systems allowing for a hands-on approach. It also gives the visitor a chance to meet with a large number of other physicians and technologists and compare the information they have gathered and their likes and dislikes. Although attending the RSNA requires the technologist to be away from their facility, it is an often overlooked opportunity to visit a great number of manufacturers in a small period of time.

The recent proliferation and the widespread use of the Internet and World Wide Web (WWW) has given the technologist compiling system information an entirely new avenue to gather information. There are many sources of good information easily accessed on the Internet. Most major manufacturers maintain their own web sites. These web sites may be a convenient location to obtain technical information, applications information, and images taken from their systems. Listserves that serve the MRI technologist and the radiological sciences allow for the candid exchange of information regarding manufacturers' systems. Who better to get information from, than the technologists actually working on those systems? By simply putting a query out over these listserves you can elicit comments not only from technologists working on systems all over the country, but worldwide.

After all the necessary information has been collected and the matrix has been completed, the vendors should be given an opportunity to check your work for accuracy. Do not send the entire matrix to the vendor. Make a copy of the matrix showing only the columns necessary for that vendor. You may also want to include the headings showing which other vendors are being considered (but none of the information). This will let the vendors know who their competition is and may make them more responsive to your needs. By allowing the vendors to check your work, you assure that you have the most current and correct information available.

As you are gathering the necessary information for the matrix, the vendors will want to know the next phase or stage of this evaluation process.

What can they do to expedite matters? Who will make the decisions and when will they be made? It would be wise to pass these questions on to your radiologists and/or administrators. Trying to answer these questions can only complicate and potentially confuse your efforts to compile and collate the information.

Table 18-5

A Sample Informational Matrix Showing Possible Setup between Two Similar MR Systems

Feature	System A		System B	
	Available	Cost	Available	Cost
Pulse sequence				
Spin echo	yes	inc.	yes	inc.
Inversion recovery	yes	inc.	yes	inc
Gradient echo, T1	yes	inc.	yes	inc.
Gradient echo, T2	yes	Inc.	yes	inc.
Gradient echo, T2*	yes	inc.	yes	inc.
Stir	yes	inc.	yes	inc.
Volume imaging	yes	inc.	yes	inc.
Fast spin echo	yes	inc./opt.	yes	opt. (35,000)
MR angiography	yes	opt. (41,000)	yes	opt. (36,000)
2D TOF	yes	—	yes	—
3D TOF	yes	—		—
Phase contrast	yes	—	no (wip)	—
Mag. trans. contrast	no (wip)	—	yes	—
Mult. thin slabs	yes	—	yes (motsa)	—
Multitasking	yes	inc.	yes	inc.
Multiangle obliques	yes	inc.	yes (mao)	inc.
Offset FOV	yes	inc.	yes	inc.
Presaturation	yes (presat)	inc.	yes	inc.
Fat saturation	yes (fatsat)	inc.	yes	inc.
Anti-alias	yes	inc.	yes	inc.

You have now spent months gathering and arranging mountains of information. You have prepared the informational matrix and given all the facts and figures to your radiologists. They should now narrow the list to two or three systems they feel will best fit their needs.

SITE VISITS

Once two or three systems have been chosen, it is time to begin to truly evaluate the operational characteristics of each system by making site visits. As the technologist that will be responsible for throughput and patient scanning, you should arrange to accompany the radiologists during their site visits. Because you are the one that operates, or will be operating, the system on a daily basis you will have different questions than theirs. As the technologist you will be able to supply your radiologists with a different perspective. For the most part, the radiologist will be concerned about final images, not about the time and steps necessary to get those images. You, however, will want to know whether the software is easy to use. Are the filming and archive functions easy to manipulate? Is it easy to communicate with the patient? Are the patient comforts adequate? Will it be easy to access the patient while in the scanner?

Before setting out on a visit call several sites that are using the type of system you are planning to look at. Talk to the technologists working on the machine. Get their comments, both on the good points as well as the bad. What type of things would they like to see changed? What could be altered to make it easier? Is there an option or feature that would help speed throughput or patient comfort that is not included in their system? Does the equipment take the stresses of everyday scanning? Has the machine and/or company lived up to its promises? Is the vendor as easy to work with after the sale as they were before?

Talk to them about applications. Did they receive adequate applications? Should the time have been longer/shorter? How could it have been better? Was there an applications person that did a superb job or one that was not quite up to par? Did the technologists at this site already have a good working knowledge of MR imaging and physics? If you have technologists at your site that are new then you might wish to push for more applications than the vendor quotes as normal. Does the company support ongoing applications, such as a hot line or timely publications? Can you get information on new scanning parameters, pulse sequences, or coils in a timely manner?

Immediately before a visit, look over your completed informational matrix and the notes from your conversations to develop a list of questions, both for the technologists at the site and the vendor accompanying you. If possible, spend a full day at the site not just a few hours. This way can you see a full range of patients and a full range of exams. Spend as much time with the technologists as possible getting to know them and the system. Arrange to operate the console, running a few scans. Are you comfortable with the operating system and is it easy to use [Figure 18-2]? Make sure you see the system stressed to maximum, such as thin slices, multi-echo, and T2 weighted images. Look at the acquisition times on their routine scans and show images; are they similar? Are the scan times

realistic and would they fit into your schedule and patient load? Take a look at as many images as you can, not just the show images. Ask them to pull random cases from their files for you to inspect. When you find what you feel are good representative images of the system's capabilities ask for copies, or originals if possible. These films can serve not only as comparisons for other systems, but also for reference films during acceptance testing at a later date.

During the day take a break from the site and meet with your radiologists. Do this someplace where you can talk openly and compare notes. Is there anything you've missed? Are the stories you

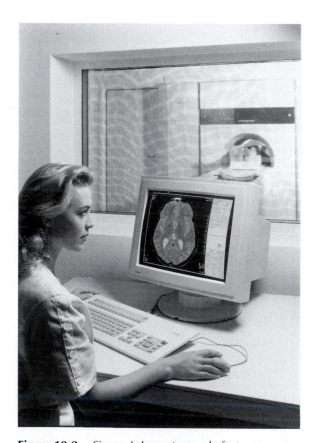

Figure 18-2. Siemen's Impact console features mouse control, which allows the operating platform to be modified via software changes. (Courtesy Siemens Medical Systems.)

are both hearing the same? Do you have any unanswered questions? This may be your only opportunity to visit a site using this particular system, so try not to miss anything.

Once back from the site visit the job of information gathering is done. Sit down and summarize your findings in writing. What did you think about the system, the applications support, the images, and everything else you saw? Was the system configuration you saw similar to the vendor's quote? Be available for your radiologists to discuss how you feel the machine will fit into their practice. Remember, you bring to the table a lot of subjective feelings and ideas about how the system would react under day-to-day use.

During the negotiation process, everything is negotiable. Suggest items or features the radiologists may have neglected but which they should consider when meeting with the vendor. There is no such thing as asking for something stupid. If you don't ask, you can be sure the vendor will not volunteer it. This is the time when you need to bring up items such as length of applications, follow-up, person performing the applications, coils, and anything you feel is important. If you had the perfect situation and money was not an object how would your ideal system be configured?

RECOMMENDATION

After the site visits are complete it is time to decide which system is to be purchased. Final negotiations can now take place. If you have taken an active part in the information gathering, the construction of the informational matrix and the site visits, you will know as much about the competing systems as the radiologists. Now is the time for you, the technologist, to make your recommendation to the radiologists. Sit down and go over all the information you have accumulated during the past months including the informational matrix and site visit summaries. More than likely, by this time, you probably have already chosen a favorite for one reason or another. Comparing top-of-the-line systems can sometimes boil down to some very subjective feelings. Although not always easy, try to analyze these feelings, summarize your thoughts about each system reviewed, listing the pros and cons briefly, then make your final recommendation to your radiologists on which system you feel would best fit the needs of the department. If necessary develop a packet of information for your radiologists to help them see the validity of your recommendation.

SUMMARY

Medical imaging is evolving at an ever increasing pace. Technology continues to outpace our ability to assimilate it. With so many new and sophisticated systems coming to market, purchasing decisions require the evaluation of a great deal of information and many similar systems. This is sometimes very difficult to do in today's world of acronyms and abbreviations. The secret of evaluation is in gathering large amounts of information in a format that allows comparison of apples to apples. Once this is done the decision becomes relatively straightforward. The role of the technologist in this process can be summed up as follows.

- Serve as the information gatherer for your radiologists.
- Give your radiologist a different perspective on site visits.
- Recommend the system you feel is best for your facility.

CHAPTER 19

Perspectives on Future MRI Technology and Applications

Joseph V. Fritz

INTRODUCTION

This chapter presents several important technical and clinical issues likely to impact on future MRI developments. Technological trends are toward systems that are more compact, easier to use, quieter, faster, and more automated[1,2]. It is important to recognize that pragmatic considerations strongly influence which promising research methodologies will be incorporated in next-generation commercial systems. Examples include the protection of intellectual property, the impact of U.S. Food and Drug Administration regulations on the pre-market approval (PMA) and marketing clearance processes, and the conduct of market research, which must financially justify every investment in new technology by demonstrating improved profitability or market share.

Today's cost-conscious healthcare environment demands that physicians and manufacturers overcome the inertia of the status quo and direct their efforts towards the development of increasingly cost-effective technologies to manage disease and significantly improve clinical outcomes. Although achieving those goals will take time, advances in diagnostic imaging, especially in MRI, should prove fascinating for years to come[3].

MAGNET TECHNOLOGY

Magnet technology has taken several interesting developmental twists since the original clinical scanners of the early 1980s [Figure 19-1]. Field strength started small with 0.15 T resistive systems and evolved to superconducting, air-core, 1.5 T scanners by the late 1980s. Experimental systems, which were initially vertical-field open configurations, quickly became the closed-bore configuration typically associated with today's MRI scanner. Huge growth occurred in this decade because MRI reimbursements were very high and expensive systems could be justified.

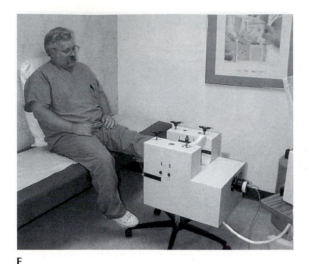

E

Figure 19-1 (*continued*).   Evolution of MRI architectures. **E** Small inexpensive portable devices represent an increasingly popular trend toward tailoring MR systems to specific applications. (Courtesy MagneVu Corporation.)

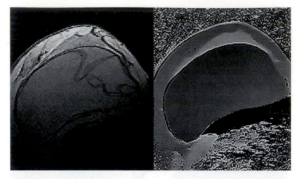

Figure 19-2.   A form of chemical shift imaging can be generated at lower field strengths by using phase reconstructions of field echo sequences. In this example, silicone, water, and fat are clearly identified in the right phase map demonstrating an intact silicone breast implant. Implant integrity is equivocal using only magnitude reconstruction on the left.

suggest that over one-third of patients have some degree of anxiety reaction while inside an MR scanner[5,6].

In 1996, the first superconducting open MRI system was introduced[7]. With the advent of open MR imagers that produce very acceptable image quality, offer a complete selection of sequences, improve patient comfort, and maintain or enhance throughput, open MRI reached a new level of acceptance. By 1998, although conventional bore 1.0 T and 1.5 T systems continued to serve as the mainstream MRI device, open scanner machines captured almost half of the MRI market share and are now seen as complementary to, and in some cases substitutes for, closed bore systems[8].

The convergence of the two technologies implies an interesting and plausible trend toward future whole body scanners becoming high-field superconducting whole-body open configurations. As a result of the growing clinical acceptance and confidence in the marketplace, manufacturers feel justified in allocating substantially larger research and development budgets to further enhance open scanner capabilities[9].

Many technical advances incorporated in closed-bore systems are also appropriate for open scanners, although field orientation, field strength, and methods of shaping the field necessitate different approaches. Gradients can certainly be made more powerful and computer hardware advances are just as applicable. Although spectroscopy in its current form will require higher field strengths, there are novel phase-mapping methods that uniquely map some tissue characteristics [Figure 19-2]. Because the magnet, gradients, and receiver and transmitter coils must assume an open geometry, field of view and spatial linearity on open scanners present unique challenges. Field strength has been limited because the open system typically uses iron to shape the field. Increasing the field strength increases the amount of iron required, thereby increasing weight and cost. Using superconducting drivers rather than permanent magnets or resistive configurations improves the homogeneity, and stability and minimizes the amount of iron required.

Clinical evaluation of open versus closed bore MRI systems will be important to determine variations in diagnostic capabilities. Differences in field strength and orientation change susceptibility artifacts caused by implanted devices, air–bone interfaces, magic angle effects, or postoperative image quality. The reduction in signal-to-noise ratio (SNR) attributable to field strength is countered by various advantages, such as faster T1 recovery and lessened vulnerability to motion artifact[10]. Whether a more comfortable imaging experience translates into an economic advantage of any kind will require further investigation. Clearly, the ability to perform interventional or joint motion studies within an open system may well expand the role of MRI.

As of early 1999, the literature on open MRI system applications and trade-offs remains sparse. Because of limitations that became evident in first-generation open scanners, many high-field MR experts have been biased against their routine use in whole-body imaging. As open systems gradually expand into additional clinical research environments, however, the pace of development and awareness of capabilities through publications will dramatically accelerate their penetration in the marketplace.

The magnet configuration battleground is not completely limited to open versus 1.5 T. There is a resurgence of interest in the small, inexpensive niche scanners that can be installed almost anywhere or hand-held[11,12]. Limitations in field of view, depth of penetration, and SNR are the primary drawbacks of this technology. Research continues into prepolarized MRI (PMRI) as a low-cost approach using a strong inhomogeneous pulsed field to create large longitudinal magnetization and a homogeneous but weak field during readout[13].

Research also continues on very-high field systems for enhancing signal-to-noise ratio, necessary for MR microscopy, imaging of very subtle signal changes such as produced by blood oxygenation changes, and multinuclear spectroscopy[14]. The negative aspects which must be overcome include weight, fringe-field containment, hazards related to RF heating and metal attraction, chemical shift, RF penetration, susceptibility artifacts, and cost[15,16]. With Medicare and third-party insurer reimbursements continuing to decline, there will need to be as much research into the potential clinical benefits and economic advantages of very high field MRI systems as in the engineering and materials that will make this development possible.

COILS

Coil and receiver design have evolved from analog to digital to an array of multiple receive channels. The receiver and coils are responsible for collecting signals associated with anatomic and physiologic data as well as introducing noise into the system. As a coil increases in size or electrical resistance, more noise is introduced. Amplifiers themselves introduce noise.

Methods of reducing the noise introduced by the receiver have as much bearing on system SNR as the magnet field strength and homogeneity. Noise reduction techniques include the use of smaller coils, implementation of new coil materials or cooling methods to reduce resistance, the use of low-noise amplifiers, and bandwidth reduction methods to filter noise before the signal is digitized[17].

While smaller coils introduce less noise, they also have less penetration. Arrays were initially built to allow a cascade of smaller, anatomically optimized coils to cover a large field of view. In the extreme, the patient would be virtually sleeved into a body cast of conformed coils for a whole body scan. Peripheral vascular coils are examples of current work-in-progress long FOV scanning. The array concept has expanded to include multichannel receivers, which digitally process each component of a quadrature coil; hence, quadrature coils may be considered array coils in some architectures.

The design of the coil differs somewhat between horizontal and vertical magnetic fields. Solenoid or loop coils are often inappropriate in closed-bore scanners because sensitivity must be perpendicular to the magnetic field. They are ideal for vertical fields, however, since the body naturally lies at a right angle to the magnetic field.

Alternatively, quadrature coils built from two pairs of saddle coils offer almost 40 percent improvement in SNR over linear coils, for many closed bore applications. Vertical field systems, however, often see much less improvement compared with linear. This is because the single solenoid coil is very efficient, but the second channel saddle or surface coil is much less so. After blending the two signals and performing uniformity correction, the improvement over a solenoid alone may not be noticeable. For similar reasons, array configurations in open vertical MRI systems require a different design approach, and is currently an active area of research.

GRADIENTS

Advances in gradient technology have been a key factor in the development of many MRI techniques. Reduction in eddy currents via shielding or insulating methods had great ramifications in pulse sequence design, the most notable being fast spin echo (FSE) in the early 1990s. Gradient slew rates are strongly related to minimum TE, acquisition speed, and improved image quality as exemplified by less blur or ringing in FSE sequences. Stronger gradients permit greater resolution through smaller fields of view and thinner slices, and are instrumental in diffusion imaging.

Historically, the drawbacks to faster gradients have been expense and safety concerns. During the 1980s, systems priced at $2 million delivered gradient slew rates of the order of 20 T/ms. By the late 1990s, double this slew rate became standard at costs under $1.5M. Advanced gradients for extreme speed imaging, such as for cardiac applications, are pushing strengths toward 50 mT/m with slew rates promised beyond 200 T/m s.

In terms of safety, physiologic stimulation only becomes an issue when high slew rates are applied over large fields of view[18]. By restricting

the gradients to operate over a smaller region, via smaller patient aperture or specialized gradient coils, faster switching can occur with reduced safety concerns.

Open magnet technology has traditionally operated at lower bandwidths (lower gradient strengths) to reduce noise, thereby regaining some of the SNR disadvantages compared with high field devices[19]. High field systems have traditionally required high bandwidth to avoid its unique artifacts. By the same token, the initial marketing strategy for open scanners was predicated on low cost, comfortable imaging in settings which would likely have little use for high-end academic capabilities requiring much stronger gradients. With the unexpectedly explosive market growth of open MRI, however, high-end applications featuring the gradient enhancements traditionally seen on high field systems will very likely be implemented on third generation open scanners.

COMPUTER TECHNOLOGY

Advances in computer software design strategies and strong competition among computer manufacturers will continue to have tremendous fallout in the diagnostic imaging industry. MRI manufacturers have become adept at developing modular software components and upgrades which almost automatically take advantage of the most recent advances in today's super-fast computing speeds.

Over the past two decades, computer speed has doubled roughly every 18 months[20]. This will result in much faster reconstruction times for both standard imaging and sophisticated postprocessing. Real-time interactive imaging will become much more prominent. Quantitative analysis, image fusion, and other visualization methods which have had slow acceptance in busy non-academic imaging centers will become much faster and generally more usable for the typical imaging practice [Figure 19-3][21].

The 1990s also witnessed enormous growth in computer networking. Network speed has

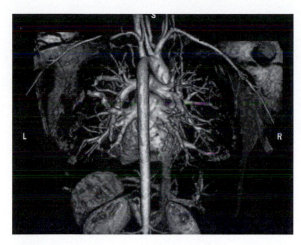

Figure 19-3. Pulmonary MR angiogram of a normal pulmonary tree acquired using contrast enhanced MRA. 3D visualization is becoming a practical means to visualize large raw image data sets from multiple modalities. Reliance on advanced display technology will increase with proven applications, computer systems' speed, ease of use, and cost reduction. (Image courtesy of Vital Images and Andre J. Duerinckx, MD, PhD, Chief of Cardiovascular MRI at the West LA VA Medical Center, Associate Professor of Radiology, & President-elect of the North American Society for Cardiac Imaging (NASCI).)

advanced from the days of slow telephone modems to the degree that home personal computers can achieve faster Internet access than most businesses and universities had in the early 1990s[22]. Together with the development and refinement of standards for data communication and internet security, the picture archiving and communication system (PACS) industry is expected to begin achieving the significant impact that has been promised for more than a decade[23-25].

SEQUENCE DEVELOPMENT

A survey of the academic literature shows MR to be a minefield of acronyms describing a wide variety of pulse sequences. Programmability of these sequences makes an MR system uniquely capable of continual and progressive evolution.

Certainly faster examinations with very high spatial and contrast resolution will continue to be a goal. Functional imaging methods and image-guided procedures will expand MRI applications[26].

The 1980s produced the basis for many of the standard scans performed on a day to day basis: spin echo, multislice, inversion recovery, gradient (field) echo, and 3D. 1980s research yielded early 1990s commercialization and acceptance of MRA. Shielded gradients which minimized eddy currents led to various echo planar imaging (EPI) and fast spin echo techniques in the mid 1990s.

Tissue-specific excitation including magnetization transfer and various fat or fluid suppression techniques are among the methods used to enhance lesion contrast. Single shot fast spin echo sequences have been applied to a growing number of applications: fast T2 weighted imaging such as MRCP and myelography; 3D imaging with reduced susceptibility artifacts such as in the inner ear or lungs; and in conjunction with gating to obtain high in-plane resolution MRA without the use of contrast[27,28].

Although anatomic relationships remain important, increased understanding of cell structure and function is rapidly moving toward diagnosis and treatment at the cellular level. By the late 1990s diffusion imaging and proton spectroscopy have become well accepted, with other forms of functional imaging (perfusion, blood oxygenation level dependent or BOLD, multi-nuclear spectroscopy) likely to become mainstream in years to follow. Key improvements will involve speed to shorten the time to diagnosis, minimize artifacts, and permit expansion of functional imaging to cardiac and abdominal applications.

Sequences optimized to various contrast agents will play a major role in future applications. Bolus-catch MRA methods offer fast, artifact-free alternatives to conventional MRA. Blood pool agents will overcome critical timing issues. Hepatocellular specific agents promise to improve liver imaging[29].

The measurement of tissue characteristics using imaging agents that target specific cells using monoclonal antibodies, liposomes, and short peptides bound to chelates containing paramagnetic atoms will be used to evaluate the chemical composition of tumors. This will have direct impact on diagnosis, therapy planning, and therapy monitoring[30,31].

As MRI manufacturers invest more resources in open MRI technology, capabilities thought to be unique to high field will gradually become incorporated on these scanners. Indeed, diffusion imaging, true fat suppression, real time inter-active imaging, and various forms of echo planar imaging have already been incorporated on lower field scanners.

NEURORADIOLOGY

The "decade of the brain" resulted in much greater awareness of stroke, now often referred to as a "brain attack." Diffusion has grown in popularity for identifying acute infarcts and helping to differentiate old versus new stroke. Diffusion is generally seen as a means of identifying irreversible stroke, while perfusion studies demonstrate at-risk brain[32]. In the future,

Expert Perspective
Neuroradiology

William W. Orrison, Jr

As a neuroradiologist, I am constantly amazed at the progress that continues to occur in modern imaging. Neuroimaging has often led the way in the development of new imaging methods, and modern neuroimaging must rank as one of the most successful stories in the history of medicine. For many of us, the memories of archaic practices such as pneumoencephalography have been overwhelmed by techniques such as computed tomography (CT), and magnetic resonance (MR) imaging. Although single photon emission computed tomography (SPECT) has been in use for almost a quarter of century, the use of this technique to provide information regarding brain function is more recent, as is the addition of positron emission tomography (PET). The most recent developments in brain functional analysis have included functional magnetic resonance imaging (fMRI) and magnetic source imaging (MSI). MSI combines MR and magnetoencephalography (MEG) into a single image or magnetic source image. It is also possible to include the more traditional information from electroencephalography (EEG) on these magnetic source images as well as the vascular detail from magnetic resonance angiography (MRA) or magnetic resonance venography (MRV).

In addition, the ever increasingly important information available from magnetic resonance spectroscopy (MRS) may also be available. One of the most exciting areas of future imaging developments involves the incorporation of multiple methods of brain assessment into a single image using high resolution MR as the template. This includes information from fMRI, MEG, EEG, SPECT, PET, CT, MRS, MRA, and/or MRV. Through the use of advanced computer techniques it is not only possible to illustrate all of this anatomic and functional information on a single image set, but it is also possible to view this information in three dimensional space and, when appropriate, in a real-time format.

Radiology in general, and MR in particular, is moving into a new era where both structure and function play an increasingly important role. As we develop higher resolution techniques that allow us to visualize smaller structures, methods are simultaneously being developed that allow us to follow bodily functions from the most mundane to the most complex. It is indeed an exciting time to be involved in medical imaging, and MR serves as the launching pad into the next millennium.

the stroke workup may also consist of fMRI[33]. Despite the foreseeable development of a complete MRI stroke package, helical multislice CT and relatively inexpensive and accessible ultrasound systems using echo-enhancing agents will rival MRI for stroke imaging[34].

Neurological applications of diffusion and perfusion beyond stroke include the assessment of tumor vascularity, demyelinating disease, pediatric brain development, trauma, and perhaps dementia. Because of their clinical utility, these techniques will likely become commonplace and manufacturers will likely increase baseline gradient specifications. Post-processing will certainly improve both in the visual presentation of complex data sets and in automation.

MR spectroscopy (MRS) is rapidly progressing into non-academic clinics, in part due to its acceptance by insurance payers and ease of use. Proton MRS applications include distinguishing between necrotic tissue, recurring tumor, brain injuries, infarct, or clarifying the nature of metabolic disorders. In epilepsy, spectroscopic studies have been useful in localizing the epileptogenic zone in intractable focal epilepsy. Future applications include its use as a means of observing the transport and metabolism of various compounds in the brain, including assessing the short-term effects of CNS targeted pharmacological interventions[35]. Although other nuclei, such as ^{13}C, $^{14/15}$N, ^{19}F, ^{39}K, and $^{35/37}$Cl facilitate the imaging of metabolites closely related to many disease states, they suffer from low abundance and very small SNR. As an alternative to very high field imaging of these nuclei, various coupling mechanisms which use proton imaging to magnify the spectrum from other nuclei are in development [Figure 19-4].

High-resolution imaging using small fields of view and special coils will expand MR neurography for evaluation of peripheral nerve pathology[36]. Acquisition improvements in speed, SNR, and contrast offer improved sensitivity and specificity for multiple sclerosis lesions[37]. Combining quantitative signal changes in brain structures of schizophrenics with neurocircuit

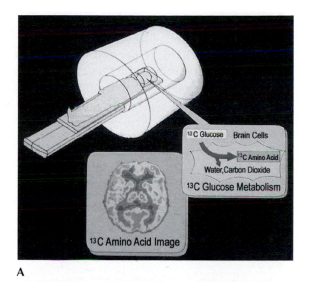

A

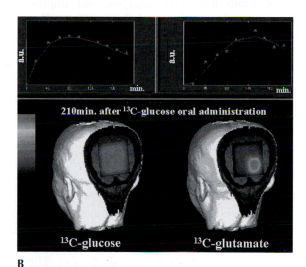

B

Figure 19-4. Imaging of synthesized amino acids using MRI after administration of carbon-13 glucose represents a highly sensitive technique to observe hydrogen-1 coupled to carbon-13. MRS followed by superimposition of functional information on anatomic MR images offers a safe, nonradioactive tool for the early diagnosis of metabolic and psychiatric disorders. (This work was performed as part of the National Research & Development Programs for Medical and Welfare Apparatus under entrustment by the New Energy and Industrial Technology Development Organization (NEDO).)

expand the clinical utility of MRA to the evaluation of the abdominal, thoracic, and peripheral vasculature. Bolus timing is critical, and has led to several new developments, such as automatic triggering or dynamic imaging. Various forms of projection or partial data update techniques allow a stream of images to be collected while the contrast is flowing through the area of interest, thereby obviating the need for bolus triggering. As interactive imaging techniques evolve, real-time subtraction methods will emerge similar to X-ray digital subtraction angiography (DSA)[48]. New coil designs will permit extended field-of-view imaging, such as aortic arch to intracranial circulation or peripheral vessel MRA.

Blood-pool agents allow for longer acquisitions, permitting higher resolution and minimizing hardware requirements, because the contrast remains in the blood vessel for a relatively long time[49]. Contrast can be eliminated altogether using gating with an in-plane acquisition and relying on the natural relaxation of blood to give vessel detail [Figure 19-5]. Both of these methods are improved by postprocessing to separate arterial and venous flow.

Endovascular coils offer intraluminal views at very high resolution and may have applications in central nervous system (CNS) aneurysms, trans-jugular intrahepatic portal shunt (TIPS) procedures, and renal artery treatment. Pulmonary imaging with hyperpolarized gases, very short TEs, and advanced fast spin echo imaging have been proposed as a means for addressing susceptibility induced signal loss.

ORTHOPEDIC MRI

Musculoskeletal imaging techniques and equipment are keen focus areas for MRI research. General improvements in MRI will likely include low-noise coil development, new ergonomic scanner designs intended to improve patient comfort and reduce siting costs, enhanced access to facilitate interventional procedures, and specialized joint imaging techniques, including the ability to apply or simulate weight loading[50]. The

Expert Perspective
Orthopedic MRI

Phillip J. Tirman

Evaluation of the musculoskeletal system has changed dramatically because of the impact of the diagnostic power of MRI, perhaps more than any other discipline. The job description for a "musculoskeletal radiologist" or technologist barely resembles that found even as late as the latter half of the 1980s. Routine MRI examinations have become commonplace around the world because of the advantages of high soft tissue contrast and spatial resolution as well as the physiologic information over other imaging modalities. A wide variety of disorders that were not detected by other modalities are well depicted by MRI and we are now to the point where MRI is essentially a screening test for many causes of pain in the skeletal system. Because of the advances in MR imaging technology, more patients that were previously excluded from MRI because of claustrophobia and size now can receive a high quality examination with state of the art pulse sequences.

As MRI has discovered the effect of some disorders on the body not previously known such as bone marrow edema in the setting of a bone trabecular injury, many more discoveries are sure to be found. Improved depiction of hyaline cartilage will allow the specialty trained orthopedic surgeon to plan cartilage repair procedures without the necessity of two surgical procedures. The increased prevalence of accurate arthroscopic procedures underscores the need for prearthroscopic evaluation.

The future of musculoskeletal MRI is very bright indeed. One can envision a more clinically oriented MRI suite where the radiologist, in concert with the referring clinician, can perform limited physical examination with MRI as the "fluoroscope", observing real-time many disorders that afflict joints and other parts of the body. In this way a type of "holistic evaluation center" can be developed. Improved imaging techniques will allow blood flow/perfusion information, motion, and other physiologic information to be obtained routinely allowing many aspects of a disease to be evaluated with a single modality thus obviating the need for other, sometimes costly, investigations.

success of low-cost, office-based, joint-imaging systems will partly depend on the role orthopedic physicians will have in imaging, which in turn depends on their ability to navigate the maze of state and federal laws regarding self-referral of patients that began with California Congressman Fourtney "Pete" Stark several years ago, as well as their knowledge about imaging techniques and business practices.

Imaging trauma patients with MRI can be invaluable due to the many soft tissue injuries that cannot be readily diagnosed with plain film X-ray. Sequences continue to be developed for cartilage imaging, with impact on both trauma evaluation and therapy for osteoarthritis, including very high resolution 3D, fat suppression, and magnetization transfer imaging[51].

The value of dynamic, or kinematic, MR imaging remains under investigation[52]. The key advantages of MRI over X-ray fluoroscopy include its soft tissue contrast and the ability to image joint motion in any plane, even curved planes using postprocessing. Stepped and real-time acquisitions each offer advantages and disadvantages. While fluoroscopic imaging more accurately represents the inertial characteristics of the joint, stepped acquisitions permit increased resolution, improved SNR, and contrast control. Research on postprocessing methods that provide detailed kinematic model parameters will require clinical validation of their usefulness before orthopedic surgeons accept them clinically.

Whole body T1 and STIR MRI has been proposed as a replacement to bone scintigraphy to confirm or exclude metastatic spread to the skeleton[53,54]. Techniques which merge individual acquisitions into a single long field of view can be used to mimic the typical bone scan film.

Joint imaging using direct intra-articular injection of contrast has proven extremely useful for rotator cuff and glenoid labrum pathology. Indirect MR arthrography is a relatively new method using intravenous injections. Current studies indicate that this less invasive form of MR arthrography may be just as accurate as direct methods[55].

Intervertebral disc disease and spinal stenosis are common application areas for MRI. Modern MRI scanners demonstrate structural status well, but the functional impact of these structural alterations, as well as treatment planning and outcomes assessment remains an active area of imaging research[56,57].

INTERVENTIONAL MRI

Interest in interventional MRI (iMRI) has grown substantially with the popularity of open MRI scanners[58-60]. The term "interventional" implies many procedures: from percutaneous approaches to open surgery, intravascular techniques to energy ablation. Although open systems appear to be the more appropriate means for conducting iMRI, conventional closed-bore systems can be used for frameless stereotactic procedures, intravascular methods, and "in-out" intraoperative mode[61]. As with any image-guided intervention, the purpose of employing MRI would be to minimize the degree of invasion by intraprocedurally providing the physician with accurate knowledge of the location and types of tissue. Applications of minimally invasive iMRI include disk surgery, vertebroplasty, nerve blocks, liver biopsy, breast biopsy, and tumor ablation[62].

X-ray, CT, and angiography have long been used for imaging based intervention. Ultrasound suffers from acoustic window limitations and less image detail. MRI avoids ionizing radiation while offering better soft tissue discrimination and acquisition in any plane. However, there are several important considerations to be addressed before MRI can achieve mainstream utility for interventional procedures.

If open surgery is the goal, cost is an enormous concern since the magnet itself represents only a fraction of the total investment. Siting a scanner and controlling its magnetic field within an operating room, the purchase of MRI-compatible devices, and the addition of in-room fluoroscopy can make the cost of an otherwise less expensive open scanner many times that of the most expensive closed-bore scanners. It can

Expert Perspective
Interventional MRI

William Bradley

Interventional/intraoperative MRI technology will be increasingly embraced by neurosurgeons and radiologists. Over the next five years, intraoperative MR systems will become as common as operating microscopes in hospitals doing sufficient volumes of neurosurgery. While such systems are usually shared by radiologists and neurosurgeons today, I suspect there will be a bifurcation in magnet technology, surgeons migrating towards higher field, short bore systems using the "in and out" approach with radiologists continuing to perform biopsies (particularly of the breast) with the patient in the magnet.

Even though we now have only a few years experience with interventional MRI in the neurosurgical environment, it has become obvious that 60–80 percent of the time surgeons leave tumor behind when they think they've gotten it all out. For low grade tumors, this can mean the difference between ultimate survival and death, since the remaining tumor tends to degenerate into a much more malignant form. The increasing availability of MR compatible breast biopsy devices will make the increased sensitivity of gadolinium-enhanced MRI more widely implemented for diagnosis of cancers which can't be seen by either mammography or ultrasound.

Similarly, interventional MRI will be used more and more to guide thermal/cryoablations for the same reasons MRI has replaced CT and ultrasound for routine diagnosis: increased tissue contrast. Interventional MRI will also be heavily utilized as we migrate from traditional surgical solutions to "minimally invasive therapies". Using MR guidance in an open architecture system, tumors, e.g., in the breast, brain, and liver will be entered under MR guidance and using various thermal techniques heated to the point of coagulation necrosis, all through a percutaneous route. At the other end of the temperature scale, MR will be used increasingly to guide cryoablations, e.g., in the prostate, where ultrasound guidance has proven to be less than adequate.

also hinder access to conventional reimbursement. When an MRI installation is planned primarily for standard imaging applications with only the occasional percutaneous procedure, fewer siting modifications are necessary[63,64].

Interactive imaging, tracking systems, and more sophisticated yet less confusing display strategies represent key works-in-progress for the MRI system itself. Although MR compatible equipment was initially a major area of concern, the number of manufacturers involved in device research and development has blossomed[65]. Alterations in the magnet architecture for the purpose of interventional ergonomics may force trade-offs in important imaging parameters, such as field-of-view, signal-to-noise ratio, and homogeneity. Robotic assistive devices offer the possibility of remote controlled approaches, with the potential for improved hand stability.

CARDIAC MRI

Cardiac MRI has become an accurate modality for diagnosis of adult and pediatric cardiac conditions[66,67]. However, the elusive goal of a single scanner able to meet all cardiac imaging needs has not been met, primarily due to the difficulties inherent in coronary imaging. Single-shot EPI, gated multishot techniques, motion correction, curved surface reconstruction of 3D data sets [Figure 19-6], and other enhancements have dramatically improved the quality of coronary imaging, but they still do not rival the consistency, accuracy, and confidence of X-ray angiography. Although more than 10 percent of cardiac catheterization procedures prove negative, if the coronary artery imaging is not reliable or extensive enough, cardiologists will be unlikely to assume the risk and will continue to perform the more invasive catheter based study. To be fully accepted by cardiologists, MRI may need to deliver high-quality coronary artery imaging[68]. Much of the development activity in attempting to image the coronary arteries may have as its primary success the "NASA factor," i.e., other as yet unknown applications will

Expert Perspective

Cardiac MRI

David Feiglin

The immediate clinical value of cardiac MRI resides in two areas: anatomic evaluation of the heart, and functional evaluation of the heart. At this time evaluation of the coronary vessels and quantitative estimates of flow and valvular disease remain more in the experimental realm.

The utility of gated fast spin echo allows for good differentiation of myocardial tissue from signal void of blood. This allows determination of myocardial and pericardial thickness as well as for discerning atrial (myxoma) or ventricular tumors. A small but significant number of patients that have unusual arrhythmias include a group of patients with abnormal fat deposition and deterioration, particularly involving the right ventricle. Diagnosis is very difficult with echocardiography and other imaging modalities but readily determined using spin echo sequences (T1 weighted) and fat suppressed inversion recovery sequences to determine the relative activity of the pathological process. Combinations of gradient echo, inversion recovery and spin echo (T1 and T2 weighted) sequences allow for accurate determination of pericardial pathology.

Current availability of fast gradient echo sequences (using breath-hold techniques) allows for multislice acquisition encompassing the whole cardiac volume. Temporal resolution of image data can be much less than 10 ms and spatial resolution with 512 matrices can allow pixel sizes that are much less than 1.0 mm in plane. The trade off of spatial resolution, temporal resolution and acquisition times are determined on a patient-by-patient basis. However, a complete volumetric data set of the heart encompassing 20–30 image sets in the cardiac cycle can be accomplished within a few minutes with current high-field magnets. Equally accurate data can be acquired on low-field magnets (e.g. 0.2 T) but involve a somewhat longer scanning time. The acquired data allows for both right and left ventricular functional data to be acquired: specifically ejection fraction. Other parameters such as contraction and relaxation times of the ventricles can also be acquired. The data is as accurate as that acquired by echocardiography and nuclear medicine, but allows for right ventricular assessment, which cannot be currently easily done with other imaging modalities. The follow-up of patients on chemotherapy as well as myopathies, not to mention patients with lung disease, can be easily performed and clinically used with cardiac MRI.

---

emerge due to the technological advances derived from demanding cardiac research.

Cardiologists' involvement in MRI will likely drive the more advanced cardiac applications. In the short-term, proven applications such as tumor imaging, pulmonary vasculature, and aorta imaging will probably dominate. As MRI post-processing continues to emulate and improve on that of nuclear medicine, the number and types of applications will expand. For example, stress cine wall visualization and ejection fraction measurements can be used to reveal chemotherapy overdosing.

Better methods for automatically segmenting the chambers from the myocardium, assisted by new pulse sequences and contrast agents which will aid in creating more discernible boundaries, will enable faster computers to quickly generate cardiac function curves and provide more sophisticated displays of 3-D dynamic movement. Although physical stress testing is more difficult with MRI, pharmacological stress should be an acceptable alternative.

Improved ECG signal acquisition and processing will improve the reliability and accuracy of cardiac gating. Image-based gating and motion correction algorithms will supplement conventional gating to further minimize artifact and permit higher resolution imaging even in the presence of severe arrhythmias. In-room control

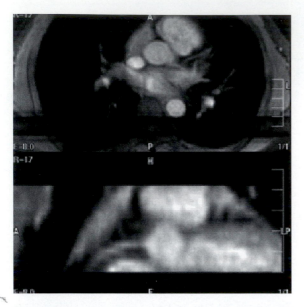

Figure 19-6. Coronary artery imaging using MRI is still not used for regular clinical imaging, but advancements in acquisition speed, motion correction, and display technologies show promise in visualizing proximal branches of the coronary tree.

will enable the physician to manipulate image acquisition in real time, as in echocardiography[69]. Simultaneous acquisition of the left and right ventricles, together with quantitative velocity estimation, will improve treatment of valvular dysfunction[70].

Cardiac care represents an enormous market, and once a critical threshold of development and applicability has been achieved, every MRI facility will want these capabilities.

BODY MRI

CT and ultrasound continue to be the dominant abdominal and thoracic imaging choices, but improvements in speed, contrast agents, and pulse sequences have led to much wider use of MR imaging. Phased-array body coils and endorectal coils have provided increased SNR, which has been applied to both higher resolution imaging and faster scans.

Expert Perspective
Body MRI

Mark Winkler

MRI of the body has matured as an imaging modality. It is no longer viewed as an adjunctive problem-solving modality. It has begun to assume the role of a primary imaging modality.

In the chest, MR is no longer limited to a problem-solving role when chest CT, echocardiography, or nuclear medicine prove insufficient due to the inability to use contrast, patient body habitus, or resolution limitations. Chest MR has assumed a primary role in evaluating cardiac anatomy and function as well as for MR angiography of the great vessels. MR shows great potential for more accurate ventilation/perfusion imaging of the lungs as well as for screening for coronary artery disease. MR will not be able to fully supplant chest CT as its evaluation of pulmonary parenchyma is limited by magnetic susceptibility.

In the abdomen MR is no longer just a problem-solving modality to differentiate hepatic hemangiomas more specifically or adrenal adenomas from malignancies. It has begun to assume a primary role in oncologic staging of the liver, adrenal glands, and lymph nodes. Abdominal MRA is now the best screening study for the evaluation of the abdominal aorta and renal arteries. Contrast-enhanced renal MRI is equivalent to contrast-enhanced CT for the evaluation of renal masses, and is the modality of choice in a patient with impaired renal function. CT will continue in its role as the strongest imaging modality for evaluation of the bowel, mesentery, and urinary calculi.

In the pelvis MRI rapidly established itself as the primary imaging modality for tumors involving the uterus and cervix. It has a competitive role in evaluation of the prostate and ovaries. The potential of MR spectroscopy could advance the role of MR in tumor evaluation in the pelvis. Pelvic sonography will continue as the most cost effective screening tool for gynecologic and obstetric workups and CT will continue in its primary role for the evaluation of bowl masses and inflammatory disease.

Clinical applications in thoracic imaging include evaluation of mediastinal masses, hilar lesions, pleura and the chest wall, pulmonary vasculature, and pretherapeutic evaluation of intrathoracic masses[71]. Pulmonary imaging improvements include the use of hyperpolarized gases and very short TE sequences to mitigate susceptibility related signal loss[72].

MR hydrography, especially MR cholangio-pancreatography (MRCP), using 2D and 3D half Fourier FSE have become competitive with ERCP[73,74]. MRCP guided intervention has the potential to limit the use of invasive transpapillary and percutaneous methods[75]. MRA techniques such as those discussed above have been used for noninvasive imaging of portal venous disease in Budd Chiari disease, before placement of trans-jugular intrahepatic portosystemic shunts (TIPS), and for pancreatic cancer staging[76]. While ultrasound dominates in the area of prostate imaging[77], improvements in intensity correction and array coils are expected to increase the utility of MRI.

Liver imaging continues to improve with the development of new intravenous contrast agents, which either darken (particulate agents) or brighten (hepatobiliary agents) the liver parenchyma[78]. These agents may be less necessary on low and mid field MRI, which exhibit sufficient natural T1 contrast between lesion and parenchyma[79].

Renal cancer is diagnosed in 27 000 Americans and accounts for 12 000 deaths per year. In addition to improvements in detection and characterization of renal masses by new MRI techniques, MRS may help provide completely new insight into our understanding of renal cancer[80]. Renal function assessment using quantitative perfusion is a promising approach for noninvasive differentiation between renovascular and renoparenchymal diseases[81].

Women's health issues, particularly screening and staging for cervical and breast cancer, have become very active areas of MRI research. Mammography and ultrasound remain the most practical and reliable procedures for routine breast

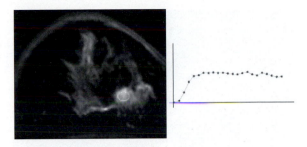

Figure 19-7. Breast cancer detection using dynamic contrast uptake analysis is greatly improved by automatically generating images representative of the dynamics (e.g., slope of the enhancement curve shown on the left) rather than expecting the user to evaluate numerical ROI graphs (right).

cancer screening[82]. However, mammography is often inconclusive due to prior surgery, dense breasts, or silicone implants[83]. High-contrast, high-resolution dynamic contrast-enhanced breast MRI has become useful in staging and determining the extent of breast cancer[84] and MR guided biopsy and intervention promise to augment X-ray guided approaches[85,86]. Improved automation in the processing and display of dynamic data will make these methods more accepted in general practice [Figure 19-7]. There is also growing evidence that MRI is superior to, and less expensive than CT and ultrasound in the workup of endometrial and cervical cancer[87]. MRI has also been shown to be a valid complement to ultrasound in fetal imaging using single shot fast spin echo [Figure 19-8][88].

Interventional and functional MRI, virtual endoscopy and cholinoscopy, and molecular activity imaging such as diffusion and spectroscopy are expected to play a significant role in future abdominal imaging[89]. Limitations in conventional histopathological tissue diagnosis coupled with improvements in MR spectroscopy motivate a growing contribution of MRS to both the clinical management of disease and the determination of disease mechanisms[90]. The human genome project has yielded the promise of correcting genetic defects through gene therapy,

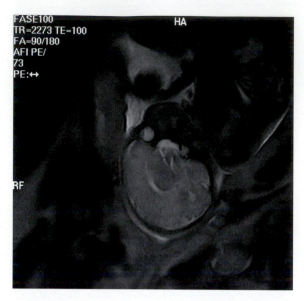

Figure 19-8. Single shot fast spin echo permits imaging of the fetal brain and is an evolving application that may allow early diagnosis and treatment of developmental defects.

and given that MR imaging of gene delivery systems has already been accomplished in animal models and cell cultures, the future of MRI in this exciting new area of medicine is extremely bright[91].

REFERENCES

1. Brice J. Industry panel reveals brave new world of MR. *Diagn Imaging* July 1998.
2. Rothenberg LN, Nath R, Price RR, et al. A Perspective on the New Millennium. *Radiology* 209:600–603, 1998.
3. Bradley WG. How to increase volume while maintaining quality. *Diagn Imaging* 27–28, April 1998.
4. Kaufman L, Arakawa M, et al. In: Margulis AR, Gooding CA, eds. *Low Field MRI in Diagnostic Radiology.* University of California, San Francisco: Radiology Research and Education Foundation, 1989.
5. Goyen M. Communication eases patient anxiety over MRI. *Diagn Imaging Eur* 15, Dec 1997.
6. Melendez JC, McCrank E. Anxiety-related reactions associated with magnetic resonance imaging examinations. *JAMA* 6:745–747, 1993.
7. Kaufman L, Carlson J, et al. Open magnet technology for MRI. *Admin Radiol J* 28–35, May 1996.
8. Domestic MRI industry heads toward billion-dollar sales year. *MR Ind Rep* 1, Sept 1998.
9. Clisham G. Strategies that optimize quality and applications will aid open-MRI growth. *MR Ind Rep* 20, Sept 1998.
10. Davis M. High- vs. low-field MR: What's the difference? *Diagn Imaging (Open MRI Supplement)* October 1998.
11. Krotz D. Dedicated MR redefines scanning of extremities. *Diagn Imaging* 49–55, Dec 1997.
12. Hand-held scanner points way to new opportunities. *MRI Ind Rep* 4, Dec 1998.
13. Morgan P, et al. A readout magnet for prepolarized MRI. *Magn Reson Med* 36:527–536, 1996.
14. Brice J. Ohio State to install world's first 8-tesla whole-body MRI. *Imaging News, Diagn Imaging*, 1998.
15. Schenck JF. MR safety at high magnetic fields. *Magn Reson Imaging Clin N Am* 6:715–730, 1998.
16. Schenk JF, Leue WM. Instrumentation: magnets, coils, and hardware. In: Atlas SW, ed. *Magnetic Resonance Imaging of the Brain and Spine*, 2nd ed. Philadelphia: Lippincott-Raven, 5, 1996.
17. Lazarus-Karaoglan T. Medical electronics. *IEEE Spectrum Technology 1999 (Analysis and Forecast Issue)* 82, Jan 1999.
18. Schaefer DJ. Safety aspects of switched gradient fields. *Magn Reson Imaging Clin N Am* 6:731–748, 1998.
19. Winkler ML, Kaufman L. Matched bandwidth technology, cost implications. *Admin Radiol*, Oct 1987.
20. Gates B. *The Road Ahead.* Penguin Books, 34, 1996.
21. Krotz D. Volumetric 3-D imaging. *Diagn Imaging* 48–53, Jan 1999.
22. Computing in the New Millennium. *PC Magazine.* 9 June, 1998.
23. Fishman EK. 3D CT angio might give PACS a jump start. *Diagn Imaging* 31–32, June 1998.
24. Gropper A. Internet approach promises cost-benefits to PACS users. *Diagn Imaging* 59–64, Feb 1999.
25. *J Digital Imaging* 11 (Suppl 2), Nov 1998.
26. Del Maschio A, Panizza P. MR state of the art. *Eur J Radiol* 27 (Suppl 2):S250–S253, 1998.
27. Kassai Y, Makita J, Sugiura S, et al. Increase in FASE speed and new applications. *Toshiba Medical Review*, No. 69, 32–40, Aug 1999.
28. Mitsuoka H, Arai H, et al. Microanatomy of the cerebellopontine angle and internal auditory canal: study with new magnetic resonance imaging technique using three-dimensional fast spin echo. *Neurosurgery* 44: 561–567, 1999.
29. Sandrick K. Newer agents contest gadolinium's dominance in contrast MR exams. *Diagn Imaging* 41, Feb 1999.
30. Calvo BF, Semelka RC. Beyond anatomy: MR imaging as a molecular diagnostic tool. *Surg Oncol Clin N Am* 8:171–183, 1999.

31. Rand SD, Frost R, Haughton V. MR spectroscopy extends MRI's diagnostic potential. *Diagn Imaging* 36–42, Feb 1998.

32. Pomeranz SJ. Mini-series on Functional Imaging – Diffusion Imaging. *CMRS Vision* V:1, 1999.

33. Berry I, Ranjeva JP, Duthil P, Manelfe C. Diffusion and perfusion MRI, measurements of acute stroke events and outcome: present practice and future hope. *Cerebrovasc Dis* 8 (Suppl 2):8–16, 1998.

34. Ringelstein EB. Echo-enhanced ultrasound for diagnosis and management in stroke patients. *Eur J Ultrasound* (Suppl 3):S3–15, 1998.

35. Novotny E, Ashwal S, Shevell M. Proton magnetic resonance spectroscopy: an emerging technology in pediatric neurology research. *Pediatr Res* 44:1–10, 1998.

36. Maravilla KR, Bowen BC. Imaging of the peripheral nervous system: evaluation of peripheral neuropathy and plexopathy. *AJNR* 19:1011–1023, 1998.

37. Filippi M. The role of non-conventional magnetic resonance techniques in monitoring evolution of multiple sclerosis. *J Neurol Neurosurg Psychiatry* 64 (Suppl 1): S52–S58, 1998.

38. Okazaki Y. Morphological brain imaging studies on major psychoses. *Psychiatr Clin Neurosci* 52 (Suppl): S215–S218, 1998.

39. Weiss KL, Figueroa RE, Allison J. Functional MR imaging in patients with epilepsy. *Magn Reson Imaging Clin N Am* 6:95–112, 1998.

40. Laughlin S, Montanera W. Central nervous system imaging. When is CT more appropriate than MRI? *Postgrad Med* 104:73–76, 81–84, 87–88, 1998.

41. Doraiswamy PM, Steffens DC, Pitchumoni S, Tabrizi S. Early recognition of Alzheimer's disease: what is consensual? What is controversial? What is practical? *J Clin Psychiatr* 59 (Suppl 13):6–18, 1998.

42. Soininen HS, Scheltens P. Early diagnostic indices for the prevention of Alzheimer's disease. *Ann Med* 30: 553–559, 1998.

43. Rosen BR, Buckner RL, Dale AM. Event-related functional MRI: past, present, and future. *Proc Natl Acad Sci USA* 95:773–780, 1998.

44. Biederman RW, Fuisz AR, Pohost GM. Magnetic resonance angiography. *Curr Opin Cardiol* 13:430–437, 1998.

45. Kauczor HU. Contrast-enhanced magnetic resonance angiography of the pulmonary vasculature: A review. *Invest Radiol* 33:606–617, 1998.

46. Ward J, Burch D, Prince M. MRA volume grows as new applications emerge. *Diagn Imaging* 56–61, Feb 1998.

47. Runge VM. Contrast Enhanced MR Angiography (CE-MRA). *CMRS Vision* V:1, 1999.

48. Reimer P, Landwehr P. Non-invasive vascular imaging of peripheral vessels. *Eur Radiol* 8:858–872, 1998.

49. Muhler A. The future of contrast-enhanced magnetic resonance angiography. Are blood pool agents needed? (Editorial). *Invest Radiol* 33:709–714, 1998.

50. Danielson BI, et al. Axial loading of the spine during CT and MR in patients with suspected lumbar spinal stenosis. *ACTA Radiol* 39:604–611, 1998.

51. Cooper JR. Drug research drives wider use of MRI in arthritis. *Diagn Imaging* 29, Dec 1998.

52. Shellock FG, Mink JH, Fox JM. Patellofemoral joint: kinematic MR imaging to assess tracking abnormalities. *Radiology* 168:551–553, 1988.

53. Bares R. Skeletal scintigraphy in breast cancer management. *Q J Nucl Med* 42:43–48, 1998.

54. Steinborn MM, Heuck AF, et al. Whole-body bone marrow MRI in patients with metastatic disease to the skeletal system. *J Comput Assist Tomogr* 23:123–129, 1999.

55. Vahlensieck M, Sommer T, et al. Indirect MR arthrography: techniques and applications. *Eur Radiol* 8:232–235, 1998.

56. Cassar-Pullicino VN. MRI of the ageing and herniating intervertebral disc. *Eur J Radiol* 27:214–228, 1998.

57. Fritz JM, Delitto A, Welch WC, Erhard RE. Lumbar spinal stenosis: a review of current concepts in evaluation, management, and outcome measurements. *Arch Phys Med Rehabil* 79:700–708, 1998.

58. Gronemeyer DH, Rainer MM, et al. Low-field design eases MRI-guided biopsies. *Diagn Imaging*, 47:139–143, 1991.

59. Jolesz FA. Genesis of interventional MRI. *JMRI* 8:2, 1998.

60. Jolesz FA. Interventional and intraoperative MRI: A general overview of the field. *JMRI* 8:3–7, 1998.

61. Gildenberg PL. Stereotactic surgery – the past and the future. *Stereotact Funct Neurosurg* 70:57–70, 1998.

62. Onik GM, Helms C. Nuances in percutaneous discectomy. *Radiol Clin North Am* 36:523–532, 1998.

63. Jolesz FA, Kettenbach J, Grundfest WS. Cost-effectiveness of image-guided surgery. *Acad Radiol* 5 (Suppl 2): S428–S431, 1998.

64. Krotz D. Interventional MR pricey but occupies unique role. *Diagn Imaging* 39–42, April 1998.

65. Jolesz FA, Morrison PR, et al. Compatible instrumentation for intraoperative MRI: expanding resources. *J Magn Reson Imaging* 8:8–11, 1998.

66. Hartnell GG. New developments in cardiac magnetic resonance imaging. *Hosp Med* 59:567–573, 1998.

67. Boothroyd A. Magnetic resonance – its current and future role in paediatric cardiac radiology. *Eur J Radiol* 26:154–162, 1998.

68. Brice J. Cardiac MR closes in on ischemic heart disease. *Diagn Imaging* 44, Aug 1998.

69. Yang PC, Kerr AB, et al. New real-time interactive cardiac magnetic resonance imaging system

complements echocardiography. *J Am Coll Cardiol* 32:2049–2056, 1998.

70. Wyttenbach R, Bremerich J, Saeed M, Higgins CB. Integrated MR imaging approach to valvular heart disease. *Cardiol Clin* 16:277–294, 1998.

71. Bittner RC, Felix R. Magnetic resonance (MR) imaging of the chest: state-of-the-art. *Eur Respir J* 11:1392–1404, 1998.

72. Harty MP, Kramer SS. Recent advances in pediatric pulmonary imaging. *Curr Opin Pediatr* 10:227–235, 1998.

73. Barish MA, Ferrucci JT. MR cholangiopancreatography challenges invasive methods. *Diagn Imaging* 32–36, April 1998.

74. Neuhaus H. The future of endoscopic retrograde cholangiopancreatography: what is necessary and what should be improved? *Endoscopy* 30:A207–A211, 1998.

75. Takehara Y. Can MRCP replace ERCP? *J Magn Reson Imaging* 8:517–534, 1998.

76. Haycox A, Lombard M, Neoptolemos J, Walley T. Review article: current practice and future perspectives in detection and diagnosis of pancreatic cancer. *Aliment Pharmacol Ther* 12:937–948, 1998.

77. Wasserman NF. Imaging benign prostate disease: prostatitis. *Contemp Urol* 27–40, Nov 1998.

78. Clement O, Iauve N, Lewin M, de Kerviler E, Cuenod CA, Frija G. Contrast agents in magnetic resonance imaging of the liver: present and future. *Biomed Pharmacother* 52:51–58, 1998.

79. Winkler ML. MR Imaging in Oncology. *Open MRI Conference, Educational Symposia*, Las Vegas, March 1999.

80. Kramer LA. Magnetic resonance imaging of renal masses. *World J Urol* 16:22–28, 1998.

81. Aumann S, et al. Quantification of renal perfusion: results of an experimental animal study. Abstract 1857. *ISMRM Seventh Scientific Meeting and Exhibition*, Philadelphia, 1999.

82. Samuels TH. Breast imaging: A look at current and future technologies. *Postgrad Med* 104:91–94, 97–101, Nov 1998.

83. Ziewacz JT, Neumann DP, et al. The difficult breast. *Surg Oncol Clin N Am* 8:17–33, 1999.

84. Harms SE. Integration of breast magnetic resonance imaging with breast cancer treatment. *Magn Reson Imaging* 9:79–91, 1998.

85. Harms SE. Breast magnetic resonance imaging. *Semin Ultrasound CT MR* 19:104–120, 1998.

86. Friedrich M. MRI of the breast: state of the art. *Eur Radiol* 8:707–725, 1998.

87. Ascher SM. Imaging issues in women's health: current challenges and potential contributions of magnetic resonance. International Society for Magnetic Resonance in Medicine, Seventh Scientific Meeting and Exhibition, Philadelphia, 22–28 May 1999, p. 288.

88. Garel C, Brisse H, Sebag G, Elmaleh M, Oury JF, Hassan M. Magnetic resonance imaging of the fetus. *Pediatr Radiol* 28:201–211, 1998.

89. Ferrucci JT. Advances in abdominal MR imaging. *Radiographics* 18:1569–1586, 1998.

90. Mountford C. Spectroscopy rediscovered: the gold standard for the next millennium. International Society for Magnetic Resonance in Medicine, Seventh Scientific Meeting and Exhibition, Philadelphia, 22–28 May 1999, p. 290.

91. Moonen CTW, Madio D, Olsen A, et al. On the feasibility of MRI-guided focused ultrasound for local induction of gene expression. Presented at the Fifth Scientific Meeting and Exhibition of the International Society for Magnetic Resonance in Medicine; Vancouver, British Columbia, April 1997.

Glossary

2DFT: Two dimensional Fourier transformation of the time domain signal.

3DFT: The signal is collected during slice selection as a "slab" instead of unique slices. During Fourier transformation, the slab is reconstructed to thin slices. The advantage of 3DFT is increased signal collected during the acquisition.

#A: Atomic mass number, the total number of protons and neutrons in a given nucleus. The atomic mass number is the superscript in ^3_1H for example.

Å: Angstrom unit, the fundamental unit of wavelength: $Å = 10^{-8}$ cm or 10^{-10} m.

Absolute zero: The temperature at which all materials have no thermal energy and some metals lose their electrical resistance. ($0\,K$, $-273\,°C$, $-459\,°F$).

AC: Alternating current.

Acquisition: The process of collecting data.

Acquisition matrix: The total number of independent data samples in the phase (ϕ) and frequency (f) encoded directions.

ADC: Analog-to-digital converter.

Algorithm: A complex mathematical process specifically used by the Fourier transformation process.

Aliasing: An artifactual wraparound image that extends beyond the image proper, caused by the misregistration of the higher frequency component being posted at the lower frequency areas.

Alloy: A substance that is a mixture of two or more metals.

Alnico: Alloy used in permanent magnets (aluminum, nickel, cobalt)

Alpha particle (α): Form of radioactivity consisting of $2n + 2p$ ejected from unstable nuclei. Can be stopped by a piece of paper.

Alternating current (AC): A current that continuously changes its direction. In the USA the current changes 120 times per second.

Ampére: Unit of measurement of electrical current – number of electron flow.

Amplitude: The signal height. The greater the amplitude, the larger the number of protons in the image and the brighter the image.

Analog: Raw undefined data, such as no hands on a clockface.

Analog-to-digital converter (ADC): Receiving general image information (analog) and assigning to it a digital value.

Angular momentum: The angle formed between a precessing object and its imaginary axis.

Antenna: A device enabling the sending and/or receiving of electromagnetic waves.

Anti-parallel alignment: Against the magnetic field in the high energy state.

Aperture: Opening of the magnet bore.

Archiving: The storage of the image data for future retrieval.

Array processor: Portion of the computer that converts raw (time domain) data, using Fourier transformation, into clinically useful information.

Arteriovenous malformation (AVM): A vascular malformation associated with an interwoven network of dilated arteries and veins.

Artifact: An error in the reconstructed image that has no counterpart in reality.

Atoms: Fundamental submicroscopic unit of all mass.

Averaging: The number of signal collection, referred to as NEX, number of excitations, and number of acquisitions.

AVM: Arteriovenous malformation.

Axial: Cross sectional images along the length of the patient's body from head to foot.

Axis: An imaginary line that passes through the center of the body of mass or field of force. Three orthogonal reference points representing length, width, and height (3D). In MRI the conventional x = sagittal, y = coronal, and z = transaxial.

B_0: Symbol representation of the static magnetic field strength generated by the electromagnetic coils within the gantry. It is this source that polarizes the responsive molecules in the immersed human body once placed within the gantry.

B_0 vector: Each of the responsive MDMs within the tissue sample precessing around the stronger B_0.

B_1: Symbol for the radio frequency (RF) coil located 90° to B_0.

B_1-RF: Symbolic reference to the externally applied RF torquing pulse originating 90° to B_0.

Bandwidth (BW): An all-inclusive term referring to the preselected frequency range which can govern both slice select and signal sampling. Range or window of frequencies over which a given signal can be extended principally to increase sampling time, thus signal.

Beta particle (β): Created whenever an electron is ejected from a neutron in an unstable nuclei.

Bipolar flow encoding gradients: The reversal of gradients for the purpose of refocusing the rapidly dispersing phases.

Bloch, Felix: American theoretical physicist who discovered and perfected the first spectroscopy experiment concurrent with and independent of Edward Purcell.

Bloch equation: A complex mathematical approach describing the motion of the magnetization vector, **M**.

BOLD: Blood oxygen level dependent; specific to fMRI.

Bolus/tracking: A method where a preselected bolus is tagged by the system and at a designated time sequence is detected and recorded.

BW: Bandwidth.

Carbon (^{12}C): The basic infrastructure of all organic material consisting of millions of bonding options and forms.

Carr/Purcell method: A method for measuring T2, following the Hahn echo, utilizing 180° RF pulses at T, $3T$, $5T$, etc., which will create echoes at $2T$, $4T$, $6T$, etc. A prelude to the train of spin echoes used in the fast spin echo sequence (FSF).

Cartesian coordinate system: Three reference points 90° relative to each other. In MR applications the $+z$-axis is longitudinal, the x-axis and y-axis are transverse but all are separated by angles of 90°.

Center frequency: A match of the system's transmit/receive frequency with the precessional frequency of the protons being imaged.

CBF: Cerebral blood flow.

CBV: Cerebral blood volume.

Chemical shift: A regional chemical difference of molecules containing a variance in its diamagnetic field, which in turn interacts causing image misregistration. This is detected in frequency values and measured in parts per million (ppm).

Cine: A series of rapidly recorded multiple images taken at sequential cycles of time and displayed on a monitor in a dynamic movie display format.

Circle of Willis: A large network of interconnecting vascular vessels resembling a circle and located at the base of the brain.

Circumference: The distance, C, around a circle given by $C = \pi d$. (Area $= \pi r^2$.)

Claustrophobia: A psychological reaction to being confined to a relatively small area, i.e., the gantry/tunnel.

CNR: Contrast-to-noise ratio.

Coaxial: Occupying the same space or time (coincident).

Coded signals: Signals that contain informative data.

Cognition: The brain's mental processes involved in knowing, thinking, learning, and judgment.

Coherence: The existence of constant phase relationships between and amongst the rotating oscillating waves (or objects) of a given sample. Effectively these phase components begin to lose their state of coherence once torqued by the B_1-RF resonant pulse.

Coil: Single or multiple loops of conductive wire, designed to create an intensified magnetic field within the looped conductor.

Coil, saddle: Specialized coil conventionally used when the static B_0 is coaxial with the coil's axis versus a surface coil.

Coils, crossed: Pair of RF coils oriented at right angles to each other and designed to minimize their mutually induced magnetic effect.

Compound: Combination, union, or bonding of two or more elements.

Conductor: Any medium that will allow the flow of electricity. Generally copper (Cu) is used for commercial electricity and niobium titanium (NbTi) for superconductive electromagnets.

Conservation law of energy: Based upon Einstein's theory of relativity law, $E = mc^2$, which states that energy can be neither created nor destroyed but can be transformed. $E =$ energy (ergs), $m =$ mass (g), and $c^2 =$ velocity of light squared.

Contraindication: Inadvisable, unsuitable; in MR contraindications exist that preclude the procedure on certain patients.

Contrast: Comparable differences; in MR, the difference between pixel signal values.

Contrast agents: Oral or injectable compounds that enhance the comparable differences of tissues.

Contrast, high: Few grays between the brightest and darkest portion of the image.

Contrast, latitude: The gray difference between the brightest and darkest diagnostic portion of an image.

Contrast, low: An image consisting of a relatively large number of grays between the brightest and darkest portion of the image.

Contrast, subjective: Contrast image scale relative to the viewers desires.

Contrast reversal: An image phenomenon where the brights become dark and the darks become bright. This is usually associated with an extended TR and is primarily governed by the regional spin density (DS).

Contrast-to-noise ratio (CNR): The perception of the distinct difference in intensities between two clinical areas of interest. The interfering of the noise factor reduces or degrades CNR.

Coordinate: One of several integrating references usually designated numerically or by letter, that collectively defines a spatial location.

Coronal slice: Cross sectional images from anterior to posterior in the patient's body

Cortex: Outer layer of an organ or an anatomical part.

Coulomb's Law: The strength of an electric field is defined as the force, in newtons, that a test charge experiences, divided by the charge.

Covalent: Bonding process – the combination two or more elements by the sharing of outer electrons, for example, H_2O.

Crosstalk: An artifactual image created by inter-slice communication between adjacent scan slices. This is resolved by increasing the interslice spacing gap.

Cryogen: A cooling agent, often used at or near absolute zero. Both liquid helium (LHe) and nitrogen (LN) are generally used in the MRI to optimize superconductivity.

Cryogenic: Freezing at or near absolute zero.

Cryostat: The assembly or component designed to maintain a constant very low temperature flow by using cryogenic LHe/LN in MRI.

Current: Flow of electrons through a conductor. Current is measured in ampères.

Davy's experiment: Illustrating the reverse perpendicular concentric lines of magnetic force created by current flow.

dB: Decibel.

DC: Direct current.

Decibel (dB): Unit of measure of intensity of sound.

Decoding: Process of making information useable.

Decoupling: A technical applicator to avoid objectionable interaction of the function of coils, i.e., the transmitter and receiver coils.

Democritus: Early Greek philosopher (approximately 400 B.C.) who first indicated that atoms were the fundamental unit of all mass and were both invisible and indivisible.

Demodulator: Synonymous with detector.

Dephase: The fanning out or separation of signals on the transverse $x-y$ plane. The greater the dephasing the greater the inhomogeneity and the shorter the corresponding relaxation time.

Dephasing: The process by which individual nuclei in tissue lose their synchronicity due to fluctuations in their precessional rates. In MR the major sources of dephasing are thermal motion in tissues and nonuniformity of field strengths.

Diamagnetic: A particular substance that possesses the innate properties which will actually decrease or oppose an adjacent magnetic field due to its outer electrons' rotation/spin properties. An example is gold.

Diameter: An imaginary line through a circle dividing it into two equal halves.

Diffusion: The process of molecular absorption as molecules mix to reach equilibrium.

Digital converter: That portion of the computer interfaced to convert the analog data into a digitized reference.

Dipole: A magnetic field characterized by its own magnetic north/south poles separated by a finite distance.

Direct current (DC): A current that flows uninterrupted in one direction.

Direct, pulsating: A current that flows in one direction while rhythmically pulsating.

Display matrix: The total number of pixels in the selected matrix, calculated by the product of its $y(\phi)$ and $x(f)$ axis.

DS: Spin density. Number of protons in the tissue sample.

DTPA: Diethylenetriaminepentaacetic acid, bound to the gadolinium molecule to serve as a detoxifying agent.

DWI: Diffusion weighted imaging.

$E = mc^2$: Conservation of energy law (see Einstein).

Echo planar imaging (EPI): The utilization of rapid gradient reversal pulses of the readout gradient(s) resulting in a series of gradient echo signals to reduce fast dephasing or signal loss.

Echo train: Relative to the fast spin echo (FSE) exhibited by a series of 180° RF rephasing pulses and their corresponding echo signals.

Eddy current: Relative to MRI it is the creation of small induced spurious electrical current within the ROI. This situation produces artifactual images created from and by metallic implants during an MRI examination.

Edema: A localized or generalized tissue area containing an excess accumulation of water.

Edge acuity: Refers to the sharpness of an edge within an area of interest which is controlled by pixel size and slice thickness.

Einstein, Albert: German/American physicist, atomic theory pioneer, discovered the theory of relativity and the energy conservation law, $E = mc^2$.

Electricity: Flow of electrons through or along a conductor.

Electrolysis: The creation of a chemical change by the passage of a current through a medium.

Electromagnetic: Having both electric and magnetic properties.

Electromagnetic spectrum: Electromagnetic waves are produced by electric charges that are undergoing accelerations and can be categorized according to their frequency and wavelength into a spectrum. The way in which the wave interacts with matter depends on its frequency.

Electromagnetic wave: Simultaneous periodic variations of electric and magnetic properties at 90° to each other.

Electromotive force (EMF): The maximum electrical potential between the negative and positive polarity (i.e., battery) measured in volts.

Electron (e): A negatively charged elementary particle that has mass, rotation, and spin. It possesses 1/1837 of the proton's mass.

Electron microscope: An electronic optical instrument where a beam of electrons is focused by electrostatic lenses to enlarge images of atoms onto a fluorescent/photographic plate.

Electron spin resonance (ESR): A phenomenon consisting of unpaired electrons creating a frequency range much higher than a conventional ω_0. ESR is relative to the type of dipole–dipole interaction between Gd and that of the regional responsive tissue atoms.

Electronegative: An element or a molecule with an excess negative charge, such as oxygen in H_2O.

Electronic: Relating to electron flow.

Electrostatics: A discipline of physics that investigates attraction and repulsion phenomena of electrical charges.

Element: One of over 100 fundamental submicroscopic identifiable substance in nature and consisting of a single atom. Its number of protons and its number of neutrons is its mass number ($\#A$) reveals its physical and chemical identity.

Elliptical: Very oblong in shape, similar to the shape of a football.

EM spectrum: See Electromagnetic spectrum.

EMF: Electromotive force.

Encoding: Decoding or deciphering coded signals for spatial location.

Endoscopy: The visualization of an internal organ or part of the body, generally by using fiber optic instruments.

Energy: Required to perform work; kinetic energy is energy of motion, potential energy is stored energy.

Energy level ground state: Stationary charged quantum energy at its equilibrium state.

Energy level, high energy state: Charged energetic particles that have absorbed an external applied force elevating them to a higher energy position.

Energy state: It is nature's command that all objects innately have a propensity to reside at ground or equilibrium (state). Relative to MRI, when the MDMs have acquired excess energy they are torqued to a higher energy antiparallel state or location. When these MDMs are at ground state they are positionally at a $+z$ antiparallel longitudinal equilibrium state.

Entrance slice phenomena: Relative to MRI, an image portraying the contrast variance created between flowing nuclei versus the stationary nuclei located in the slice select.

EPI: Echo planar imaging.

Equilibrium: A state of balance existing between two opposing forces or divergent forms of influence.

Erg: A minute form of energy measurement embodied in Einstein's formula $E = mc^2$. It requires about 70–100 ergs to softly phonate an Ah!

Ernst angle: Professor R.R. Ernst perfected the RF pulse angle in conjunction with optimum signal saturation (see fast scanning).

Erythrocytes: Bicave nonnucleated cells found in the blood, numbering 4.5 to 4.8 million per cubic millimeter. Generally referred to as red blood cells (RBCs), their primary function is to transport oxygen bound to hemoglobin.

ESR: Electron spin resonance.

Excitation: Adding energy into a given mass, i.e., the atomic spins of the tissue sample.

Exponential decay: Graphically depicting the relaxation decay process in an exponential format.

Extracellular: Fluids located outside the cell, i.e., blood plasma.

Extrinsic: Coming from or without.

Faraday cage: A six-sided cage constructed of a low resistance metal, such as copper or aluminum, which is used to shield against radiofrequencies that may interfere with the production of an MR signal.

Faraday, Michael: Founder of the phenomenon electromagnetic induction.

Faraday's Law: A changing magnetic field causes the induction of an electric potential; the change can be either in amplitude or direction. The greater and/or faster the change, the larger the induced potential (voltage).

Fast Fourier transform (FFT): An accelerated computational procedure to obtain a Fourier transform analysis.

Fast spin echo (FSE): A fast spin echo process characterized by rapidly applied 180° RF refocusing pulses.

Fat suppression: Pulsing an ROI usually with the frequency of fat or H_2O to remove its deleterious effect from the resultant image.

FDA: Food and Drug Administration.

Ferromagnetic metals: Those metals which have the inherent ability to highly concentrate magnetic lines, therefore interacting with the magnetic field. Examples are iron, cobalt, and nickel.

FFT: Fast Fourier transform.

FID: Free induction decay with specific reference to T1 and T2*, i.e., decay uninfluenced by external RF.

Field echo: Pulse sequence that uses a gradient reversal technique to re-phase the hydrogen particles. Any flip angle between 1 and 90 degrees may be used depending on clinical indications.

Field of view (FOV): Defined as the size of the 2D or 3D spatial encoding area of the image.

Filter: Any process or procedure to remove deleterious frequencies so as to avoid or reduce an alteration of the image quality.

Five gauss exclusion zone: An important limitation barrier for persons with electronically or magnetically activated implants. Such devices may be rendered inoperable by strong magnetic fields in excess of the 5 gauss line. Examples of such devices are pacemakers, hearing aids, and neurostimulators.

Fleming's right-hand rule: Curl the fingers in direction of the electron flow and the thumb will point in the direction of its magnetic north pole.

Flip angle: The angle through which the bulk magnetization vector (**M**) has been torqued or mutated by the resonant B_1-RF pulse.

Flow compensation: The strategic application of reversal gradient pulses to compensate the objectionable spin phase effects of flow motion.

Flow-related enhancement: The process by which enhanced signal intensity of flows is a result of the unsaturated spin entering a saturated slice.

Flux: A flow of energy, i.e., magnetic field flowing from its north to south pole.

Flux, magnetic: Pattern of the magnetic lines of forces.

fMRI: BOLD based imaging technique that can aid in the detection of blood volume changes, flow, and saturation that accompany focal activation of brain cells.

Force: The ability to create work or create change (often measured in horsepower).

Fourier transform (FT): Algorithms process for integrating the signal frequency and phase values to convert the raw image data (k-space) into its spatial location on the matrix.

FOV: Field of view.

Frame of reference: There are two conventional frames of reference used in MRI for viewing a spinning process: static and rotational.

Free-induction decay (FID): The measurable magnetic resonance signal that occurs as the transverse magnetism (produced by the application of the 90-degree RF pulse) decays toward zero.

Frequency: The number of repetitions of rhythmic periodic processes in a given length of time. For MRI in the EM spectrum, time is measured in hertz (Hz) or cycles per second.

Frequency encoding: Spatial encoding where the coded signals contain frequency-related spatial data.

Fringe field: The intensity of a force or source of energy characteristically indicated by a series of isobar intensity curves.

Fringe magnetism: The magnetic field strength measured on the outer borders of the magnet

FSE: Fast spin echo.

FT: Fourier transform.

Functional imaging: Broadly defined as the assessment of anatomy-specific function.

G_x, G_y, G_z: Conventional symbols for the three orthogonal gradients. The subscripts denote the conventional spatial direction and, based upon their functional position in the selected pulsing system, will denote the spatial application.

Gadolinium (Gd): Gadolinium is a paramagnetic contrast enhancement agent generally invasively applied in MRI. Gadolinium unpaired electrons undergo dipole–dipole interaction with outer electrons in the receptive tissue.

Gamma ray (γ): An electromagnetic wavelength of energy emanating from an unstable nucleus that has the power to penetrate lead.

Gauss: CGS unit of magnetic flux, 1 gauss = $1-10^{-4}$ T.

Gaussometer: An instrument to measure gauss magnetic flux fields of force.

GE: Gradient echo.

Ghosting: An image artifact primarily associated with phase direction.

Gibbs: A unique type of truncation artifact.

GMN: Gradient moment nulling.

Golay coil: A gradient coil designed to create magnetic field gradients located perpendicular to B_0.

Gradient amplifier channel: One of three channels that functions to amplify gradient power.

Gradient coils: Three paired orthogonal coils located within the gantry which collectively and sequentially generate their magnetic field onto B_0 for the prime purpose of selective spatial excitation. Gradients are also used for reversal pulses in fast scanning pulsing techniques.

Gradient echo (GE): Gradient echo pulsing creates a gradient echo image. It refocuses spins by reversing the last gradient pulse.

Gradient moment nulling (GMN): A specialized gradient sequence to rapidly null or cancel out dephasing spins to rephase them, thus a flow/phase compensator.

Gradient, rephasing: Brief magnetic gradient rephasing that occurs after the selective excitation pulse. The result is the rephasing of the out-of-phase spins along the direction of the selection gradients, thus forming a gradient echo. This process is employed to improve the sensitivity of the imaging and follows the selective excitation pulse.

Gradient reversal: Used in place of a 180-degree refocusing pulse to cause phase shift and refocusing of the nuclei to produce an echo. The polarity of the gradient is reversed but the strength of the gradient is the same as before the reversal.

Gradient reversal pulse (GRP): Use of gradient reversal pulses to reduce the effects of signal loss.

Gradients (G_x, G_y, G_z): Three orthogonal external magnetic fields designed to torque B_0 into a predesignated gradient slope for spatial excitation.

Graduated fields: Magnetic fields that are produced by gradient coils.

Gray matter (gm): Nervous tissue of the brain, grayish in color due to its lack or reduction of myelinated neuronal fibers.

GRP: Gradient reversal pulse.

Gyromagnetic ratio: A constant for a particular nucleus that relates its precessional frequency to a field strength of 1.0 tesla. For hydrogen, it is 42.58 mHz/T.

Hahn, Erwin Lewis: Founded the spin echo pulse sequence in 1949.

Hahn echo: An echo of the T2* FID created by a 90° RF torquing pulse followed by an RF 180° refocusing pulse.

Half FT imaging: A technique characterized by sampling the latter part of an echo for the purpose of reducing the echo/sampling time. (See Fourier transform.) Also known as HFI.

Hardware: A generic term for the main computerized mechanical and electrical components.

Helix: A looped coil of conductive wire.

Helmholtz coils: A pair of current-carrying coils specifically designed to produce a uniform magnetic field to the tissue sample located between them.

Hemodynamics: Moving fluids – the basis of MRA.

Hertz (Hz): A measure of one complete frequency (360°) which passes a given reference in one second.

Homogeneous: Similar in composition; in MR the homogeneous magnetic field is a field that has very small calculated variations in the magnetic field.

Hydrated: Characterized by possessing relatively large amounts of water.

Hydrogen density: The composition of a structure based on hydrogen content.

Hyperintense: Optimum signal intensity generally characterized by a bright T1 image. Opposite of hypointense.

Hz: Hertz, measure of frequency oscillations.

I: Nuclear spin number.

Image acquisition time: The image or scan time for 2DFT is equal to the product of TR, number of signal averages or excitations (NEX), and phase (ϕ) encoding steps. The total time to acquire all the image acquisition data.

Image artifacts: See 'artifacts'.

Image quality: Can be defined by contrast, spatial resolution, and signal-to-noise ratio.

Image reconstruction time: The time required to assimilate all the data acquisition until the image is visualized.

Imaginary: The complex number defining the y component of the vector that is 90-degrees out of phase with the reference vector.

Imaging sequence (protocol): Scanning parameters that are usually selected by the radiologist, which are based on the patient history, and should provide the most useful information for diagnosis.

Indivisible: Unable to be divided by ordinary means (e.g., atoms are indivisible).

Inductance: The coupling effect of two current-carrying loops. Initially established by Michael Faraday in 1831 and is the basis of the resonant frequency MR signal detection circuitry.

Induction: The act of causing or creating a specific action, i.e., magnetic induction, as discovered by Michael Faraday in 1831.

Induction, electromagnetic: Creation through a phenomenon of persuasion. The application of electromagnetic waves traversing a receiver conductor coil at 90° will create a voltage/current within that coil.

Inertia: The property of a mass at rest which tends to keep it at rest; and the property of a mass in motion which tends to keep it in motion.

Infarct: A tissue that is undergoing necrosis due to deprived blood flow.

Inflow enhancement: A specialized MRA technique utilizing a gradient echo pulse sequence where the bolus is excited, detected, and recorded in the same slice.

Inhomogeneity: The reduction of homogeneity or uniformity.

In-plane resolution: The resolving power perpendicular to the slice, i.e., the pixel dimensions.

Insulator: Any medium that prevents the flow of electrons.

Integer: Any of the natural numbers, the negatives of these numbers, or zero.

Integrals: An essential volume or position necessary for completeness, i.e., to the values of the electron spins in a given element which fulfils the innate balance of force.

Interface/interfacing: Computerized integration of images from various imaging modalities, e.g., PET, MRI, CT.

Interleaving: A pulsing technique which sequentially staggers the collection of data (1–3, 2–4, etc.) so there is no interslice gap.

Interpulse time: The time between successive RF pulse sequences.

Intravoxel phase dispersion: Coherence loss suffered by phases within the imaging voxel. The consequent reduction in signal intensity can usually be minimized by using smaller voxels and/or less flip angle.

Intrinsic: Within or originating from inside.

Inversion: The macroscopic magnetization vector oriented opposite or 180° to the B_0 field. Inversion is generally related to the inversion recovery technique and is generally used to produce a heavily weighted T1 image.

Inversion recovery (IR): A specialized pulsing technique where the bulk MDMs are inverted 90° below the transverse $x–y$ plane. This process usually produces a T1 weighted image but can produce T2-like images and contrast reversal images.

Ionization: Atoms or molecules that have gained or lost a charge.

Ionizing radiation: Radiation that removes an electron from an atom, resulting in a free electron which is then available to participate in some physical or chemical process. X-rays are a form of ionizing radiation.

IR: Inversion recovery.

Isotropic motion: A motion which is uniform in all its dimensional directions.

***k*-space:** A spatial frequency domain where the raw MR signals are collected in the computer system before being processed for reconstruction.

Kelvin: Unit of temperature where absolute zero is at $0\,K$ or $-273\,°C$.

Kilogauss: One thousand gauss.

Kinematic scan: Scan procedure where a given joint is moving in a flexed/extended position during the scanning process.

Larmor equation: $\omega_0 = \gamma B_0$, where ω_0 is the Larmor frequency, B_0 is the strength of the static magnetic field, and γ is the gyromagnetic ratio of a given element.

Larmor frequency: The frequency at which the nuclei precess within a unique field strength.

Lattice: A general term relating the magnetic and thermal environs comprising the nuclear energy exchange activities; it is solely related to the longitudinal $+z$ signal relaxation process.

Law: A reproducible and predictable event.

Leukocyte: A general term representing the five types of white blood cells (WBCs), measuring approximately $20\,\mu$ in diameter, and numbering 5000–10,000 per cubic millimeter of normal blood. The primary function of WBCs is to combat inflammation and disease.

Linear: Straight-line.

Lipid: Any of the fatty acid fractions normally located in the body.

Lipoma: A tumor of fatty tissue.

Lodestone: A piece of magnetite iron ore containing natural magnetism.

Longitudinal relaxation: Returning of the net magnetization vector to $+z$ equilibrium.

Long scale: Large gray scale latitude.

Longitudinal plane (Z): The axis of the magnet in which the patient lies, that is oriented with the magnetic field.

Lorentzian line: The conventional shape of the graphic lines comprising the MR spectrum.

Luminar: Related to blood flow patterns.

m: Meter.

M: Mega, one million, 10^6.

M: Net macroscopic magnetization vector, usually shown as a positional vector arrow.

M_0: The designated equilibrium value of the magnetization of the MDMs; it is always oriented along or with B_0.

M_{xy}: The torqued MDMs residing on the transverse x–y plane. From this point, they begin to relax spontaneously and in the process will characteristically emit T1 and T2 signals.

Macromolecules: Very large molecules some of which may be seen under powerful microscopes. A macromolecule can be several thousand times larger than an unbound water molecule.

Macroscopic magnetization vector: The net magnetic dipole moments per given volume, represented as a relatively large vector quantity and designated by an arrow.

Magnet, permanent: A substance whose magnetic properties have been induced naturally by the earth's magnetic field.

Magnetic cloud: The orbiting electrons create a magnetic shielding which modestly impedes the proton MDMs as they exit from the nucleus. Extreme cases will cause image misregistration called chemical shift.

Magnetic dipoles: Magnetic domains exist in pairs know as dipoles.

Magnetic dipole moment (MDM): The minute magnetic properties of a given nucleus, as opposed to the net (bulk) magnetization vector, which is generally symbolized as a larger black arrow. The MDM is the composite of three magnetic properties: nucleus, electron orbit, and electron spin.

Magnetic field: A vector quantity consisting of both a north and south pole; it exerts an induction force on ferromagnetic and paramagnetic substances.

Magnetic field, energy levels in: Each spin exists in a distinct energy state and has an identifiable spin quantum number.

Magnetic field gradients (MFG): Superimposing a weaker magnetization on B_0 to create a linear slope for spatial excitation.

Magnetic induction: See induction.

Magnetic lines of force: The magnetic lines of force forming a given magnetic domain or field of force.

Magnetic moment: The net strength and orientation of a magnetic field.

Magnetic resonance angiography (MRA): MR image visualization of selected vascular structures.

Magnetic resonance imaging (MRI): The integration of the minute magnetic properties of the tissue atoms with the static magnetic field (B_0), to be in a resonant state with an applied external RF pulse, and will in turn produce MR signals that are converted into an exquisite tissue image.

Magnetic retentivity: The innate ability of a magnetized substance to resist demagnetization.

Magnetic susceptibility: The measurement of a given substance in becoming magnetized through the process of magnetic induction.

Magnetism: The power or force created by a substance having the property of creating or inducing magnetic dipoles.

Magnetization vector, M: The integration of all the individual nuclear magnetic moments which have a positive magnetization value at equilibrium versus those in a random state.

Magnetohemodynamic effect: An artifactual effect produced when blood crosses a magnetic field.

Magnetometer: An instrument for measuring magnetic force.

Magnitude: Quantity or amount; often exhibited by an MRI spectral peak.

Mass: A quantity of matter without a definite shape.

Matrix: The x and y dimensions of the image region of interest defined by phase encode steps and frequency or readout steps.

Matter, brain: Approximately 1350–1500 grams (g) of nerve-related soft tissue divided into cerebrum, cerebellum, pons, medulla oblongata, and midbrain.

Maxwell coils: A special type of gradient coil that generates a changing magnetic field in the B_0.

MDM: Magnetic dipole moment.

Mega (M): One million, 10^6.

Melanin: The pigment giving color to certain parts of the body, e.g., skin, eyes, brain.

MHz: Megahertz, or a million wavelengths traversing a given reference in one second of time. The hydrogen proton has a precessional rate of 42.58 MHz or 42,584,000 Hz/sec.

Micron (μ): $1\,\mu = 10^{-1}\text{m} = 1/1,000,000$ m.

Microsecond (μsec): $10^{-6} = 1/1,000,000$ sec.

Milli (m): Divided by one thousand, 10^{-3}, or $1/1000$.

Mobile unit: An MRI system that may be moved at random.

Modulations: Radio frequency variations.

Molecule: Any atom (element) or group elements that cannot be broken down any further by ordinary means without losing their identity.

Moment: A magnetic field created by the positively charged particle within the nucleus, which has an angular momentum or spin. A current loop therefore exists which results in a moment.

Morphology: Cellular structure interest versus functional interest.

MR signal: An electromagnetic signal in the RF resonant range, generally between 1–100 meters in length.

MRA: Magnetic resonance angiography.

MRI: Magnetic resonance imaging.

MTT: Mean transit time maps generated via perfusion imaging techniques.

Multiple echo imaging: A fast spin echo technique utilizing many spin echoes. This pulse sequence is characterized by a series of 180° refocusing pulses.

Multiple slice imaging: An imaging technique involving the formation of multiple images from a single volumetric acquisition.

Multi-slice imaging: The process of incorporating multiple slice acquisition during "dead" time of a TR.

#N: Symbol for the number of neutrons in the nucleus: $\#N = \#A - \#Z$.

Necrosis: Dead tissue or bone primarily due to deficient blood flow.

Net magnetization vector: The MDMs surviving from the flip-flop self-annihilation process and precessing around B_0 before being torqued by the resonant B_1-RF pulse.

Neutron: An uncharged neutral component located in the nucleus which serves as a stabilizer. The neutron mass is slightly greater than the proton mass and has an enormous effect on the quantum spin value of an element.

NEX: Number of excitations.

Noise: An undesirable background interference or disturbance that affects image quality.

NSA: Number of signal averages (see signal averaging).

Nuclear species: An atomic structure.

Nuclear spin number (I): A quantized property relating to spin quality.

Nucleon: A general term for the neutron and proton in the nucleus.

Nucleus: The center of an atom, it contains the positive (+) protons and neutral neutrons, and occupies one hundred million billionth of the 3D atom, yet consists of more than 99.99 percent of the total atomic mass in nature.

Number of excitations (NEX): How frequently each k-space line is scanned.

Nyquist limit: The optimum frequency where aliasing will not occur.

Oersted, Hans: Discovered in 1819 that electricity produces magnetism.

Ohm's law: $E = IR$, where E = volts, I = amperage, and R = ohms.

Oil-filled phantom: QA is performed initially on oil-filled phantoms which yield the most homogeneous signal intensity for evaluation.

Orientation: A conventional positional standard, i.e., M_0 is oriented to $+z$ at equilibrium, which is coincident with the north pole of the magnet.

Orthogonal: Coordinates that are 90° to each other.

Oscillation: Rhythmic periodic motion.

P/N: Proton/neutron ratio.

Parallel alignment: Alignment of the net magnetic vector with the magnetic field (longitudinal plane or z axis).

Parallel versus antiparallel energy state: An energy state where the parallel is at the lower equilibrium state and the antiparallel is positionally at 180° and in a higher energy state.

Paramagnetic metals: Those materials in which some of the electrons are unpaired so that there is a net spin magnetism. When an external magnetic field is applied, alignment of the atom with the magnetic field occurs thereby increasing the field strength. Paramagnetism has a small effect compared to that of ferromagnetism. Examples are titanium, platinum, and gadolinium.

Paramagnetism: Substance with weak magnetic properties due to its unpaired electrons. Researchers have developed certain paramagnetic materials as MRI invasive contrast media.

Parenchyma: The essential and distinctive tissue of an organ.

Partial flip (gradient reversal): Pulse sequence that uses less than the conventional 90-degree RF flip to resonate the spins to the transverse plane; flips less number of spins therefore longitudinal relaxation is decreased requiring decreased TR; scan time is diminished.

Partial saturation (SP): An image where the 90° RF excitation pulse are rapidly reapplied. A series of repeated RF pulses following the initial torquing pulse.

Partial volumning: A loss of resolution due to excessively large voxels.

Passive shimming: Iron is placed on the magnet itself, in order to shape field flux lines in the desired configuration.

Patency: Lumen opening integrity.

PC: Phase contrast in MRA.

Perfusion: Brain hemodynamic assessment in MRI using techniques which evaluate cerebral blood volume, cerebral blood flow, and mean transit time.

Periodic table: A categorical listing of the elements corresponding to their physical and chemical properties.

Permanent magnet: The simplest of all magnets, whose magnetism is based on the property of ferromagnetism, possessed by certain elements, alloys, and ceramic substances.

Permeability: How readily a substance can become magnetized. The lower the permeability, the greater the retentivity, and visa versa.

Phantom: A simulated object of specific size and composition to check or monitor a system's homogeneity and general imaging integrity.

Phase: A position relative to a periodic function such as a cyclical movement. An in-phase situation relates the relative positions as being consistently uniform; an out-of-phase situation relates the relative positions as varying from one moment to another.

Phase contrast (PC): An MRA technique utilizing the change in the phase shifts of the sample flow protons to create an image.

Phase cycling: A strategic signal execution process where phase components of the refocused RF pulses are summarily varied. This reduces and/or eliminates certain phase-related image artifacts.

Phase encoding: Sequentially encoding MR signals by their phase values; it conventionally occurs along the G_y (view) axis. As each component in their respective vertical view position has experienced a different phase encoding gradient pulse, its exact spatial reconstruction can be specifically and precisely located by the Fourier transformation analysis.

Phase encoding gradient: That gradient whose function is to identify phase relationships of rows of data accumulated in the y direction of the matrix. It is applied in a precise manner during the acquisition of a scan.

Phase reversed pulse: RF pulses designed to reverse the M_{xy} magnetization.

Phosphorus (^{31}P): A natural element of cellular protoplasm that plays a significant role in ATP–ADP cellular energy transformation.

Pixel: The smallest discrete two-dimensional picture element of a digital image display.

Planar: The imaging process of a selected plane.

Planar spin imaging: A specialized technique where the MR planar image is created sequentially. Conventionally each G_y column

SI units: I
and me

Signal av
given
purpos

Signal-to-
of true

Sine wav
sinuso
charac
of the

Slice: Sy
image

Slice enc
encod

Slice sel
appli
uniq

Slice se
func
an i
of
acqu

Slice th
ima
(m

SNR (

Sodiur
boc

Softw
du
wit

Solend
th
ide
G

SP: P

Spati
si

Spati
ac
n

Spec
t
t

experiences a different ϕ and each G_x a different f.

Polarity: An intrinsic separation of charges, i.e., magnetic north and south pole; the gradient negative and positive polarity. Negative electricity is where it is stored, and positive where it is going.

Poles: Either of two opposed forces, as at the end of a magnet.

Population: The number of sampled nuclei; image brightness is directly proportional to population size.

Position dependent phase shift: Accumulated gradient influences on phase values of spins within and around the ROI; they are detrimental to the image quality due to their gradient-dependent positional state. Image degradation is effectively reduced by applying reverse gradient pulses just before and just after the RF refocusing pulse.

Potential: Stored energy.

Precession: The phenomenon of a magnetic field (or any object) spinning or gyrating around an imaginary axis of its own creation.

Precessional angle: Often referred to as angular momentum; it is the angle created by an object precessing around its unwavering vertical axis.

Precessional frequency: The frequency of precession of the hydrogen nucleus determined by the Larmor equation (also known as the Larmor frequency).

Presaturation (pre-sat): A specialized technique employing repeated RF bombardment of adjacent structures to the ROI for the purpose of reducing or eliminating their artifactual phase effects.

Processed data: Reconstructed time domain data using Fourier transformation.

Projection profile: An NMR spectrum that is varied by the gradients and viewed on the monitor.

Protein: A large molecule of hydrogen, oxygen, nitrogen, phosphorous, sulfur, and iron, and found throughout the plant and animal kingdoms. Essential for growth, repair, and energy.

Proton: A positively charged nucleon; the number of protons ($\#Z$) governs the chemical properties of a given element. The proton is 1847 times more massive than the electron but has a charge of equal magnitude, but opposite sign.

Proton density weighted image: An image influenced more by the number of protons in the tissue sample than by T1 or T2.

Proton, mobile: Protons that have a tendency to move when exposed to the static magnetic field.

Pseudo: A false image or process.

Pulse programmer: The component of a computer system that controls the pulse features such as time, amplitude, phase, and frequency.

Pulse sequence: A preselected set of parameters, usually consisting of RF, gradient magnetic field pulses, and time spacing of TR/TE.

Purcell, Edward: Invented spectroscopy independently of and concurrently with Felix Bloch.

PWI: Perfusion weighted imaging.

Q: Quality factor.

Quality factor (Q): The resonant circuit integrity, usually related to the coils.

Quantum: An indivisible unit of energy on a submicroscopic level.

Quantum physicist: One who views mass by its energy levels or subatomic parts.

Quench: When a system has a malfunction of its electronics and/or there is a significant loss of cryogenic coolants, the magnetic field becomes excessively incoherent causing it to malfunction or go inoperative – thus a quench.

Radio frequency: The number of oscillations or cycles per unit time generated by radio waves.

Readout gradient: Conventionally refers to the frequency encoding gradient activated during the echo pulse.

Real: Complex number defining the x component of a vector that is in phase with the reference vector.

Receiver dead time: A segment of time after the excited RF pulse where the FID cannot be detected due to saturation of the RF receiver circuitry.

Spin relaxation: Formation of T1 signal from one RF pulse.

Spin–spin relaxation: Formation of T2 signal indicating that the RF resonant pulse was activated at least twice (90° and 180°) during a given TR.

Spin tagging: A brief time (equal to T1) where nuclei retain their magnetic orientation, allowing them to be tagged in fluid flow imaging.

Spoiler gradients: Applied gradients used to electronically destroy residual M_{xy} before energizing the subsequent RF torquing pulse.

SR: Saturation recovery.

Static: Stationary or nonmoving, i.e., B_0.

Static frame of reference: Depicted by a magnetization vector, **M**, which relates to the location of its net (bulk) relaxation state at a given time.

Stochastic: Probabilities in the sampling process, random or statistically chosen.

Substance: Any mass that has a definite composition.

Superconducting magnets: Electromagnets whose circuitry is supercooled to near absolute zero thereby decreasing electrical resistance within the system. Once current is applied and the desired field strength is reached, no further power is required.

Superconductivity: Flow of electrons free of any molecular resistance.

Suppression: A specialized pulsing technique used to minimize or cancel out the adverse effects from adjacent dephasing protons by RF bombardment onto the ROI.

Surface coil: A circular coil is placed directly on or over the ROI for increased magnetic sensitivity. The imaging depth is $r/2$ from the midpoint of the coil's diameter.

Susceptibility: See magnetic susceptibility.

Syringomyelia: Chronic progressive disease of the spinal cord resulting in cavities.

T: Tesla.

T1: The relaxation process of the T1 MDMs to recover 63 percent of its original signal value. T1 relaxation is exponentially expressed and

often referred to as spin relaxation and/or longitudinal relaxation.

T1 weighted: An image created by predominantly T1 signals and associated with decreased TR/TE.

T1 relaxation: The time constant for a given tissue's MDM B_0 vector components to repolarize to $+z$ longitudinal equilibrium; solely governed by the thermal energy content within the tissue lattice structure.

T2: Signals occurring immediately following a 180° refocusing B_1-RF resonant pulse and consisting of very rapidly dephasing T2 components and magnetic inhomogeneities created by the B_0 magnetic field.

T2*: Signals occurring immediately following the 90° RF torquing pulse and consisting of both magnetic inhomogeneities and rapidly dephasing T2 signals (FID).

2-T2: A second spin echo characterized by less image contrast. 2-T2 is significantly affected by its spin density (DS) (protons) and its amplitude will be less than the previous 1-T2. System software governs how many multiple spin echoes can be imaged within a given TR.

T2 signals: After **M** is torqued to M_{xy}, those components undergoing the 180° RF refocusing pulse will subsequently produce T2 signals during the dephasing/rephasing process.

T2 weighted: An image consisting of more T2 relaxation data and conventionally obtained by using a long TR/TE.

Tau (τ): Designated time segment in the pulse sequence.

TE: Echo time, the time frame from the 90° B_1 RF pulse to the midpoint of the TE echo.

Tesla (T): Unit of magnetic field measurement 1T = 10,000 gauss.

Theory: An educated guess that some act or process will create a predictable result or conclusion.

Thermal: Relating to heat energy.

Thermal equilibrium: The condition where the system or tissue sample experiences the same effective temperature. In MRI, thermal equilibrium means relative alignment of spins with B_0.

Thermal motion: The movement of molecules and atoms of an object determines the amount of kinetic energy of that object.

Three-dimensional imaging (3DFT): A specialized imaging technique that uses a computer to sandwich together slice acquisitions for an image representation of length, width, and height. $3DFT = N_p \times N_f \times G_z \times NEX$.

TI: Inversion time.

Time domain data (TD): Unprocessed time domain data obtained during acquisition (frequency and phase information).

Time of flight (TOF): An MRA technique relying solely on the flow of unsaturated blood into a magnetized presaturated slice. The difference between unsaturated and presaturated spins creates a bright vascular image without the invasive use of contrast media.

Time to echo: TE or echo time is the time between the middle of the 90° pulse and the middle of the resulting spin echo in a single slice.

Time to repetition: TR or repetition time is the time that a pulse sequence is repeated for a given slice.

Time-varying magnetic field: The magnetic field strength is varied linearly over time by the application current to the gradient coils.

Torque: The application of an external resonant B_1-RF pulse that will mutate or create a sufficient force to increase its angular momentum (γ) from $+z$ longitudinal orientation.

TR: Repetition time.

Transaxial: A plane 90° to the long axis of the human body.

Transformer: A device or induction process which steps electromotive force (voltage) either up or down.

Translate: Move from side to side.

Transreceiver coil: An MRI surface coil that serves as both a transmitter and a receiver.

Transverse (XY) plane: The plane that orients perpendicular to the magnetic field (which is in the longitudinal plane); the net magnetic vector is transferred to the transverse plane following excitation by an RF pulse.

Truncation: An image artifact characterized by a multiple ring-like effect caused by adjacent high and low signal intensity areas.

Tuning: Adjustment process of the B_1-RF resonant pulse; it must equal W_0 for the tissue sample.

Two-dimensional imaging (2DFT): The FT mathematically encodes the frequency and phase values of the detected signals at 90° to each other. $2DFT = N_p \times N_f \times NEX$.

Ultrasonic frequency: Frequency that is above the range of sound audible to the human ear (approximately 3 kHz).

Valence: The combining power of a given element/molecule based upon the number of its outer electrons. The valence governs the ability of elements/compounds to bond, as indicated in the Mendeleev periodic table.

Vector: A mathematical entity characterized by magnitude and direction. Vector quantities can be added or subtracted from one another.

Velocity: Speed in a particular direction.

Velocity encoding (VENC): Specialized technique for encoding flow velocities.

VENC: Velocity encoding.

Viscosity: A property of a fluid or semifluid that affects its mobility, thus its image intensity.

VMRI: Vascular magnetic resonance imaging.

Volt: Unit of electrical pressure; 1 kilovolt (kV) = 1000 volts.

Volumetric imaging: A specialized technique where all the MR signals are collected from the entire tissue samples and imaged as a whole entity. Compare with slice select.

Vortex flow: Area within a blood vessel where the blood is suddenly accelerated then rapidly decelerated, i.e., blood passing through a vascular stenosis.

Voxel: A 3D volumetric portion of an image where viewing face is the pixel and whose depth is the third dimension.

Watt: Unit of electrical power, the product of volts and ampères.

Wave: The propagation of a wavelength of energy that has the dimensions of period, frequency, and amplitude.

Wavelength: The distance measured in the direction of progression of a wave, from one point to another in the same phase.

White matter (wm): Nervous-related tissue or fiber located in the brain and sheathed in myelin.

Window: A range of values considered together (looked at).

WM: White matter.

Work: Moving mass through space by overcoming the resting inertia. Work $(W) =$ force $(F) \times$ distance (d).

X axis: The axis in the magnet that corresponds to the width of the magnet or from patient's shoulder to shoulder.

Y axis: The axis in the magnet that corresponds to the vertical direction of the magnet or anterior/posterior orientation of the patient.

#Z: Atomic number, the number of protons in a given nucleus. It is the subscript in $^{16}_{8}O$, for example.

Z axis: The longitudinal axis of the magnetic field.

Zero, temperature: Water freezes at $0°$ Celsius $= 32°$ Fahrenheit. Absolute zero, when all molecular motion ceases, is equivalent to $0\,K$ or $-273\,°C$.

Symbols and Abbreviations

α	Flip of B_1-RF torquing excitation pulse		ΔE	Energy difference
γ	Angular momentum		EM	Electromagnetic (spectrum)
γ	Gyromagnetic ratio or magnetogyric ratio		EPI	Echo planar imaging
			EPR	Electron paramagnetic resonance
θ	Angle formed between the M_0 and B_0		ESR	Electron spin resonance
μ	Magnetic moment vector		ETL	Echo train length
ϕ	Phase or phase angle		f	Frequency
ω	Angular frequency measured in radians/second		fMRI	BOLD-based imaging technique that will aid in the surgical planning of the brain
ω_0	Angular resonant frequency expressed as Larmor equation ($\omega_0 = \gamma B_0$)		FSE	Fast spin echo
			FFT	Fast Fourier transform
τ	Time (tau) segment		FID	Free induction decay
2DFT	Two-dimensional Fourier Transform = $N_2 \times N_y \times$ NEX		FOV	Field of view
			FT	Fourier transform
3DFT	Three-dimensional Fourier Transform = $N_x \times N_y \times N_z =$ NEX		G	Gauss
			Gd	Gadolinium
AC	Alternating current		GMN	Gradient moment nulling
ADC	Analog-to-digital converter		Hz	Hertz
B	Magnetic field		I	Spin
B_1	RF torquing pulse		IR	Inversion recovery
B_0	Static magnetic field		k-space	Where raw MR data is stored before reconstruction
BOLD	Blood oxygen level dependent; specific to fMRI		M	Magnetization
BW	Bandwidth		M_0	Magnetic dipole moments at equilibrium
CBF	Cerebral blood flow		MHz	Megahertz
CBV	Cerebral blood volume		MR	Magnetic resonance
CNR	Contrast-to-noise ratio		MRA	Magnetic resonance angiography
DC	Direct current		MRS	Magnetic resonance spectroscopy
DTPA	Diethylenetriaminepentaacetic acid		MTT	Mean transit time maps generated via perfusion imaging techniques
DWI	Diffusion weighted imaging			
E	Photon energy			

M_{xy}	Magnetic dipole moments in the transverse $x-y$ plane	SAR	Specific absorption rate
NEX	Number of excitations	SE	Spin echo
NMR	Nuclear magnetic resonance	T	Tesla
N_f	Number of frequency encoding rows	T1	Longitudinal relaxation time, MR signal
N_p	Number of phase encoding views	T2	Transverse relaxation time, MR signal
N_x	Number of frequency encoding steps on the matrix	T2*	T2 star signal, rapidly dephasing components consisting of T2 + inherent inhomogeneities
N_y	Number of phase encoding steps on the matrix	TE	>Echo time
PC	Proton : neutron ratio	TI	Inversion time
PPM	Parts per million	TOF	Time-of-flight
PS	Partial saturation	TR	Repetition time
PWI	Perfusion weighted imaging	VENC	Velocity encoding
RF	Radio frequency	$x-y-z$	Cartesian axes at 90° to each other

Index

Page numbers in **boldface** indicate tables and illustrations

401